ACLS – 2013

Arrhythmias

(*Expanded Version*)

Ken Grauer, MD
Professor Emeritus in Family Medicine
College of Medicine, University of Florida
Founder of KG/EKG Press

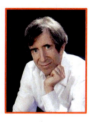

☞ *Dr. Grauer can be reached by:*

- **Mail** — KG/EKG Press; PO Box 141258
  Gainesville, FL 32614-1258
- **E-Mail** — ekgpress@mac.com
- **Web site** — www.kg-ekgpress.com
- **Fax** — (352) 641-6137
- **ECG Blog** — www.ecg-interpretation.blogspot.com

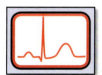

KG/EKG Press
Gainesville, Florida

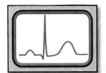

KG/EKG Press
Gainesville, Florida

- **Sole Proprietor** — Ken Grauer, MD
- **Design of All Figures** — Ken Grauer, MD
- **Printing** — by Renaissance Printing (*Gainesville, Florida*)
  - ▶*Special* Acknowledgement to Colleen Kay (*for making this book happen!*) and to Jay (*for all things technical!*).

▶ *Additional* Acknowledgements:
- Sean Smith, RN, BSN, NREMT-P — for his feedback, clinical wisdom, and *on-the-scene* insights. *Thank you Sean!*
- Harsha Nagarajarao, MD, FACC — for his cardiology pearls.
- John Gums, Pharm.D. — for his incomparable assistance on *all* matters pharmacologic.
- Rick & Stephanie of Ivey's Restaurant (*great food, staff and atmosphere that inspired my 'ACLS creativity'*).
- Abbas, Jane, Jenny & Gerald of the Haile Village Bistro (*for great food at my other 'writing space'*).

♥ *Special* Dedication — to Cathy Duncan (*who is my wife, my best friend, and the LOVE of My Life!*).

ISBN # 978-1-930553-34-7 (*# 1-930553-34-X*)

About ACLS – 2013 – Arrhythmias
(Expanded Version)

● Treatment of **cardiac arrest** (*and other acute cardiac arrhythmias*) demands *prompt* attention to clinical protocols with emphasis on *prioritizing* care. Herein lies the "beauty" of **ACLS-2013-Arrhythmias**: It facilitates understanding of *KEY* concepts in ACLS/Arrhythmia management <u>and</u> *lightens* the "**memory load**" — by providing *ready* reference to the most commonly used drugs and doses in emergency cardiac care.

- This is a *new* book.

- We have taken the ACLS-2013 PB (*Pocket Brain*) book — and substantially added to it. There are more than 100 new pages and figures on arrhythmia interpretation. Numerous explained and illustrated *Practice* Tracings have been added. Regardless of whether you are new to arrhythmias — intermediate — <u>or</u> highly experienced — your interpretation ability will advance to the *next* level!

- All content has been updated from previous editions of our work. In addition to actively incorporating *current* ACLS Guidelines — We venture **"Beyond-the-Textbook"** with commentary on each of the major algorithms that contains practical *management* pearls <u>and</u> important *clinical* insights.

 How to Use this *Expanded Version* Book:

☞ Our goal is *to provide key information fast*. Use of the **Rapid-Find Contents** (on the *front-inside* cover) facilitates finding the info you need *within* seconds. **Enhanced** features of this *new* book include:

- *User-friendly* organization into 20 major Sections.
- Numerous cross-referencing to *specific* pages for overlapping topics.
- *Summarizing* Algorithms on the *back-inside* cover.
- *Spiral* binding to enhance ease of use.
- Lots of *Practice* Tracings with detailed explained answers.

● **NOTE:** The content of this book is available electronically for *kindle-nook-kobo* and *ibooks*. This work is entitled, **"ACLS-2013-ePub"**.

- In the event you would like additional practice with a series of case studies in cardiac arrest — the new (*5th Edition*) of our companion ACLS book (**ACLS: Practice Code Scenarios-2013**) is out!

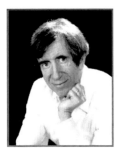

● **Ken Grauer, MD** has taught ECG inter-pretation for more than 3 decades. Author of more than 10 books (*which have sold half a million copies*) — he is a family physician educator whose medical passion is cardiology. His other "passions" are foreign languages (*Fr./Sp./Ger.*) — as well as dancing (*ballroom/2-step/Argentine tango*).

• Amazon Author Page: amazon.com/author/kengrauer

— *Other* Material by this *Author* —
(www.kg-ekgpress.com)

• ECG-2011 Pocket Brain (*our best selling PB book*)

• ECG-2011-ePub (*for nook/kindle/kobo/ibooks*)
  o *Expanded* ECG pdf File
  o ECG Practice Exercises booklet

• ACLS-2013 Pocket Brain (*the pocket-sized version of this book*)

• ACLS: Practice Code Scenarios-2013

• ACLS-2013-ePub (*for nook/kindle/kobo/ibooks*) — the *elec-tronic* version of this book.

• *For Those Who* **Teach** — *Please* check out:
  o My ECG-PDF Course (*lecture slides – learner notes – for any level of learner*)
  o ECG Competency (*objective documentation of primary care ECG interpretation ability*).

 Details on *my* **Web Site** (www.kg-ekgpress.com)
  • I'll *welcome* your feedback! (ekgpress@mac.com)

  • Please check out my **Free** *On-Line* **Resources:**
    o ECG Blog: www.ecg-interpretation.blogspot.com
    o ACLS Comments: www.kg-ekgpress.com/acls_comments

Section 01 – VFib (*pp 1-11*)

 Ventricular Fibrillation

● The patient is *unresponsive* in the following rhythm. *No* pulse. *No* spontaneous respiration:

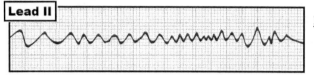

Figure 01-1:
Ventricular
Fibrillation.

• **Rhythm Description** — chaotic, completely *disorganized* waveform (*reflecting the fibrillating heart*).
• **Bedside Pitfalls** — IF a *pulse* is felt with a rhythm similar to the one shown above, you should *suspect* artifact! Potential causes of artifact include signal gain turned way down *and/or* disconnected leads (*easy to happen during the activity of cardiopulmonary resuscitation*).

KEY Clinical Points — VFib is a *potentially* treatable cause of cardiopulmonary arrest (*it is a "shockable" rhythm*). **Survival** from cardiac arrest due to V Fib can be optimized by: **i)** Finding (and *fixing*) the **cause** of arrest if at all possible; <u>and</u> **ii)** Minimizing the **time factors** (*minimizing* time to *recognize* patient collapse — *access* EMS — *initiate* CPR — and deliver a **shock**).

• Practically speaking, there is *little* that can be done to save those patients who arrest from a *'fate'* factor (ie, *from massive pulmonary embolus, ruptured aortic or ventricular aneurysm, etc.*). <u>Regardless</u> of how quickly you defibrillate these patients — they will *usually die* despite treatment ...
• Much more can be done <u>IF</u> the cause of V Fib is *potentially* reversible (*See pg 10*) — <u>IF</u> optimal BLS is performed — <u>and</u> the patient is *rapidly* defibrillated.
• *Ongoing* monitoring *during* CPR with **Capnography** may provide *useful* prognostic information (*See Addendum D on pp 18-20*).
• *Therapeutic* **Hypothermia** — may improve neurologic outcome in comatose survivors of cardiac arrest (*See Addendum A on pp 12-13*).

Ventricular Fibrillation

 ➡ **Suggested *Initial* Approach:**

Note: — **Pulseless** VT is treated the **same** as **VFib** (ie, *with defibrillation ASAP — and the identical algorithm!*).

• *Verify* **VFib** (ie, *that the patient is <u>truly</u> pulseless and unresponsive*) — Call for help! — Get a defibrillator.

- *Begin* **BLS** *as soon* as this is possible. Strive to *optimize* BLS performance and technique (*pp 5-6*).

▶ Possibility #1: IF arrest **witnessed** or thought to be *short-lived* (ie, *not more* than 4-5 minutes) — deliver **single** **shock** ASAP! (typically **Defibrillate** with **150**-200 **joules** for *biphasic* defibrillator or AED — or 360 joules for *monophasic* defibrillator).

▶ Possibility #2: IF arrest **not** **witnessed** (*especially* IF *thought to be more than ~4 minutes in duration*) — an option is to **perform** BLS for a **brief** **period** (*up to a minute or so*) until the defibrillator is ready for shock (*See pp 9-10*).

- Resume **BLS** *immediately* after each shock attempt. (*Minimize interruptions in chest compressions!*).
- Intubate/Achieve **access** for drug delivery (**IV**-**IO**-*or* ET).

☞ Drug Delivery: *What is the Optimal Access Route?*

ACLS Guidelines now advocate for *either* **IV** (*IntraVenous*) – or – **IO** (*IntraOsseous*) **access** as the optimal route for drug delivery during cardiopulmonary resuscitation.

- ACLS-PM *no longer* recommends giving drugs by the **ET route** during CPR (*higher doses are needed; absorption is far less reliable*). That said – there is *some* absorption by the ET route. The best approach in 2013 is probably to *reserve* ET dosing as a *last* resort only to be used if *neither* IV *nor* IO access is available.
- The **ET dose** for **Epinephrine** = **2-3 mg Epi** (*of 1:10,000 soln.*) down the ET tube, to be followed by several insufflations of the Ambu bag.
- IF a **peripheral** **IV** is used — Give drugs by bolus injection followed by a 20ml bolus of IV fluid (*also elevating the extremity*) to facilitate drug flow into the central circulation.
- **IO Route** — provides access into a *noncollapsible* venous plexus resulting in comparable drug delivery and dosing as by the IV route (*vs 2-3X more drug needed via the ET route*). Use of commercial kits makes IO use fast/easy/safe (*minimal complications*) and reliable.
- **Adenosine** is one drug that should probably not be given via the IO route (*because time for absorption may exceed the <10-second half-life of this drug*).
- *Central* **IV Drug Delivery** — recommended only for experienced providers (*with advantage that peak drug concentrations are superior to those from use of peripheral IV*) — BUT the central route is *not* necessarily favored if chest compressions need to be interrupted ...

☞ Epinephrine for VFib

Give **Epinephrine** (*See pg 8*) — *still* the drug we feel is 1st choice for cardiac arrest. Try to *give* **Epi** IV or **IO**.

- **IV** (*or* IO) **Dose**: Give **1.0 mg** of Epinephrine (*or 10 ml of a 1:10,000 soln.*) by **IV bolus**. May <u>repeat</u> every 3-5 minutes (*as long* as patient *remains* in V Fib).
- The **IO route**: — is *safe* to use — fast (*and easy*) to establish – <u>and</u> – provides *reliable* absorption with *minimal* risk of complications.
- **ET Dose**: Give **2-3 mg** Epinephrine (*of 1:10,000 soln.*) down the ET tube, followed by several insufflations of the Ambu bag (*Only give Epinephrine via the ET route if <u>no</u> <u>other</u> route available – page 2*).

☞ VFib *Initial* Approach: *After* Epi – *Consider* Vasopressin

- *Continue* **BLS**. *Minimize* interruption. Limit pulse checks (*unless the rhythm changes or capnography suggests ROSC*).
- Consider **Vasopressin** (*See pg 9*) — as an *acceptable* alternative to the 1st dose of Epinephrine — *and/or* may be *additive* to Epi. Give **40 U IV** (*or* IO) as a *one-time* dose (*whereas Epinephrine should be repeated every 3-5 minutes*).
- *Continue* **BLS**. *Minimize* interruption. Limit pulse checks (*unless the rhythm changes or capnography suggests ROSC*).
- *Repeat* **Shock** as appropriate (*usually not more often than every 2 minutes unless rhythm changes*). Use **150**-200 **joules** for *biphasic* defibrillator or AED <u>or</u> 360 joules for *monophasic* defibrillator.

☞ Amiodarone for VFib

    Give **Amiodarone** (*See pg 11*) — now *clearly* the antiarrhythmic agent of 1st choice for VT/V Fib!
- Give a **300 mg IV**/IO bolus for cardiac arrest. May give *repeat* boluses (*usually of **150 mg IV**/IO*) if/as needed for *persistent* V Fib (*max cumulative dose ~2,200 mg over 24 hours*).
- Follow Amiodarone bolus by *maintenance* **IV infusion** <u>IF</u> the patient converts *out of* V Fib (*at a rate of **1 mg/minute** = 60 mg/hour for 6 hours* — then *at a rate of **0.5 mg/minute** for the next 18-72 hours*).

☞ If VFib Persists: *Measures to Consider*

    A number of considerations arise if VFib persists. These include certain *ongoing* actions throughout the code, as well as *other* measures.
- Continued *high-quality* CPR (*with minimal interruption!*).
- **Search** for a *Predisposing* **Cause** of VFib (*Reexamine patient; Review chart; Body temperature; O2 status; Lab; Echo; 12-lead ECG; Ongoing Capnography; etc. — See pp 10-11*).
- Periodic Defibrillation (*as necessary/appropriate*).
- Repeat Epinephrine (*every 3-to-5 minutes*).
- **Magnesium** — Dosing is empiric (*pg 11*). Give **1-2 gm IV** for cardiac arrest. May repeat (*up to 4-6 gm IV*).
- An **IV Beta-Blocker** — Most likely to work <u>IF</u> excess *sympathetic* tone caused the arrest (*pg 11*).

- Might *consider* **Lidocaine** — 75-100 mg IV (*pg 11*).
- **Sodium Bicarbonate** (*See pg 9*) — is generally <u>not</u> indicated for the first 5-10 minutes of arrest (<u>*unless*</u> *patient had severe preexisting metabolic acidosis*). Thereafter may *empirically* try 1-2 amps of Bicarb <u>IF</u> pH remains *very* low (ie, <7.20) *despite* good ventilation.
- *Clarification* of **Code** **Status** if this has not yet been done (*advance directives if any; realistic goals for the resuscitation effort*).

☞ In the Event that ROSC is Attained ...

It is good to anticipate and contemplate interventions to initiate (*or at least consider*) in the event ROSC is attained. Among others – these include:

- ***Reassessment*** of the patient's overall condition (*including review of as much prior history as possible; serial physical exam; important lab tests/X-rays; assessment of intravascular volume status, dose and need for ongoing pressor agents and/or other medications*).
- Consideration of **Cooling** (*if not already started and the patient is not alert – See Addendum A on pp 12-13*).
- **IV Amiodarone infusion** – especially if felt that IV Amiodarone facilitated conversion out of VFib (*may help to prevent VFib recurrence over ensuing hours*).
- Is patient a **candidate** for ***immediate*** **cardiac catheterization?** (*See Addendum B on pp 14-16*).
- ***Transfer*** to **ICU** for ongoing *post-resuscitation* management.

☞ When ROSC is <u>*Not*</u> Attained: *When to STOP the Code?*

Practically speaking, the chance for *long-term* survival (*with intact neurologic status*) becomes much *less* — <u>IF</u> VFib persists *beyond* 20-30 minutes <u>*despite*</u> appropriate treatment.

- This is especially true <u>IF</u> capnography monitoring shows persistently *low* ET CO_2 values (*<10 mmHg*).
- Exceptions to the above generality exist (ie, *when prolonged resuscitation is more likely to work*). These include pre-code hypothermia, pediatric patients, and victims of drowning (*especially cold water drowning*).
- Unfortunately – initial neurologic exam (*including pupillary response*) is notoriously inaccurate in predicting outcome for victims of cardiopulmonary arrest.
- Clarification of code status (*that may not have been known at the time resuscitation began*) may add perspective.
- All the above said – sometimes *"ya just gotta be there"* to best determine *when* to stop the code (*though consideration of the above will hopefully help in decision-making*).

Ventricular Fibrillation

  ⇨ _Beyond-the-Textbook_ ...

● The incidence of **VFib** as the mechanism (*initial rhythm*) of cardiac arrest has been **decreasing** in recent years. This holds true for _both_ in-hospital _and_ *out-of-hospital* arrests. Implications of this trend are obvious — since the chance for successful resuscitation (*with intact neurologic status*) is far greater IF there is a **"*shockable*" rhythm** (*VT/VFib*) vs PEA/Asystole for the initial rhythm.

• In 2013 — decidedly *less* than 1/3 of all cardiac arrests *both* in- and out- of the hospital manifest VFib as the initial rhythm (*the majority being PEA/asystole*). In the past — VFib accounted for up to 2/3 of all cases.

• A number of reasons may account for this frequency change in the initial mechanism (*rhythm*) of cardiac arrest. The incidence of VFib during the early hours of acute infarction is significantly *less* than in years past because patients with acute STEMI (*ST Elevation Myocardial Infarction*) are routinely catheterized and promptly reperfused (*with angioplasty or thrombolytics*) in an ever increasing number of institutions. Patients seek help at emergency departments sooner for chest pain, and are generally admitted to the hospital. Among those who rule out for acute infarction — a diagnostic test is invariably done prior to discharge. Given that the risk of sudden death from coronary disease is greatest among patients not previously diagnosed — the above tendency toward hospital admission and workup for chest pain with resultant earlier diagnosis of coronary disease has decidedly reduced the incidence of malignant arrhythmia. Finally — use of the ICD (*Implantable Cardioverter-Defibrillator*) is increasingly widespread. Especially among patients with end-stage heart failure — far fewer die from VFib than ever before.

• At the same time as the overall incidence of VFib is decreasing — the **incidence** of a **nonshockable rhythm** (ie, *PEA or Asystole*) as the mechanism of cardiac arrest is **increasing**. PEA and asystole have become especially common as the *terminal* event in chronically ill patients with multiple underlying co-morbidities, who have often been kept alive only by extraordinary treatment measures (*long-term use of ventilators, pressor drugs, hyperalimentation, and extended use of broad spectrum antibiotics*).

• BOTTOM Line: The overall incidence of VFib as the mechanism of cardiac arrest is *less* than it used to be. This clinical reality has important prognostic implications because **prompt defibrillation** of **witnessed VFib works!** Assuming the patient does *not* have an underlying untreatable condition — the *sooner* one defibrillates a patient with *new-onset* VFib — the *better* the chance for survival (ie, *>90% of VFib episodes in cardiac rehab centers survive due to prompt recognition and shock*).

- In contrast — When the *precipitating* mechanism of cardiac arrest is PEA or asystole in a chronically ill patient — the likelihood of *successful* resuscitation that is sustained to the point that the patient will be able to *leave* the hospital with intact neurologic status becomes *exceedingly* small.

☞ Assessing/Improving *Realistic* Chance for Recovery

Realistic chance for *recovery* from VFib is enhanced by the *presence of* or *attention to* the following:
- *Prompt* recognition of VFib. Getting help fast. Rapid initiation of **high-quality CPR**. *Prompt* defibrillation.
- Identification of a readily *treatable* cause of VFib (*pp 10-11*).
- ***Minimizing*** **interruptions** in **CPR**. *Immediately* resume chest compressions after *each* shock. <u>Unless</u> the rhythm changes on the monitor or ET CO2 rises abruptly — it is best to wait ~2 minutes (~5 BLS cycles) *before* checking for a pulse. Limit intubation attempts to *less* than 10 seconds. (*Intubation is <u>not</u> necessarily needed for oxygenation to be adequate*).
- ***Awareness*** that <u>unless</u> you count — there is a tendency to compress *less* rapidly than 100/minute — <u>and</u> to ventilate *more* rapidly than 8-10/minute.
- Insight to the likelihood that a patient will respond to treatment may be provided by **Capnography**. Prognosis is exceedingly poor — IF **ET CO2** (*End-Tidal CO2*) values **persist** **<10mm Hg** after more than 20 minutes of CPR. In contrast — progressively *rising* ET CO2 values with ongoing CPR is indication to *continue* intensive therapy (*See Addendum D on pp 18-20*).

☞ What is *High-Quality* CPR?

A major focus of ACLS Guidelines is performance of *high-quality* CPR. Poorly performed BLS (*excessive interruptions — suboptimal technique — compressing too slow — ventilating too fast*) — are major contributors to poor outcome. We need to do better. Among the **most important** features of *high-quality* **CPR** are the following:
- Increase compression RATE to *at least* 100/minute (*was previously "approximately" 100/min*). We surmise the optimal compression rate is *between* 100-to-125/minute (*tendency for depth of compression and therefore quality to decrease IF compression rate faster than 125/min*).
- Increase compression DEPTH to *at least* 2 inches in adults (*was previously 1.5-to-2 inches*).
- Revise sequence to "**C**-**A**-**B**" (*from A-B-C*). Early on — rescue breaths are *less* important than chest compressions for cardiac arrest (*low flow rather than apnea the key limiting factor*).
- *"Hands-Only CPR"* for the untrained lay rescuer (*or rescuer unwilling to give rescue breaths*).
- *Compression-to-Ventilation* Ratio is still 30:2 for *single* rescuers of adults and children.

• *Rescue* Breaths — still given over ~1 second to produce visible chest rise (*avoid large/forceful breaths that increase risk of gastric insufflation IF no advanced airway yet placed*).

• Once *Advanced* Airway <u>is</u> in Place — Chest compressions need *no longer* be cycled. Instead 2 rescuers provide *continuous* compressions (*at least 100/minute*) <u>and</u> regular (*asynchronous*) delivery of 8-10 rescue breaths/minute (*=1 breath every 6-8 seconds*). Must *count* breaths!

● **SUMMARY of *High-Quality* CPR:** Coronary flow during CPR is optimized by pushing hard (*at least 2 inches*) <u>and</u> fast (*at least 100/minute*) — allowing *full* chest recoil — and *minimizing* interruptions. Be sure to *avoid* hyperventilation (*which increases intrathoracic pressure thereby reducing flow*).

• The importance of absolutely *minimizing* interruptions in chest compressions *cannot* be overstated!

• **KEY:** We use the example of **trying to bicycle uphill.** It is incredibly difficult to get started. Eventually (*once you get going uphill on a bicycle*) — it goes much better – <u>BUT</u> – if you have to stop — it will once again take you substantial time to get going again from a standstill ...

• **So it is with CPR:** Studies suggest that after each interruption of CPR (*no matter how brief that interruption may be*) — that it takes ~7-8 compressions (*or more*) until you once again begin to generate some effective cardiac output. **MORAL:** *Minimize* interruptions!

☞ Is Intubation *Essential* in Cardiac Arrest?

The answer to the question of whether intubation is "essential" in cardiac arrest is **no longer yes.** ACLS Guidelines state that ventilation with a bag/mask (*BVM*) – or – with bag through an advanced airway (ie, *ET tube* – <u>or</u> – *supraglottic airway*) — "is acceptable" during CPR.

• **Bag-Valve-Mask** (*BVM*) **ventilation** — is adequate initially during CPR (*should be done with 2 providers to ensure optimal seal of mask-to-face and optimal tidal volume delivery*).

• ***Endotracheal* Intubation** — offers advantages of optimal airway control; prevents aspiration; allows suctioning and high-flow O2 — <u>BUT</u> – complications common if performed by inexperienced providers — <u>and</u> intubation may be *detrimental* IF it results in interruption of compressions ...

• ***Supraglottic* Airways** — are easier to insert than an ET tube (*the glottis need not be directly visualized*) — there are *fewer* complications — you *don't* have to stop CPR! – <u>and</u> – they *are* effective!

☞ Use of Epinephrine in Cardiac Arrest

ACLS-PM still recommends Epinephrine *and/or* Vasopressin as "pressors of choice" during cardiac arrest. That said — there has been recent controversy on the Pros and Cons of using Epinephrine:

- Pharmacologically — the alpha-adrenergic (*vasoconstrictor*) effect of Epinephrine increases cerebral and coronary flow (*the latter by increasing aortic diastolic pressure*).
- There is to date *no evidence* that use of Epinephrine in cardiac arrest increases survival to hospital discharge.
- There <u>is</u> evidence that **Epinephrine** *increases* the chance of **ROSC** (*Return of Spontaneous Circulation*) with initial resuscitation.
- A number of recent studies question if Epinephrine may have detrimental effect. *These studies are flawed.* Nothing will save a patient if the rhythm is flat line on EMS arrival. Use of Epi *does* increase the chance of getting back a pulse in such patients — but irreversible brain damage has most probably *already* occurred. This does <u>not</u> constitute "proof" that Epi "caused" neurologic injury — but rather raises the more important question of whether patients with unwitnessed *out-of-hospital* arrest who are found by EMS in PEA/asystole should be resuscitated in the first place. (For **more discussion**: https://www.kg-ekgpress.com/acls_comments-_issue_10/).
- The final answer regarding optimal use of Epinephrine in cardiac arrest is *not* yet known. The dilemma is *What to do in the meantime?* **ACLS-PM *still* recommends** use of **Epinephrine** for cardiac arrest. Results of studies in which a majority of subjects had *out-of-hospital* PEA/asystole should <u>not</u> be generalized to all cases of cardiac arrest with VFib as the initial rhythm. As a result — We still favor initial use of Epinephrine for arrests when the patient is found in VFib.
- ACLS-PM does *not* recommend use of higher dose Epinephrine. That said — The **"*maximum dose*"** of **Epi** is really unknown. A **1mg IV bolus** peaks in ~2-3 minutes. Studies of *out-of-hospital* arrest have *not* shown benefit from **HDE** (*Higher-Dose Epinephrine*) — however, the number of study subjects was probably inadequate to rule out possibility of benefit from HDE in certain subsets of patients not responding to shock.
- ***OUR THOUGHTS:*** We do <u>not</u> favor routine use of HDE. That said — a case can be made for *empiric* trial of increasing Epinephrine dose (*2,3,5mg*) in *selected* nonresponding patients for whom the clinician believes the chance for successful resuscitation with intact neurologic function still exists.
- **P.S.:** Whether ***therapeutic* hypothermia** will increase the chance of neurologic recovery for some *out-of-hospital* arrest victims achieving ROSC with Epinephrine is the subject of intense *ongoing* study. Current criteria to initiate cooling include *persistent* coma post-ROSC. *Stay tuned ...*

Use of *both* Epinephrine *and* Vasopressin?

ACLS-PM allows for *substitution* of Vasopressin for *either* the 1st or 2nd dose of Epinephrine in cardiac arrest. Given the longer duration of action of Vasopressin — administration of a single 40IU dose essentially lasts for the duration of most codes:

- ACLS-PM describes Vasopressin as a *nonadrenergic* peripheral vasoconstrictor with efficacy in cardiac arrest that is "no different from that of Epinephrine".
- Data are lacking regarding *potential* for **synergistic effect** using *both* **Epi** *plus* **Vasopressin** in cardiac arrest.
- We feel use of both drugs <u>is</u> reasonable (*slightly differing mechanisms of action*) — <u>and</u> that little is lost by *adding* Vasopressin if patients fail to respond to Epinephrine alone. That said — We do <u>not</u> favor routine Epi *plus* Vasopressin for all cases <u>IF</u> arrest is prolonged, prognosis appears dismal, and irreversible brain damage appears likely.
- Realistically — it will be difficult to design a study that "proves" synergistic benefit from use of both drugs — so bedside decision to add Vasopressin or not is empiric.

Use of Bicarb?

ACLS-PM *no longer* routinely recommends Bicarb in the cardiac arrest algorithm. The initial acidosis in cardiac arrest is primarily respiratory (*especially during the first 5-10 minutes*). Giving Bicarb during these initial minutes may paradoxically *worsen* intracellular acidosis (*despite improving ABG pH values*). That said — there <u>are</u> select circumstances when **empiric BICARB** (~1 mEq/kg = ~1-1.5 amps) may be reasonable and should *at least* be considered. These include:

- **Hyperkalemia** (*Bicarb is a treatment of choice!*).
- **Tricyclic Overdose** — to alkalinize to pH ~7.45-7.55 in select severe cases.
- ***Preexisting* Metabolic Acidosis**.
- Perhaps (?) for **refractory** cardiac arrest *after* ~5-10 minutes of resuscitation — <u>IF</u> pH is *still* low (<*7.25*) and *nothing* else is working ...

Immediate <u>vs</u> *Delayed* Shocked for VFib?

Delayed defibrillation of VFib may <u>not</u> work. It may even be deleterious — by *reducing* the chance that defibrillation will successfully convert the VFib rhythm. The obvious difficulty lies with determining **how much delay** (?) becomes *too long* for recommending defibrillation as the immediate *initial* action when VFib is found on EMS arrival.

- 2005 Guidelines favored *delaying* defibrillation — <u>IF</u> it was likely that *more* than 4-5 minutes had passed since onset of cardiac arrest. More

recent studies are *inconclusive* about benefit or not from defibrillating prior to CPR for VFib present more than 4-5 minutes.
- *New* Guidelines in ACLS-PM now allow the option to *immediately* shock VFib of *uncertain* duration <u>without</u> a preceding period of CPR.
- **Witnessed** **VFib** should be **promptly** **shocked** (*as soon as an AED/defibrillator is available*).
- Assuming time until arrival is not excessive — many (*if not most*) hospital providers routinely shock *newly-discovered* VFib as soon as they are able to do so.
- Data is *inconclusive* for the optimal approach to **unwitnessed** **VFib** that occurs ***out-of-hospital***. New Guidelines allow for performance of 1.5-to-3 minutes of BLS (*~5 cycles of 30:2 CPR*) <u>before</u> the 1st shock is given. Alternatively (*our preference*) — it may be most practical to **perform** CPR for a **brief** period just <u>until</u> the **defibrillator** is **ready** for shock delivery!

☞ *Correctable* Cause of Cardiac Arrest?

Finding a cause of VFib you can "fix" offers the *greatest* chance for survival. Potentially ***treatable*** **causes** of *persistent* VFib **include:**
- Acute MI (*electrical instability during initial hours of MI*);
- Drug overdose (*which may precipitate respiratory arrest in a patient with an otherwise normal heart*);
- Hypoxemia (*respiratory arrest; drowning; etc.*);
- Hypothermia (*easy to miss if you don't check body temperature*);
- Hyperkalemia/Hypokalemia/Hypomagnesemia (*or other marked electrolyte imbalance of calcium, phosphorus, sodium*).
- Acidosis / Sepsis / Heart Failure.
- Hypovolemia (*including blood loss*);
- A **complication** from **CPR** (*tension pneumothorax, pericardial tamponade, ET in right mainstem bronchus*).

☞ ACLS-<u>PM</u> summarizes ***treatable*** **causes** of cardiac arrest (*be this from VT/VFib — Asystole/PEA*) by use of **6 H**'s and **5 T**'s:
- **6 H's:** — **H**ypoxia; **H**ypovolemia; **H**ypothermia; **H**+ ion (*acidosis*); **H**ypoglycemia; <u>and</u> **H**yper- or **H**ypoKalemia.
- **5 T-s:** — **T**oxins (*including drug overdose*); **T**amponade (*cardiac*); **T**ension Pneumothorax; **T**hrombosis *that is* **Pulmonary** (*embolus*) or **Coronary** (*acute MI*).

☞ *Work-Up* looking for a *Correctable* Cause of Arrest

Lab Tests to order during (or *after*) the arrest are in large part based on *looking* for a potentially *treatable* cause. While clearly not a complete list — We mention some basic tests to consider below:
- Vital signs (*temperature?*).
- Chest X-ray (*Is ET tube/central line placement OK?*).
- 12-lead ECG (*acute infarction? / rhythm diagnosis?*).

- Echocardiogram (*if relevant to assess for tamponade; pulmonary embolus; LV function*).
- CBC; Chem profile with electrolytes (*including Magnesium, Calcium, Phosphorus, etc.*).
- Toxicology Screen (*if relevant*).
- Arterial Blood Gases/*ongoing* O2-Sat monitoring / Capnography.

☞ Role of *Antiarrhythmic* Drugs in VFib?

Use of antiarrhythmic drugs (*Amiodarone* — *Lidocaine* — *Procainamide*) has <u>never</u> been shown to improve *longterm* outcome for patients in cardiac arrest.

- **Amiodarone** — has been shown to improve *short*-term survival to hospital (*but <u>not</u> beyond*).
- ACLS-PM — *still* recommends **Amiodarone** for **refractory VFib** that *fails* to respond to Shock/Epinephrine. Although reasonable — this recommendation is <u>not</u> evidenced based (*there is no evidence Amio improves longterm outcome from VFib*).
- <u>IF</u> converted *out* of VFib — then *prophylactic* **IV infusion** of **Amidarone** is recommended (*for the next ~24 hours*) to *minimize* the chance of VFib recurrence.
- **Lidocaine** — has been relegated as a *2nd-line* agent for *refractory* VFib (*after Amiodarone*). Give **1.0-1.5 mg/kg** (*~50-100mg*) as an initial **IV**/IO **bolus**. Repeat boluses of ~50-75mg may be given every 5-10 minutes (*up to a total loading dose ~225mg = up to ~3mg/kg*).
- **Procainamide** — is <u>not</u> recommended for VFib (*it is <u>not</u> a good antifibrillatory agent*).
- **Other Drugs** — There <u>are</u> selected *special* circumstances for which Beta-blockers and Magnesium may prove to be *lifesaving* agents. For **Beta-Blockers** — this includes *refractory* VT/VFib and acute *anterior* MI with increased *sympathetic* tone. For **Magnesium** — this includes *Torsades de Pointes*). That said — decision to use these agents during cardiac arrest is to be *individualized* based on clinical circumstances.
- ACLS-PM — does <u>not</u> routinely recommend Magnesium in cardiac arrest <u>unless</u> there is Torsades. That said — **Magnesium** is clearly indicated if **K+/Mg++** are *low*; <u>and</u> there is data supporting *empiric* **use** for arrhythmias *not* responding to other measures (*1-2 gm IV; may repeat*). There would seem to be little harm and potential benefit from empiric trial of Magnesium for VFib not responding to other measures ...

☞ VFib: *Summary*

⬤ *Overall* prognosis for VFib is potentially good <u>IF</u> there is *no* irreversible underlying disorder <u>and</u> VFib is *promptly* recognized/defibrillated.
- What role **therapeutic hypothermia** will ultimately assume for *optimizing* survival and neurologic outcome in patients who remain *unresponsive* post-ROSC is actively evolving. *Stay tuned!*

➡ **Addendum A: *Who to Cool?***

● Recent years have seen marked increase in use of **Therapeutic Hypothermia** in hope of improving meaningful (*neurologically intact*) survival from cardiac arrest. Initial results from **TH** (*Therapeutic Hypothermia*) are increasingly encouraging. As a result, in 2013 — **Cooling** should be **routinely considered** ASAP *after* ROSC is attained in arrest survivors who do not wake up ...

• **BACKGROUND** — Overall survival from cardiac arrest both *in-* and *out-of-hospital* remains poor. Most victims who develop ROSC but eventually die, do so from *anoxic* brain injury. The proposed mechanism of TH is based on its attenuating effect on *"post-arrest syndrome"* with the accompanying cerebral edema, inflammatory response and reperfusion injury that occurs. Post-arrest cooling *reduces* metabolic demands <u>and</u> *slows* the sequence of adverse events.

• **WHICH Patients Qualify?** — *Any* patient resuscitated from cardiac arrest (ie, *attaining ROSC*) <u>regardless</u> of the initial mechanism of arrest (*VT/VFib/Asystole or PEA*). Cooling should be started ASAP after ROSC is attained — with goal of achieving target temperature within 3-6 hours. Post-arrest patients alert enough to follow simple commands do <u>not</u> need or benefit from being cooled! (*Most centers use a Glasgow Coma Score =* **GCS** *of <7-8/15 as qualifying criteria*).

 Glasgow Coma Scale

Eye Opening Response:
● Spontaneously open and blinking (4 points)
● Opens in response to verbal stimuli or command (3 points)
● Opens in response to pain (2 points)
○ NO response (1 point)

Verbal Response:
● Oriented (5 points)
● Confused - but able to answer questions (4 points)
● Inappropriate speech (3 points)
● Incomprehensible speech (2 points)
○ NO response (1 point)

Motor Response:
● Obeys command when asked to move (6 points)
● Purposeful movement in response to pain (5 points)
● Withdraws in response to pain (4 points)
● Flexion (*decorticate*) in response to pain (3 points)
● Extension (*decerebrate*) in response to pain (2 points)
○ NO response (1 point)

<u>NOTE</u>: You get 3 points on GCS just for showing up (*open circles*)!

- **WHEN to Start Cooling?** — Answer = *ASAP after ROSC* achieved in appropriate patients.
- **WHO to Cool?** — *Any* post-arrest patient with ROSC who is admitted to the ICU but is as yet <u>unable</u> to follow simple commands (ie, *"Lift your arm"*).

🐭☞ **KEY *Clinical* Points** — Realizing that prognosis will be poorer for cooled *post-arrest* patients who were initially found in asystole (*rather than VFib*) — <u>IF</u> decision is made for truly intense treatment (*defined by decision to treat in an ICU*) — then *post-arrest* cooling should be part of the regimen.

- **Prognostic Indicators** — Although finding a patient in asystole suggests longer "down-time" (*and correspondingly less chance of responding to resuscitation*) — <u>neither</u> asystole <u>nor</u> PEA rule out possibility of neurologically-intact survival. Initial neurologic exam (*including pupillary response*) is notoriously inaccurate in predicting outcome for victims of cardiac arrest. This explains expanded inclusion criteria for "Who to Cool?" (*See above*).
- **Exclusion Criteria** — Patients who should <u>not</u> be cooled include: **i)** Patients with a valid DNR (<u>D</u>o <u>N</u>ot <u>R</u>esuscitate) order; **ii)** Recent major surgery (*within 14 days*); **iii)** Severe systemic infection (ie, *sepsis*); **iv)** Known bleeding disorder; <u>and</u> **v)** Patients who *can* follow commands (*since alert patients do not benefit from cooling*).
- **Cooling Protocols** — are variable from one institution to the next — but most aim to *maintain* cooling at ~32-34 degrees C (*89.6-93.2 degrees F*) for ~24 hours — followed by *slow* rewarming (~*0.25 degrees C/hour*).
- **Complications** — include arrhythmias; sepsis; fluid overload; coagulopathy; hyperglycemia.
- **PEARLS:** — The *sooner* cooling is started — the *better* the response is likely to be (*ideally beginning within 30-60 minutes post-ROSC — and idelly attaining goal temperature within 3-to-4 hours*). Iced IV Saline works great (*and can usually lower temperature faster than cooling devices*). Optimal core temperature monitoring is by esophageal probe (*rectal probe lags behind changes in core temperature*).

01 – Addendum B: *Who to Cath?* (*pp 14-16*)

 ⇨ Addendum B: *Who to Cath?*

● One of the *KEY* questions to answer when working a code is IF there is a potentially *"fixable"* precipitating cause? (*pp 10-11*). Acute occlusion of a major coronary vessel is among the most important causes that might be found. We emphasize the following points:

• The most common cause of sudden cardiac death in adults over 30-35 years of age is coronary artery disease (CAD). Unfortunately, in many cases — the very first "symptom" is the patient's last (ie, *fatal VT/VFib*). Other sudden death victims have a prior history of CAD — while yet others may not know they have CAD, but were having *prodromal* chest pain over *days-to-weeks* prior to the event that they denied or ignored. Thus, the history *preceding* the event for victims of *out-of-hospital* VT/VFib is diverse.

• *Not* all victims of sudden cardiac death who have underlying significant CAD die of acute occlusion in a major coronary vessel. Awareness of this clinical reality is important — since emergent *post-resuscitation* PCI (*PerCutaneous Intervention*) will *not* necessarily improve outcome if performed on a VFib survivor who has underlying CAD but *not* acute coronary occlusion.

• In contrast — **emergent PCI may be *lifesaving*** — IF performed on a VFib survivor in whom the cause of arrest was acute occlusion of a major coronary artery.

• The importance of the ***post-resuscitation* 12-lead ECG** — is that it may help identify which patients had their VT/VFib episode precipitated by acute coronary occlusion. Thus, the finding of **acute STEMI** (*ST Elevation Myocardial Infarction*) **on *post-resuscitation* ECG** is clear indication for immediate cath with goal of acute PCI (*reperfusion*) <u>unless</u> there is clear contraindication to performing this procedure (**Figure B-1**).

• That said – the clinical reality is that ***post-resuscitation* ECGs are often _not_ normal**. Rather than acute STEMI — much of the time one may see the gamut of QRS/QT prolongation with diffuse nonspecific ST-T wave abnormalities. ST depression is common (*and may be marked*). How specific such immediate *post-resuscitation* tracings are for acute coronary occlusion as the precipitating cause of cardiac arrest is another matter …

• **QT prolongation** is **common** in *post-resuscitation* tracings. This should not be surprising given the CNS insult associated with cardiac arrest (*especially in patients who do not immediately wake up after resuscitation*).

• ***Repeating* the ECG** may be helpful. This is illustrated in the two tracing sequence shown in <u>Figure B-2</u> and <u>Figure B-3</u>. These 2 ECGs were obtained just 9-minutes apart in a victim of out-of-hospital cardiac arrest who was successfully resuscitated.

☞ **_KEY_ Points** — The issue of **WHO to Take to the Cath Lab?** following successful resuscitation is rapidly evolving. Definitive answers are *not* yet in.

- Obviously — *all* viable VFib survivors with *acute* STEMI *on post-resuscitation* ECG merit a trip to the cath lab (Figure B-1). However, consensus is lacking as to what should be done when the *post-resuscitation* ECG is less definitive. Opinions vary.
- At one end of the spectrum are advocates of "acute cath for <u>all</u> VFib survivors".
- At the other end are those who <u>only</u> favor acute cath for VFib survivors with acute STEMI on *post-resuscitation* ECG. Many institutions are somewhere in between.
- Time will tell what the *best* answer is. In the meantime — the sequence of *post-resuscitation* tracings seen in Figures B-2 and B-3 (*on page 16*) will hopefully increase awareness of a common situation in which a *"non-STEMI"* ECG may nonetheless argue strongly in favor of need for acute catheterization and potentially lifesaving PCI.

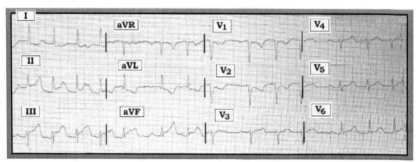

Figure B-1: Acute STEMI on ECG. If this ECG was seen in a viable *post-resuscitation* patient — acute cath would be *immediately* indicated. Goal of such cath would be acute reperfusion of the "culprit" artery — which most likely is the RCA (*Right Coronary Artery*) given *inferior* ST elevation that is *greater* in lead III than in lead II; *reciprocal* ST-T wave abnormalities in leads aVL,V1,V2 — <u>and</u> probable AV Wenckebach for the rhythm.

- Two additional <u>beyond-the-core</u> clues to *acute* RCA occlusion on this tracing are: **i)** More ST depression in lead aVL > lead I (*in this patient with more ST elevation in lead III > II*); <u>and</u> **ii)** associated *posterior* involvement (*suggested by the shape of ST depression in leads V1,V2 = positive "mirror test"*).

☞ **Example of *sequential* non-STEMI *post-resuscitation* ECGs**
— Should this *post-resuscitation* patient be taken to the cath lab?

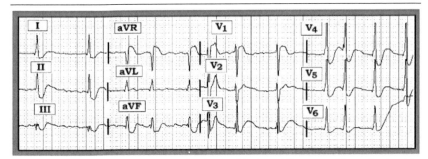

Figure B-2: Initial *post-resuscitation* ECG in a 50-year old patient with *out-of-hospital* cardiac arrest. The rhythm is relatively slow AFib. There is at least slight QRS widening of uncertain etiology (*nonspecific IVCD*). Although scooped ST depression is seen in a number of leads *with* ST coving and ST elevation in leads aVR,V1,V3 — the overall pattern is *not* specific for any particular "culprit lesion" (*and the picture is a bit different than is usually seen with left-main or severe 3-vessel disease*). This *grossly abnormal* ECG is typical for what one may see post-resuscitation. That said — the picture is clarified with the *follow-up* tracing below obtained just 9-minutes later (Figure B-3).

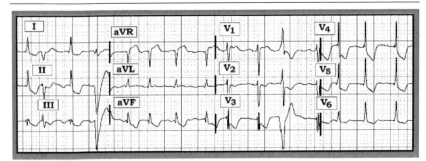

Figure B-3: Follow-up *post-resuscitation* tracing obtained 9 min-utes after the ECG in Figure B-2. The rhythm is again AFib, now with PVCs. The QRS looks to have narrowed slightly — and there is now much *more* conventional deep, diffuse ST depression in numerous leads (*still with ST elevation in leads aVR and V1*). The picture is now *more* worrisome for ischemia, consistent with what is often seen with severe 3-vessel or left-main disease (*diffuse ST depression with ST elevation in aVR and V1*). Acute cath *confirmed* this clinical suspicion, which was treated with *multi-vessel* angioplasty/stenting in this VFib survivor.
BOTTOM Line: The *post-resuscitation* ECG may be challenging to interpret. It may suggest *potential* for benefit with reperfusion, even when ECG changes of *acute* STEMI are *not* seen. *Serial* tracings help.

⇨ Addendum C: *Use of Echo*

● Reasons to consider *stat* **Echocardiogram** on a patient in cardiac arrest of *uncertain* cause (*especially when the patient is in PEA*) include:

• Determination <u>IF</u> there is *meaningful* cardiac contraction (*albeit inadequate contraction to produce a pulse*).

• Ready detection of pericardial (*or pulmonary*) effusion. *Moderate-to-large* pericardial effusions are easy to see on stat Echo as abnormal fluid collection within the pericardial space. More subtle small effusions are unlikely to be clinically significant during an *ongoing* resuscitation attempt. Motion abnormalities (ie, *"swinging heart"*) may be seen if there is spontaneous contraction. Stat Echo (*if available*) may be invaluable to identify cardiac tamponade as the cause of PEA.

• ☞ Suspicion of *acute* **PE** (*pulmonary embolism*) that might be treatable as the *precipitating* cause of arrest. **Echo findings** suggestive of hemodynamically significant PE include: **i)** Severe RV dilatation (*especially when found in association with small LV cavity size*); **ii)** Impaired RV contractility; **iii)** RV pressure overload; **iv)** Positive McConnell's sign (*which is akinesia of the mid-RV free wall, but normal motion of the apex*); <u>and</u> **v)** Identification of thrombus. Admittedly — several of these Echo findings are difficult to assess during ongoing resuscitation. That said — the *unexpected* finding of severe RV dilatation in association with normal (*or small*) LV cavity size in a coding patient should strongly suggest the possibility of acute PE as the precipitating cause. This is particularly true <u>IF</u> clinical circum-stances leading up to the arrest are consistent with *acute* PE as the potential cause (*See* <u>Figure C-1</u>).

• Detection of regional wall motion abnormalities (*might suggest acute MI that could benefit from immediate cath/acute reperfusion*).

• Diagnosis of acute dissecting aneurysm (*that might be amenable in certain select centers to emergency surgery*).

• <u>OR</u> — The Echo may be normal (*which may be comforting to know by supporting the unfortunate reality that there is little more to be done*).

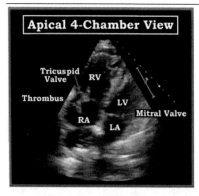

Apical 4-Chamber View

Tricuspid Valve • RV • Thrombus • LV • Mitral Valve • RA • LA

Figure C-1: Apical 4-Chamber View on Echo obtained from a patient with acute PE. Note disproportionately *increased* RV chamber size in association with a relatively *small* LV. Mobile thrombus (*seen on video as shuttling back-and-forth between the RA and RV*) is noted on this still-frame view. Unanticipated *severe* RV dilatation in association with a *smaller* LV is *highly* suggestive of *acute* PE as the cause of PEA.

01 – Addendum D: *Capnography / ET CO2 (pp 18-20)*

 ⇒ **Addendum D:** *Capnography Primer*

● Physiologic monitoring done *before/during/after* resuscitation — may be of invaluable assistance! In particular — ACLS Guidelines now endorse use of **Quantitative** *Waveform* **Capnography** *throughout* the periarrest period. We briefly review the basics of Capnography (*ET CO2 monitoring*) with goal of illustrating HOW this tool may be used:
- **Capnography** — is merely measurement of CO_2 in the *exhaled* breath. The principle is simple: *Inspired* air contains *negligible* CO_2 (*0.03%*) – vs – a percentage of 4.5% CO_2 in *expired* air.
- The amount of CO_2 can be measured — as shown in Figure D-1 which illustrates the **normal** *Waveform* **Capnogram**:

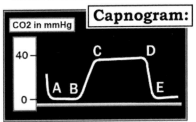

Figure D-1: Normal *Waveform* Capnogram. Note that the waveform *begins* with expiration (*at Point A*). Normal *End-Tidal* CO_2 = 35-40 mm Hg (*attained at Point D*) — after which *"inspiration washout"* begins.

- **Phase A-to-B** (*in* Figure D-1) — is the **Post-Inspiration** **Phase**. This phase occurs at the very beginning of expiration. It initially involves the 'dead space' — which explains why CO_2 remains zero!
- **Point B** – is the start of alveolar exhalation.
- **Phase B-to-C** – is the **Exhalation** Upstroke (*dead gas now begins to mix with CO2-rich alveolar gas — which explains why CO2 shows a very steep rise*).
- **Phase C-to-D** — reflects continuation (*until the end*) of expiration. The slope of Phase *C-to-D* is usually fairly flat, with perhaps a *slight* incline (*as 'slow alveoli' empty*). This phase takes on a peculiar **"shark fin" appearance** (Figure D-2) when there is delayed mixing with alveolar air (*as occurs in obstructive pulmonary disease or asthma*).

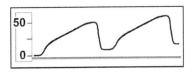

Figure D-2: Delayed mixing with alveolar air results in a *"shark fin"* appearance during Phase C-to-D (*which is characteristic of patients with COPD or asthma*).

- **Point D** (*in* Figure D-1) — is **ET CO2** (*End-Tidal CO2*) – which is *peak* CO_2 concentration (*which is normally between 35-45 mmHg*).
- **Phase D-to-E** (*in* Figure D-1) — is the **Inspiration "Washout"** (*inspired air contains negligible CO2 — so CO2 concentration rapidly drops toward zero as soon as inspiration begins*).

KEY Points — Think of *Capnography* as an *additional* "vital sign". It is far more helpful than pulse oximetry (*which provides information about oxygenation – but tells us nothing about ventilation*). A waveform will be seen with respiration *as soon as* an ET CO2 monitoring device is placed. In the *non-breathing* patient — You'll see a waveform as soon as you have intubated.

- The capnogram in Figure D-3 shows 2 normal ventilations. Note the normal *rectangular* waveform (*with ET CO2 ~35-40 mm Hg*) indicating successful placement of the ET tube in the trachea — *until* the ET tube comes out (*arrow in Fig. D-3*).

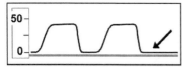

Figure D-3: Capnogram showing 2 normal ventilations until the ET tube comes out (*arrow*).

Clinical Uses of Capnography (*ET CO2 Monitoring*)

Capnography has benefit in intubated or non-intubated patients:
- In the **NON-Intubated** Patient — **i)** May help assess degree of broncho-spasm (*shark fin*) and response to bronchodilator therapy; **ii)** Rapid detection of hypoventilation (*increasing CO2*) and of need to intubate; **iii)** Detects hyperventilation (*better than counting breaths*).
- In the **Intubated** Patient — **i)** Verification of ET tube placement (*a CO2 reading = zero implies you are in the esophagus!*); **ii)** Assists in EMS monitoring during transport (*tells if you need to ventilate faster or slower based on whether CO2 is accumulating or not*).
- In the **Cardiac Arrest** Patient – many uses! (*See Examples below*).

● *Capnography During Cardiac Arrest:* Example #1 (*Figure D-4*):

ET CO2 = zero at the onset of cardiac arrest. There is *definite* correlation between ET CO2 and cardiac output:
- ET CO2 increases from zero to ~5-10 mmHg with *initial* CPR.
- Values then increase to the ~10-25 mmHg range with *effective* CPR.

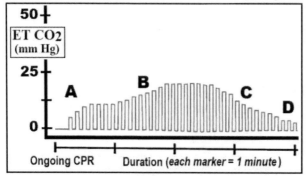

Figure D-4: Capnography Trend Analysis for Example 1 (*See text*).

- The **Capnogram** Trend (*over time*) — provides *KEY* insight on many aspects of CPR. This is evident in **Figure D-4** – which covers a period of about 4 minutes (*during which there are ~8-10 ventilations/minute; compressions are not seen on the capnogram*).
- **Period A** (*in* Figure D-4) — shows an initial short flat line (*until the airway is in place*) — after which ET CO2 attains ~10 mmHg (*which is consistent with initial CPR during cardiac arrest*).
- **Period B** — shows *gradual* increase in ET CO2 up to 15-18 mmHg (*consistent with increased flow from effective CPR*).
- **Period C** — The rescuer doing chest compressions may be tiring (*gradual drop in ET CO2 values*). An alternative explanation for the low values for **D** in Figure D-4 (*to below 10 mmHg*) — may be poor likelihood for survival (*vs a ventilator problem or pulmonary embolus*).

⬤ *Capnography During Cardiac Arrest:* **Example #2** (*Figure D-5*):

ET CO2 monitoring *during* resuscitation may predict **ROSC** (*Return Of Spontaneous Circulation*) even *before* you are actually able to feel a pulse (*IF there is sudden marked rise to >35 mmHg*).
- BUT — *Poor* outcome is likely IF ET CO2 is still *less* than 10 mmHg after ~20 minutes of *high-quality* CPR.
- The capnography trend in **Figure D-5** tells a "story" as to what occurred during this resuscitation effort. Initially (**A**) — the patient is in full arrest (*No pulse; no respiration*). Chest compressions are started (*not seen on the capnogram*).
- The patient is intubated (***B*** *in* Figure D-5). A waveform is now seen.
- ET CO2 drops back to zero by **C** (*the tube must have come out; reintubation is needed*).
- There is successful reintubation in **D**.
- Increasing ET CO2 readings by **E** (*up to ~15-20 mmHg*) suggest CPR is effective with ROSC by **F** (*sudden rise to an ET CO2 >40*).
- There is return to a normal ET CO2 of ~35-40 mmHg after ROSC (**G**).
- ET CO2 drops (**H**) — as the patient again codes.
- Prognosis is poor due to persistently low ET CO2 (**I**).

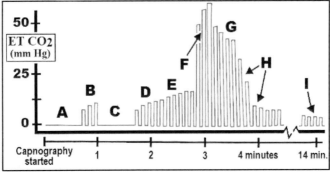

Figure D-5: Capnography Trend for Example 2 (*See text*).

Section 02 – *Clinical* Rhythm Diagnosis (*pp 21-35*)

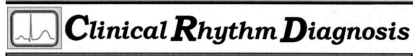

Clinical **R**hythm **D**iagnosis

● **Systematic Approach: *Watch Your Ps, Qs and 3Rs***
   The *KEY* to effective rhythm interpretation is to utilize a **Systematic Approach**. The system we favor is based on routinely assessing for the following **5 Parameters:**

- Presence (*and nature*) of **P** waves?
  - **Q**RS width?
    - **R**egularity of the rhythm?
      - IF P waves are present — Are they **R**elated to the QRS?
      - Heart **R**ate?

NOTE: It matters *not* in what sequence you look at the 5 parameters – as long as you *always* assess *each* of them!
- We often *change* the sequence in which we look at these parameters — depending on the tracing. Thus, we do not always assess atrial activity first (*especially if P waves are not overly obvious, or seem to be changing in morphology*). Instead — we may look first at QRS width — or regularity of the rhythm — depending on what seems easiest (*and most definitive*) to assess on the particular tracing. BUT — We *always* make sure we assess *all* 5 parameters.

☞ **MEMORY AID:** — We find it easiest to recall the 5 parameters by the saying, ***"Watch your Ps and Qs – and the 3Rs"***.

- **Clinical Reality:** You will <u>not</u> always be able to definitively diagnose the etiology of an arrhythmia from a single rhythm strip. *Even the experts will not always know for sure!* That said — Use of the **5 Parameter** (*Ps,Qs,3Rs*) **Approach** will allow you to: **i)** Rapidly <u>and</u> accurately assess *any* arrhythmia; **ii)** Prevent you from *missing* any major findings; **iii)** *Narrow down* differential possibilities, even if you are not sure of the rhythm diagnosis; <u>and</u> **iv)** Sound intelligent as you go through the process (*even if you don't know the answer*). We model application of this approach with a series of Practice Examples beginning on page 36.

☞ **The 6th Parameter: *Is the Patient Stable?***

   We discuss in detail assessment for hemodynamic stability in Section 03 (*pp 48-50*) <u>and</u> Section 04 (*pp 51-52*). For now — Suffice it to emphasize that the ***1st thing*** to do (*even before you begin to assess the 5 Parameters*) — is to determine <u>IF</u> the patient is hemodynamically stable. For example — ***Look at*** the rhythm in **Figure 02-1**. Clinically — *What would you do first in managing this patient?*
- **Scenario #1:** — The rhythm in Figure 02-1 is obtained from a *hypotensive* patient with shortness of breath and chest discomfort?

- **Scenario #2:** — The patient is alert, *asymptomatic* — <u>and</u> has a BP = 150/90 mmHg?
- ***Additional* QUESTIONS:** What is the rhythm in **Figure 02-1**? With regard to your *initial* intervention — *Does it really matter* what the rhythm is?

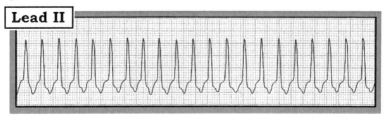

Figure 02-1: Tachycardia (*See text*).

☞ ***KEY* Point:** — Much *more* important initially than diagnosing what the rhythm in <u>Figure 02-1</u> is — is assessment of the patient's clinical status (ie, *Is the patient hemodynamically stable?*).

- We actually can <u>not</u> tell for sure what the rhythm in <u>Figure 02-1</u> is. By the **5 *Parameter* Approach** — We can say that the rhythm is fast (*~210/min*) – regular – <u>and</u> *lacks* P waves. However, we are *uncertain* about QRS width from assessment of this single monitoring lead.
- We'll soon discuss in detail how to approach such arrhythmias. That said — the point to emphasize is that clinically ***it doesn't really matter*** what the rhythm is <u>*until*</u> you've assessed hemodynamic status! For example — <u>IF</u> the patient with this rhythm is acutely hypotensive with dyspnea and chest discomfort (***Scenario #1***) — then *immediate* synchronized cardioversion will be indicated <u>*regardless*</u> of whether the rhythm turns out to be VT (<u>*Ventricular Tachycardia*</u>) – <u>or</u> — some type of SVT (<u>*SupraVentricular Tachycardia*</u>).
- On the other hand — <u>IF</u> the patient with the rhythm in <u>Figure 02-1</u> is alert and *asymptomatic* with BP = 150/90 (***Scenario #2***) — then by definition, there is at least *some* time to more accurately assess what the rhythm is likely to be (*and what specific treatment will be best*).
- **BOTTOM LINE:** Always ensure the patient is stable <u>*before*</u> you proceed with assessing the 5 Parameters. Sometimes (ie, *in cases such as Scenario #1 in* <u>Figure 02-1</u>) — you may need to begin treatment <u>*before*</u> knowing for sure what the rhythm is.

☞ *How to Define Sinus Rhythm?*

By definition (*under normal circumstances, assuming the heart lies in the left side of the thorax*) — the **P wave** should always be **upright** in standard **lead II** when the mechanism of the rhythm is **sinus**. This is because the overall direction of the electrical depolarization wavefront as it travels from the SA node toward the AV node and the ventricles is oriented *toward* standard lead II, which lies at +60 degrees in the frontal plane (**Panel A** *in* <u>Figure 02-2</u>).

- The *only* 2 exceptions to the above stated rule (ie, *when the rhythm may be sinus despite a negative P wave in lead II*) are: **i)** if there is dextrocardia; or **ii)** if there is lead misplacement.

In contrast, when the electrical impulse originates from the AV node — the P wave will *not* be positive in lead II (**Panel B** in Figure 02-2). Instead — spread of atrial activation is now directed *away* from lead II with junctional beats or junctional (*AV nodal*) rhythm.

- *Beyond-the-Core:* Although we schematically depict a *negative* P wave *preceding* the QRS as representing what happens with junctional beats (*Panel B in* Figure 02-2) — this negative P wave in lead II could be seen *after* the QRS, or might even be *hidden* within the QRS (*depending on the relative speed of retrograde conduction back to the atria compared to forward conduction down to the ventricles*).

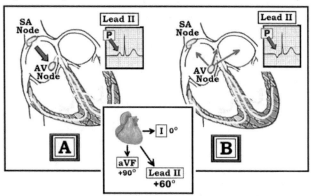

Figure 02-2: Panel A (*left*) shows the situation for normal sinus rhythm — which is defined by the presence of an *upright* P wave in lead II. Panel B shows that when the impulse originates in the AV node (*as it does with junctional beats or junctional rhythms*) — the direction of atrial activation is *away* from lead II. The P wave in lead II will therefore be negative.

☞ **Bottom Line:** (*regarding Sinus Rhythm*): Assuming there is no dextrocardia and the leads are *not* misplaced — **IF the P wave in lead II is *not* upright — then sinus rhythm is *not* present**.

- PEARL: The very *1st thing* we routinely do when assessing the cardiac rhythm in *any* tracing (*12-lead or single-lead rhythm strip*) is — Look to see IF there is a *longer* **lead II rhythm strip**. It requires *no more* than a *focused* 2-second look to determine if *upright* P waves with *fixed* PR interval regularly *precede* each QRS complex. IF they do — then the rhythm is **sinus** (Panel A in Figure 02-3).
- IF upright P waves do *not* regularly precede each QRS with fixed PR interval — then something *other than* normal **sinus** rhythm is present (Panel B and Panel C in Figure 02-3).

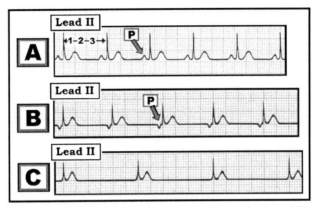

Figure 02-3: Panel A shows NSR (*Normal Sinus Rhythm*). The P wave is *upright* in lead II — and each QRS is preceded by a P wave with *fixed* PR interval. Assuming *no* dextrocardia or lead misplacement — We can tell at a glance that **Panels B** and **C** do *not* represent sinus rhythm because the P wave is *negative* in Panel B and absent entirely in Panel C. Presumably — Panel B represents a slightly *accelerated* AV nodal escape rhythm — and Panel C an appropriate AV nodal escape (*rate between 40-60/minute*) — although we *can't rule out* the possibility of a low atrial rhythm or escape from the Bundle of His, respectively for B and C. That said, what matters most — is that **lack** of an **upright P wave** in the **lead II** rhythm strips seen in Panels B and C *immediately* tells us that **a rhythm *other than* sinus is operative!**

🖝 *Sinus Mechanism* **Rhythms**

Once the mechanism of the rhythm is defined as "sinus" — the rate (*and regularity*) of the rhythm determine our terminology. There are 4 principal *sinus* mechanism rhythms:

- **NSR** (*Normal Sinus Rhythm*) — regular rhythm with a rate *between* 60-99/minute in an adult (*Norms for rate differ in children* — page 27).
- **Sinus Bradycardia** — regular sinus rhythm at a rate *below* 60/min.
- **Sinus Tachycardia** — sinus rhythm at a rate of ≥100/minute.
- **Sinus Arrhythmia** — an *irregular* rhythm *despite* the presence of a sinus mechanism (Figure 02-4).

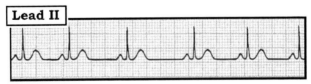

Figure 02-4: Sinus arrhythmia. Despite *irregularity* in the rhythm — sinus mechanism is present as defined by regularly-occurring *upright* P waves with *fixed* PR preceding *each* QRS complex.

☞ *Sinus Arrhythmia*

Sinus Arrhythmia is a common normal variant in infants and young children. At times, variability in sinus rate may be marked — in which case one might initially think *some other* arrhythmia is present.

- **Sinus Arrhythmia** — is confirmed by the finding of *identical-appearing* P waves that are *upright* in lead II with *fixed* PR interval (Figure 02-4). In contrast — *other* phenomena will manifest changes in P wave morphology *and/or* in the PR interval.
- Sinus arrhythmia often exhibits **respiratory variation**. This is especially true in healthy young children — for whom some variation in sinus regularity is the norm rather than the exception. Sinus "arrhythmia" is a *normal* cardiac rhythm in this setting.
- Some degree of sinus variability (ie, *sinus arrhythmia*) may persist in young *and even* older adults. This is *not* necessarily abnormal.
- The **technical definition** of sinus **"arrhythmia"** — is that *sinus-initiated* R-R intervals **vary** by **at least 0.08-0.12 second** (*2-3 little boxes*). That said, most of the time — the presence of sinus "arrhythmia" (*vs sinus rhythm*) is of *little-to-no clinical* significance.
- An **exception** to the statement that sinus arrhythmia is benign occurs in *older* patients with **SSS** (*Sick Sinus Syndrome*). Among the many manifestations of SSS (*which include sinus pauses, sinus arrest, tachy- as well as bradyarrhythmias*) — **sinus bradycardia *with* sinus arrhythmia** is the most common (*See pp 280-284*). The usual course of SSS is prolonged over years (*if not decades*). Many patients who go on to develop full-fledged symptoms (*with need for a permanent pacemaker*) manifest *no more* than sinus bradycardia/sinus arrhythmia for a period of many years. Therefore — the finding of an *inappropriately* slow and *variable* sinus rhythm in an older patient with symptoms of fatigue, worsening heart failure *and/or* syncope/presyncope *is* cause for potential concern. IF not due to rate-slowing medication — *Consider SSS* as the possible cause.

▶ *Beyond-the-Core:* Another type of sinus arrhythmia that is associated with a pathologic condition is **ventriculophasic sinus arrhythmia**. Some patients with significant AV block manifest obvious variability in the rate of their underlying sinus rhythm. This is thought to be due to variations in cardiac output as a result of the AV block. The importance of this rhythm is simply to be aware that the P-P interval may vary with certain forms of AV block (*discussed more in Section 20*).

- **BOTTOM Line:** For most patients — the clinical significance of sinus arrhythmia is the same as for sinus rhythm – BUT – **Clinical correlation to the case at hand is everything!** The ECG diagnosis of sinus rhythm or sinus arrhythmia is made in the same way that all arrhythmias are diagnosed: *By use of the Ps, Qs, 3R Approach.* The presence of *similar-appearing* P waves that regularly precede QRS complexes with a *fixed* PR interval defines the rhythm as sinus. IF the P-P interval varies — then by definition there is **sinus arrhythmia**.

 Other *Irregular* Sinus Mechanisms

In addition to sinus arrhythmia — there are other variations of *irregular* sinus mechanism rhythms. Two common ones are illustrated in **Figure 02-5**. Consider these **Questions**:
- For **A** and **B** in <u>Figure 02-5</u>: Is there **underlying sinus rhythm?**
- What happens for beats #4,5,6 in **Tracing A** of Figure 02-5?
- What happens for beat #5 in **Tracing B**?

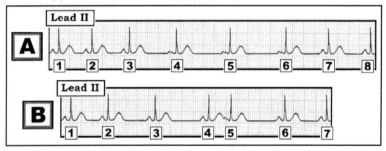

Figure 02-5: *Irregular* Rhythms with *Underlying* Sinus Mechanism. What happens *with* beats #4,5,6 in A? — *with* beat #5 in B? (*See text*).

● **Answer to <u>Figure 02-5</u>:** More important than the specific rhythm diagnosis for Tracings A and B is the process for rhythm assessment using the ***Ps,Qs,3R* Approach**:
- **Tracing A** — The overall rhythm is *not* regular. The QRS complex is narrow — and each QRS <u>is</u> preceded by a P wave. That said — there are 2 *different* shapes for P waves seen on this tracing. A taller *peaked* P wave with fixed PR interval precedes beats #1,2,3; and #7,8. The 2nd P wave shape is of smaller amplitude and notched — and is seen to precede beats #4,5,6 with fixed PR interval. Thus, the **underlying rhythm** is **sinus *arrhythmia*** — with *transient* change to *another* atrial focus for beats #4,5,6 — followed by resumption of the original sinus focus at the end of the tracing.
- **Tracing B** — The overall rhythm is again *not* quite regular. The QRS complex is narrow — <u>and</u> each QRS is preceded by a P wave. The **underlying rhythm** is again **sinus arrhythmia** (*as determined by the presence of upright, identical-looking P waves with fixed PR interval preceding beats #1,2,3,4,6,7 — albeit with slight variation in the P-P interval*). Only one P wave looks different. This is the P wave preceding beat #5. This P wave appears *earlier-than-expected* and is notched, deforming the terminal portion of the T wave of beat #4. Beat #5 is a **PAC** (*Premature Atrial Contraction*).

 ***Key* Points about <u>Figure 02-5</u> – *Wandering* Pacer**

An important principle in rhythm interpretation is to look first for the **underlying rhythm**. This may not always be obvious when more than one rhythm abnormality is present. Thus, despite irregularity of the rhythm in *both* Tracings A and B — a majority of P waves in each tracing are of *identical* morphology with *fixed* PR interval and *upright* deflection in this lead II monitoring lead. Therefore — the **underlying mechanism** is **sinus** in each case.

- Whether the change in P wave morphology for beats #4,5,6 in Tracing A represents a *single* switch to an alternate atrial focus <u>or</u> true *wandering* pacemaker (*with frequent transition in-and-out of sinus rhythm*) cannot be determined from this brief rhythm strip. Regardless, what matters is that the *underlying* mechanism is sinus.
- **Wandering** pacemaker — is a common rhythm variant that is most often benign in patients without significant heart disease. Typically one sees a series of beats with one P wave morphology that *gradually* changes to another P wave morphology (*as the site of the pacemaker shifts from the SA node to elsewhere in the atria*). As might be imagined — diagnosis of "wandering" pacemaker requires more than the "snapshot" of a single brief rhythm strip (*as was seen in* **Tracing A** *of* Figure 02-5).
- **Tracing B** in Figure 02-5 manifests *sinus* **arrhythmia** *with* a **PAC**. Additional tracings and clinical correlation is needed to determine the significance (*if any*) of this finding.

☞ Norms for Rate: *Different in Children*

Normal limits for heart rate are *different* in children. While we primarily concern ourselves in this book with rhythm disturbances in adults — it is nevertheless helpful to be aware of some differences between pediatric and adult arrhythmias.

- On page 4 — We defined **normal *sinus* rhythm** in **adults** by a rate range *between* 60-99/minute. Sinus rhythm rates *above* this range are termed sinus **tachycardia** — and below this range, sinus **bradycardia**.
- Rate limits are *different* **in children** — with "norms" depending on the age of the child. Much more important than specific "cut-off" points for each age category — is appreciation of the general concept that *slightly* faster rates (say ~110/minute) may be normal for a crying but otherwise healthy young child. Similarly — a rate within the "seemingly normal" range of 65/minute might be relatively *slow* for an active young child. *Clinical context is everything!*

● **"*Escape*" rate ranges** are also different for children than they are in adults. Whereas the normal **AV nodal *escape* rate** in an **adult** is *between* **40-to-60/minute** — it is *between* 50-80/minute in a young child. This concept is illustrated in **Figure 02-6** — in which we see an AV Nodal (*junctional*) rhythm:

- <u>IF</u> the patient with the rhythm in Figure 02-6 was an **adult** — this should be interpreted as an **"*accelerated*" junctional rhythm** (*with attention to the possibility of pathologic conditions such as Digoxin toxicity that are known to cause accelerated junctional rhythms*).

• <u>BUT</u> — IF the rhythm in <u>Figure 02-6</u> was from an otherwise *healthy child* — it should then be interpreted as a *junctional* **rhythm** with *appropriate* **escape rate** (*which is <u>not</u> necessarily abnormal as an occasional rhythm in an otherwise healthy child*).

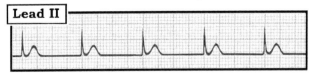

Figure 02-6: AV nodal escape rhythm, as defined by the presence of a regular, narrow-QRS rhythm at 75/minute *without* P waves in this lead II rhythm strip. <u>IF</u> the patient was an adult — this would be an "accelerated" junctional rhythm (*given that it exceeds the usual 40-60/minute range*). <u>BUT</u> in a child — this might simply represent a normal AV nodal escape rhythm (*See text*).

☞ *Is the QRS Wide or Narrow?*

The QRS interval represents the time it takes for ventricular depolarization to occur. With sinus rhythm in adults — the process of ventricular activation should **normally** be complete in **no more** than **0.10 second**. *KEY* Points to consider include the following:

• QRS duration can be measured from *any* of the 12 leads of a standard ECG. **Select** the **lead in which** the **QRS** complex **appears** to be **longest**.

• Practically speaking — all that matters is whether the QRS is normal or wide. Precise measurement of QRS duration for a complex that is clearly *within* the normal range is *not* necessary. We do <u>not</u> care if the QRS is 0.08, 0.09, or 0.0999 second in duration — since all of these values are normal. We <u>do</u> care if QRS duration is normal or long.

• *12 leads are Better than One* for measuring intervals. A part of the QRS may lie on the baseline in one or more leads — leading to false conclusion that QRS duration is "normal", when in reality the QRS is prolonged.

• Given that 0.10 second is the upper normal limit for QRS duration in adults — the QRS is said to be *WIDE* — IF it measures *more* than *HALF* a *large* **box** in duration (<u>Figure 02-7</u>).

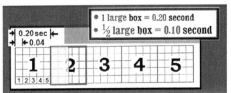

Figure 02-7: In adults — the QRS complex is said to be "wide" IF it clearly measures *more* than *half* a large box in duration (ie, *more than 0.10 second*).

● <u>NOTE:</u> The upper limit for QRS duration in children may be less than it is in adults. Children have smaller hearts (*which require less time for ventricular depolarization to occur*). Age-dependent tables exist

to assist in determining QRS duration limits in children. For example — a QRS of 0.09 second might be long in a newborn.
• Although we primarily address rhythm disturbances pertaining to adults in this book — awareness of some differences compared to arrhythmias in children <u>is</u> clinically insightful.

☞ Figure 02-8: *Is the QRS Wide or Narrow?*

To illustrate the essential points in this Section about assessing the rhythm for QRS duration — We reproduce below in **Figure 02-8** the tachycardia previously shown on page 22:
• Is the rhythm in <u>Figure 02-8</u> a *narrow* <u>or</u> *wide-complex* tachycardia?
• Why does this matter?
• <u>Clinically</u> – How can you tell?

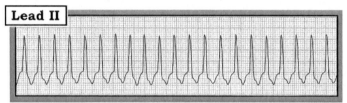

Figure 02-8: Is this a *narrow* <u>or</u> *wide-complex* tachycardia? (*See text*).

● **KEY Point:** As previously emphasized — <u>IF</u> the patient whose rhythm is shown in <u>Figure 02-8</u> is unstable — then *immediate* cardioversion is indicated. However, <u>IF</u> the patient is **hemodynamically stable** — then definitive determination of QRS duration can be accomplished by obtaining a **12-lead ECG *during* the tachycardia**.
• The importance of determining QRS width for a *regular* tachycardia such as that shown above *cannot* be overstated. <u>IF</u> the QRS is *truly* narrow in *all* 12 leads — we have virtually *eliminated* VT from diagnostic consideration. Prognosis and treatment of SVT (<u>S</u>upra<u>V</u>entricular <u>T</u>achycardia) is vastly different than it is for VT.
• **Clinical PEARL:** QRS duration on a bedside monitor may be deceptive. We have seen QRS duration at times look wider *or* narrower than it really is when a hard copy ECG is printed out. Whenever possible — *hard copy* documentation (*ideally by 12-lead during* tachycardia) is the optimal way to determine QRS duration.

● **Answer to Figure 02-8:** In **Figure 02-9** (*on page 30*) we add a *simultaneously* recorded lead V1 to the *single-lead* rhythm strip initially shown above in Figure 02-8. The answer to the question regarding QRS width *during* the tachycardia is now obvious:
• Vertical red *time lines* highlight how the terminal portion of the QRS complex in lead V1 *looked like* the initial part of the ST segment in lead II. Simultaneous viewing of leads II and V1 now leaves little doubt that the QRS is wide and the rhythm is **ventricular tachycardia**.

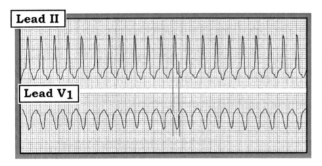

Figure 02-9: *Simultaneously* recorded leads II and V1 for the rhythm on pg 29. There is now *no doubt* that the QRS is wide (*and the rhythm is VT*).

☞ *Regularity of the* **Rhythm** (*the 1st of the 3Rs*)

Using the **Ps,Qs,3R Approach** — the 1st of the 3 Rs that we usually assess is *regularity* of the rhythm. This parameter pertains both to regularity of P waves as well as of QRS complexes. We illustrate some commonly encountered patterns below in **Figure 02-10**. For each *narrow-complex* rhythm — Contemplate the following:

• Do QRS complexes *regularly* occur? If not — Is there a *pattern* to the irregularity?
• If P waves are present — Is the *P-P interval* regular?

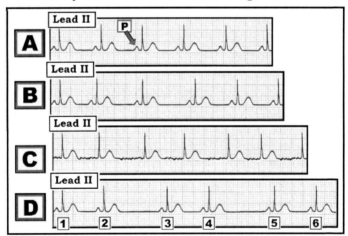

Figure 02-10: Assessing QRS and P-P interval regularity (*See text*).

● **Answer** to **Figure 02-10:** Applying the **Ps,Qs,3R Approach** to the 4 rhythms shown in Figure 02-10 — We note the following:

• **Tracing A** — The QRS complex is narrow. The rhythm is regular at a rate just over 75/minute. The P-P interval is also regular. Upright P waves regularly precede each QRS with fixed PR interval. This is **normal *sinus* rhythm**.

• **Tracing B** — The QRS complex is narrow. The overall rhythm is *not* regular. That said — the mechanism is still sinus, because upright P

waves regularly precede each QRS complex with fixed PR interval in this lead II monitoring lead. This is *sinus* **arrhythmia.**
- **Tracing C** — The QRS complex is narrow. The rhythm is *irregularly irregular*. That is — *no* pattern exists to the irregularity. P waves are not seen in this lead II. This is **AFib** (*Atrial Fibrillation*) — seen here with a *controlled* ventricular response.
- **Tracing D** — The QRS complex is narrow. Although the rhythm is clearly *not* regular — a ***pattern*** does exist to the irregularity. That is – an alternating pattern of *short-long* intervals is seen. Duration of each *shorter* interval (*the interval between beats #1-2; 3-4; and 5-6*) is approximately equal. Similarly — the duration of each *longer* interval (*between beats #2-3; 4-5*) is also approximately equal. This is unlikely to be due to chance. Otherwise — upright P waves precede each QRS with fixed PR interval, confirming an underlying sinus mechanism. *Beyond-the-Core:* Recognition of ***patterned*** **beating** (*also known as* ***"group"*** **beating**) — should suggest the possibility of some type of Wenckebach conduction. In this case — the rhythm is **SA Wenckebach** (*Wenckebach and group beating are discussed in detail in Section 20*). ● BOTTOM LINE: Much more important than the specific type of conduction disturbance in this case is awareness that although the overall rhythm in **Tracing D** is *not* regular — a *pattern* does exist <u>and</u> there is an underlying *sinus* mechanism.

☞ *How to Calculate* **Rate?** (*the "Rule of 300"*)

The 2nd "R" that we usually assess is calculation of heart rate. The easiest way to estimate rate is by the ***"Rule of 300"*** (Figure 02-11):
- Provided that the rhythm is regular — the heart rate can be estimated IF you ***divide*** **300** by the **number** of *large* **boxes** in the **R-R interval**.
- With the ECG machine set at the standard recording speed of 25 mm/second — the time required to record each *little* **box** on ECG grid paper is **0.04 second.** (*Vertically, each little box is 1mm in amplitude*).

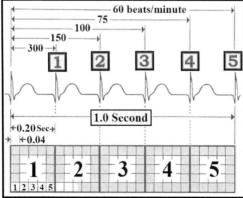

Figure 02-11: Calculation of rate by the Rule of 300 (*See text*).

◉ *Using* <u>Figure 02-11</u> (*on pg 31*) to *Explain* the "**Rule of 300**" — It can readily be seen that the time required to record **5** *little* **boxes** will be **1/5 of a second** (*5 X 0.04* = **0.20 sec**).
- The time required to record **5** *large* **boxes** on <u>Figure 02-11</u> will therefore be one *full* second (*0.20 X 5* = **1.0 second**).
- IF a QRS complex occurs each large box (*as in Figure 02-11*) — then the R-R interval will be 0.20 second — and the *rate* of the rhythm will be **300 beats/minute** (ie, *5 beats occur each second **X** 60 seconds/ minute* = a rate of 300/minute).
- IF the R-R interval is *half* as fast (ie, **2** *large* boxes) — then the *rate* will be 300 ÷ 2 = **150** beats/minute;
- IF the R-R is **3** boxes — the rate will be **100**/minute (*300 ÷ 3*); — *and so on* . . .

☞ <u>**Figure 02-12:**</u> *What is the Rate?*

As practice in rate calculation — We reproduce in **Figure 02-12** the 3 rhythms previously shown on page 24:
- Calculate the rate for each of the 3 rhythms in <u>Figure 02-12</u>.

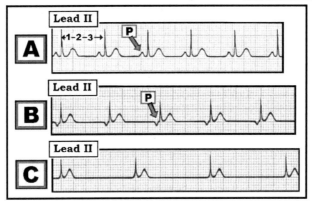

Figure 02-12: Apply the Rule of 300 to calculate heart rate. What is the rate for the 3 rhythms shown in this Figure (*See text*).

◉ **Answer** to **Figure 02-12:** Applying the *Rule of 300* to the 3 rhythms shown in Figure 02-12 — We calculate rate as follows:
- **Tracing A** — The rhythm is regular with an R-R interval just *under* 4 large boxes in duration. IF the R-R interval was *precisely* 4 large boxes in duration — then the rate would be 300/4 = 75/minute. Since the R-R interval is slightly *less* than 4 large boxes in duration — the rate must be slightly *faster* than 75/min, or about **78/minute**.
- **Tracing B** — The rhythm is regular with an R-R interval of 4 large boxes in duration. Therefore the rate = 300/4 = **75/minute**.
- **Tracing C** — The rhythm is regular with an R-R interval of 6 large boxes in duration. Therefore the rate = 300/6 = **50/minute**.

☞ *Estimating Rate when the Rhythm is Regular and Fast*

As will be discussed in detail in Sections 13 and 14 — accurate determination of heart rate is essential for assessment and differentiation of the various SVT (*SupraVentricular Tachycardia*) rhythms. When the rhythm is regular and the rate is fast — calculating rate is most *easily* accomplished using the ***Every-other-Beat* Method**. The method is best explained by example:

- To ***estimate*** the **rate** of the *regular* tachycardia in **Figure 02-13** (*previously shown on pages 22 and 29*) — We first determine the R-R interval of *every-other-beat*. This allows calculation of *half* of the actual rate.
- Select a QRS complex that begins *or* ends on a *heavy* line. Then count 2 beats over, noting the number of *large* boxes in this R-R interval for *every-other-beat*. It can be seen from Figure 02-13 that the **R-R interval** of *every-other-beat* is **just *under* 3 large boxes**. Therefore — *half* the rate is a little bit *more* than 300/3 = ~**105/minute**.
- We estimate the **actual rate** is **210/minute** (*105/minute X 2*).

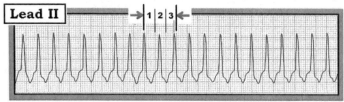

Figure 02-13: Using the ***Every-other-Beat* Method** – we estimate the rate of this *regular* tachycardia is ~210/minute (*See text*).

☞ *Are P Waves "Married"* (*= Related*) *to the* **QRS?**

The last of the 5 Parameters seeks to determine when P waves <u>are</u> present — whether some or all P waves are **related** to a **neighboring QRS** complex. We need to determine <u>IF</u> P waves are being *conducted* to the ventricles.

- The easiest (*and most common*) relationship to establish is that of **normal *sinus* rhythm**. A *brief* look in front of each QRS complex in a **lead II** rhythm strip *confirms* sinus rhythm — IF ***each* QRS** is ***preceded*** by a **upright P wave** with ***fixed* PR interval** (*See Tracing A in* Figure 02-14 *on page 34*).

● **PEARL:** The very *first* thing we do when assessing <u>any</u> cardiac rhythm or 12-lead ECG is to look for a lead II rhythm strip. It takes *no more* than 2 brief seconds to look in front of *each* QRS in lead II.

- Assuming there is *no* dextrocardia or lead misplacement — IF an *upright* P wave with *fixed* PR interval does not precede *each* QRS complex in lead II — then *something other than* normal sinus rhythm is occurring. *Forgetting this simple step is by far the most common oversight we see even experienced interpreters committing.*

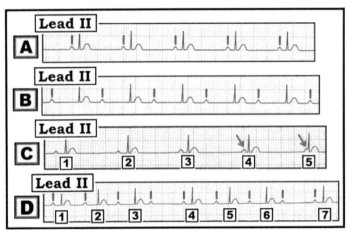

Figure 02-14: Are P waves "married" to the QRS? Determining if P waves are related to a *neighboring* QRS is most easily accomplished by looking for atrial activity *before* each QRS (*See text*).

☞ When P Waves are *NOT* "Married" to Each QRS

The *KEY* to interpreting many complex arrhythmias lies with assessment of atrial activity and determining IF P waves are **related** to a **neighboring QRS?** We illustrate basic principles of this concept in Tracings B, C, and D in Figure 02-14:

• **Tracing B** (*in Figure 02-14*) — The rhythm is regular at a rate of 75/minute. The QRS complex is narrow. Each QRS is preceded by a regularly occurring P wave (*short vertical lines in B*). However, the PR interval is markedly prolonged (*to 0.43 second*). This is **sinus rhythm** with **1st degree AV block**. We *know* sinus rhythm is present (*and that each P wave in B is being conducted to the ventricles*) – because the PR interval preceding each QRS is fixed (*at 0.43 sec*).

⬤ Clinical PEARL: Although the PR interval with 1st degree AV block is not usually as long as seen in Tracing B — on occasion, PR intervals *as long as* 1.0 second (*or more*) have been recorded.

• **Tracing C** – The rhythm begins with at least 2 sinus-conducted beats (*beats #1 and 2 in C*). Each of these initial 2 beats in Tracing C manifest an upright P wave with fixed and normal PR interval that precedes the QRS. **Something changes** with beats #4 and 5! As indicated by the *arrows* in Tracing C — the PR interval preceding beats #4 and 5 is simply **too short** to conduct. Therefore — these P waves are *not* related to the QRS (*they can't be – because there is not enough time for the electrical impulse to travel from the SA node through the atria to the AV node*). As a result — there is **transient AV dissociation** (*which simply means that for a period of time, P waves are not related to neighboring QRS complexes*).

● *Beyond-the-Core:* As will be discussed in Section 20 — full interpretation of Tracing C would be sinus rhythm with AV dissociation by default (*slowing*) of the sinus pacemaker <u>*with*</u> resultant appropriate AV nodal escape. There is *no* definite evidence of AV block on this tracing. It is likely that beat #3 in Tracing C is also *not* conducting — because the PR interval preceding beat #3 is *shorter* than the normal sinus PR interval seen preceeding beats #1 and 2.

• BOTTOM LINE: For now — it is more than enough to recognize that the P waves preceding beats #4 and 5 in **Tracing C** are <u>*not*</u> related (*and therefore <u>not</u> being conducted to the ventricles*).

• **Tracing D** (*in* <u>Figure 02-14</u> *on page 34*) — The QRS complex is narrow. Upright P waves are seen at a *regular* atrial rate of 100/min (*vertical lines in Tracing D*). The ventricular rate is <u>*not*</u> regular. That said — a P wave <u>*does*</u> precede each QRS. Thus, there <u>is</u> a relationship between each QRS and the P wave that precedes it – namely, that the PR interval *progressively* increases (*from beat #1-2 to #2-3 — and from beats #4-5 to #5-6*) until a P wave is dropped (*P waves following the T wave of beats #3 and #6 are not conducted*). This is **2nd degree AV block, Mobitz Type I** (*AV Wenckebach*).

● BOTTOM LINE: AV blocks will be covered in Section 20. The point to emphasize here is that with Mobitz I 2nd degree AV block — P waves *may* be related to the QRS that follows them even though the PR interval is *not* necessarily fixed. Instead — the "relationship" is that the PR interval *progressively* increases until a beat is dropped, after which the cycle begins again (*the PR interval after each dropped beat and relative pause in Tracing D shortens as the next Wenckebach cycle begins with beats #4 and #7*).

• With most notable exception of Mobitz I — *most* of the time you can *instantly* recognize <u>IF</u> P waves are related or not to a neighboring QRS simply by looking to see <u>IF</u> a P wave with *fixed* PR interval precedes *each* QRS.

Section 02A – *Clinical* Rhythm Diagnosis (*pp 36-47*)

 ⇨ **PRACTICE** Examples:

🔴 What follows is a series of **Practice** **Rhythm Strips** with goal of reinforcing the essential arrhythmia concepts covered in pages 21-35 of this section. Although clearly *not* an exhaustive compendium of arrhythmia tracings — our hope is that review of key principles in clinical interpretation will facilitate comfort in assessing the more common arrhythmias seen by acute care providers. (*Lots more to follow on specific arrhythmias throughout the rest of this book!*).

 • For each of the Practice Tracings on pp 36-47 — *Assess* the rhythm using the **Ps,Qs,3R Approach**. Our answers follow.

🔴 *Practice* **Tracing #1:** The patient whose rhythm is shown below was *hemodynamically* stable. Interpret the rhythm.

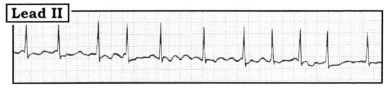

Lead II

Answer to Tracing #1: The rhythm is *irregularly* irregular. The QRS complex is narrow (*clearly not more than half a large box in duration*). No P waves are present. Instead there are a series of undulations of various amplitude in the baseline. These are *"fib waves"* — and the rhythm is **AFib** (*Atrial Fibrillation*).
• Rather than simply saying "AFib" — it is best to qualify this rhythm based on the **ventricular response**. *Untreated* AFib is most often rapid (*ventricular rate over 110-120/minute*). "Slow" AFib is said to be present when the overall rate is *less* than 50-60/minute. When the rate of AFib is in between (ie, *between ~70-110/min*) — the ventricular response is said to be "controlled".
• The R-R intervals in the above tracing are *between* 2-to-4 large boxes. The rate therefore ranges between ~80-to-120/minute, which we qualify as **AFib** with a **relatively *rapid* ventricular response**.
• Undulations in the baseline are seen with AFib as a result electrical activity from the fibrillating atria. These "fib waves" may be relatively coarse (*as they are here*) — fine — or sometimes *not* seen at all. When fib waves are absent – the diagnosis of AFib will need to be made from the irregular irregularity of the rhythm and absence of P waves in any of the 12 leads.
• Although fib waves in the middle of this tracing superficially resemble atrial flutter — the rhythm is AFib. The diagnosis of AFlutter (*Atrial Flutter*) requires regular atrial deflections (*usually in a "sawtooth pattern"*) at a rate of ~300/minute (*which is not seen here*).

Practice **Tracing #2:**

 ⇨ **PRACTICE** Tracing:

● Interpret the rhythm below using the ***Ps,Qs,3R* Approach**. The patient is *hypotensive*.

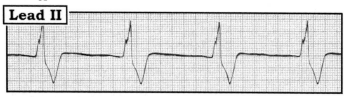

Lead II

☞ **Answer to Tracing #1:** The QRS complex is wide. The rhythm is regular at a rate of ~40/minute (*the R-R interval is ~7 large boxes in duration*). P waves are absent. This is therefore a **slow *ventricular* escape rhythm**.

• We surmise a *ventricular* site of origin for this rhythm by the presence of QRS widening in the absence of P waves. Although technically we can't rule out the possibility of a slow junctional escape rhythm with QRS widening from *preexisting* BBB (*Bundle Branch Block*) — this is far less common an occurrence than ventricular escape. In the absence of a prior 12-lead ECG for comparison — ventricular escape should be assumed until proven otherwise.

• The usual rate of an **AV nodal *escape* rhythm** in adults is *between* **40-60/minute**. It is slightly faster than this in children.

• If something happens to the AV nodal escape focus — a **ventricular *escape* focus** will hopefully take over, usually at a rate *between* **20-40/minute**. Technically — we call the above rhythm a *slow* **IVR** (*IdioVentricular Rhythm*). This rhythm is commonly seen rhythm in the setting of cardiopulmonary resuscitation.

⇨ *Clinical* **PEARL:** One may often surmise the *probable* site of an escape focus by: **i)** QRS width; *and* **ii)** The escape rate.

• IF the QRS is wide — the site of escape is likely to be ventricular (*unless there is preexisting bundle branch block*). As noted above — the usual IVR escape rate is *between* 20-40/minute.

• IF the QRS is narrow — the site of escape is *within* the conduction system (*usually at the level of the AV node — though it may be lower in the bundle of His or in one of the fascicles*). Thus, a *narrow* QRS escape rhythm at a rate *between* 40-60/minute is probably arising from the AV node. *Slower* narrow escape rhythms are more likely to be arising from the His or fascicles.

NOTE: Exceptions exist to the above rate ranges (ie, *escape rhythms may be accelerated*) — but the above generalities at least provide a starting point for suggesting the probable site of an escape focus.

Practice Tracing #3:

 ➡ **PRACTICE** Tracing:

● Interpret the rhythm below using the **Ps,Qs,3R Approach**. The patient is *hemodynamically* stable.

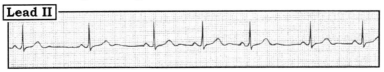

☞ **Answer to Tracing #3:** The rhythm is irregular. The QRS is narrow. Upright P waves with fixed PR interval precede each QRS complex in this lead II rhythm strip. Therefore, the mechanism of this rhythm is sinus. This is **sinus arrhythmia**.

• Sinus arrhythmia is a common normal finding in healthy children and young adults. It is the rule, rather than the exception — for there to be some variability in the rate of sinus rhythm in young children. There will often be variation of the rhythm with respiration. In some cases (*as seen here*) — variation of the rhythm with sinus arrhythmia may be marked.

• Regarding the above rhythm — the overall is relatively slow (*since several of the R-R intervals are over 5 large boxes in duration*). As a result — one might more properly call this **sinus bradycardia _and_ arrhythmia**. There will very often be at least *some* irregularity in patients with sinus bradycardia.

➡ **PEARL:** The clinical significance of sinus arrhythmia depends on the setting in which it occurs.

• As noted — Sinus arrhythmia is a **common *normal* variant** in healthy children.

• In contrast — Sinus *bradycardia* _and_ *arrhythmia* may be the first manifestations of **Sick Sinus Syndrome** when seen in older individuals (*once ischemia/infarction; medication effect; and hypothyroidism have all been ruled out*).

NOTE: Distinctly *lacking* from the information we were given about the about rhythm was the patient's age _and_ a brief clinical scenario ...

Practice Tracing #4:

 ➡ **PRACTICE** Tracing:

● Interpret the rhythm below using the **Ps,Qs,3R Approach**. The patient is *hemodynamically* stable.

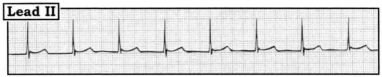

Answer to Tracing #4: The rhythm is regular at a rate of ~65/minute. The QRS complex is narrow. P waves are absent in this lead II rhythm strip. Therefore — this is an **AV nodal** (*junctional*) **rhythm**.

• When the rhythm is sinus — there should *always* be an *upright* P wave in lead II. Assuming there is *no* dextrocardia or lead misplacement — the complete *absence* of atrial activity in lead II defines this as an **AV nodal rhythm**.

• The *usual* AV nodal escape rate in adults is **between 40-60/minute**. Therefore, if this patient was an <u>adult</u> — the above rhythm would represent an **"accelerated" AV nodal rhythm** (*since it is slightly faster than the usual AV nodal escape rate*).

• The usual rate range for an AV nodal escape rhythm is somewhat *faster* in children — typically between 50-80/minute. Therefore, if this patient was an asymptomatic <u>child</u> — this would be a *normal* AV nodal escape rhythm, and there would be no need for concern.

➡ *Clinical* **PEARL:** *Accelerated* AV nodal escape rhythms are relatively uncommon. Conditions associated with this rhythm include *digitalis* toxicity, *recent* infarction, *post-operative* state, <u>and</u> sometimes extremely ill patients with *multisystem* disease.

• <u>IF</u> a patient with an *accelerated* junctional rhythm is taking digoxin — assume digitalis toxicity <u>until</u> proven otherwise.

• *Beyond-the-Core:* There appears to be slight ST segment elevation in the above tracing. This may or may not be clinically significant. Having said that — one should <u>*never*</u> draw conclusions about ST-T wave appearance based on a *single-lead* rhythm strip. Instead — concern about QRS morphology or possible ST-T wave changes on a *single-lead* rhythm strip is indication to obtain a **complete 12-lead ECG** to determine what really is happening.

Practice Tracing #5:

 ➡ **PRACTICE Tracing:**

● Interpret the rhythm below using the **Ps,Qs,3R Approach**. The patient is *hemodynamically* stable.

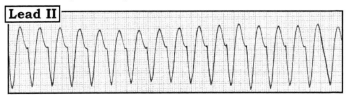

Lead II

🐾 **Answer to Tracing #5:** The QRS complex is obviously wide. No P waves are seen. The rhythm is regular at a rate of ~165/minute. Therefore — we have a regular wide tachycardia. **Assume VT** (*Ventricular Tachycardia*) **until** **proven otherwise**.

• We cover ECG diagnosis and clinical management of *wide-complex* tachycardias (*including VT*) in detail in upcoming Sections 3-*thru*-9. For now — suffice it to say that VT must be assumed <u>until</u> proven otherwise. The patient should be treated accordingly. This is true <u>regardless</u> of whether the patient remains stable or not during the tachycardia.

• Some patients may remain alert and *hemodynamically* stable for *long* periods of time despite being in *sustained* VT. This is why knowledge that the above patient is "stable" should <u>not</u> dissuade us from the *presumed* diagnosis of *sustained* VT.

• *Marked* QRS widening (*to at least 0.17 sec.*) with *all negative* QRS morphology in this lead II rhythm strip just *"looks like"* VT. Further support of this diagnosis would be forthcoming from knowing the clinical setting, seeing a 12-lead ECG *during* tachycardia, and awareness of this patient's previous medical history. So although we cannot completely rule out the possibility of SVT with preexisting bundle branch block or aberrant conduction — **the odds overwhelmingly favor VT** as the diagnosis, <u>and</u> the patient should be treated accordingly <u>until</u> proven otherwise.

➡ **KEY Point:** The <u>best</u> answer for interpretation of the above lead II rhythm strip is that there is a **regular WCT** (<u>Wide-Complex Tachycardia</u>) at ~165/minute **without** clear sign of **P waves**. This description is all encompassing.

• As noted — VT should be assumed <u>until</u> proven otherwise.
• It is still possible that the above rhythm is supraventricular (*with QRS widening due to either preexisting bundle branch block or aberrant conduction*). That said — the odds that this rhythm is VT *exceed* 90% - <u>and</u> – the patient should be treated as if this was VT.

Practice Tracing #6:

  ➡ **PRACTICE** Tracing:

● Interpret the rhythm below using the **Ps,Qs,3R Approach.** The patient is *hemodynamically* stable.

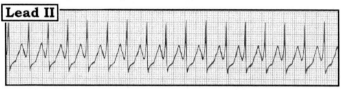

☞ **Answer to Tracing #6:** The above rhythm is fast and regular. By the *every-other-beat* method (*pg 33*) — we estimate the rate to be **~170/minute** (*since the R-R interval of every-other-beat is between 3-to-4 large boxes in duration*). The QRS complex appears to be narrow (*not more than half a large box in duration*). No definite P waves are seen. Therefore — the rhythm is a regular *narrow-complex* tachycardia *without* clear evidence of sinus P waves. This **most likely** is **PSVT** (*Paroxysmal SupraVentricular Tachycardia*).

• We cover ECG diagnosis and clinical management of *narrow-complex* tachycardias (*including PSVT*) in detail in Sections 13 and 14.

• Essential to the diagnosis of a *"narrow"* tachycardia is confirmation that the QRS complex is indeed narrow. Such confirmation can *only* be forthcoming from obtaining a **12-lead ECG *during* tachycardia.** Thus, although we *think* the QRS complex in the above tracing is narrow — we do *not* know this for sure on the basis of the *single-lead* rhythm strip shown above.

• Although we are unable to clearly identify P waves in the above rhythm — we *cannot* rule out the possibility that the peaked upward deflection preceding each QRS complex *could be* a P wave. It is possible that this peaked deflection could represent the *combination* of a T wave *and* a P wave.

• Clinically — there are **3 entities *to consider*** whenever one encounters a **regular** **SVT** (*SupraVentricular* or *narrow-complex* Tachycardia). These are: **i)** Sinus tachycardia; **ii)** Atrial flutter; and **iii)** PSVT. That said — the rate of ~170/minute is *faster* than is usually seen for either sinus tachycardia or atrial flutter. This leaves **PSVT** as the **most likely** diagnosis (*Full discussion of this concept is found in derivation of our List #2 in Section 13 on pp 117-118*).

➡ ***Clinical* Note:** Another name for the above rhythm is **AVNRT** (*AV Nodal Reentry Tachycardia*) — in acknowledgement of the almost certain role of AV nodal *reentry* in initiating <u>and</u> maintaining this *regular* tachyarrhythmia.

Practice Tracing #7:

 ➡ PRACTICE Tracing:

● Interpret the rhythm below using the **Ps,Qs,3R Approach**. The patient is *hemodynamically* stable.

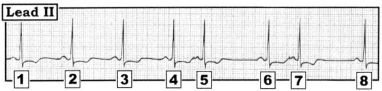

☞ **Answer to Tracing #7:** The *underlying* rhythm is **sinus** — as determined by the presence of a regular R-R interval at a rate of **65/minute** for the first 4 beats in the tracing. The QRS complex is narrow — and each QRS is preceded by an *upright* P wave with *fixed* PR interval in this lead II rhythm strip.

• **Beat #5** occurs early. Its QRS is narrow and *identical* in morphology to normal sinus beats. Beat #5 is preceded by a notched P wave that clearly looks *different* than normal sinus P waves. This defines **beat #5** as a **PAC (**<u>P</u>remature <u>A</u>trial <u>C</u>ontraction**)**.

• A second PAC follows with beat #7. Therefore, the rhythm shown above is best described as **sinus** <u>*with*</u> **PACs**.

• Note that the R-R interval following each PAC is different than the R-R interval during the normal sinus rhythm seen for the first 4 beats in the tracing. This is because the occurrence of a premature atrial impulse *resets* the sinus node.

➡ *Clinical* **Note:** The significance of PACs depends on the clinical setting in which these beats occur. They may normally occur in otherwise healthy individuals. They may also be markers for a variety of pathologic conditions (*some cardiac; some not*) — as well as serving as the precipitating event that initiates a reentry tachycardia.

• It is impossible to assess the true "frequency" of PACs from a *single-lead* rhythm strip.

• *Much more* on PACs is found in Sections 18 and 19.

Practice Tracing #8:

 ⇒ PRACTICE Tracing:

● Interpret the rhythm below using the **Ps,Qs,3R Approach**. The patient is *hemodynamically* stable.

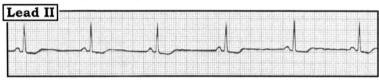

☞ **Answer to Tracing #8:** The rhythm is slow and fairly regular at a rate just under 50/minute. The QRS complex is narrow. Upright P waves with fixed PR interval precede each QRS in this lead II rhythm strip. Therefore — the rhythm is *sinus* **bradycardia**.

• Technically — we define a regular sinus rhythm with a rate *below* 60/minute as sinus "bradycardia". That said — the presence of sinus bradycardia is commonly seen as a normal variant in otherwise healthy adults. This is especially true in athletic individuals who exercise regularly.

• On the other hand — sinus bradycardia may reflect overuse of certain rate-slowing drugs *and/or* it may be the first manifestation of sick sinus syndrome. *Clinical correlation* is everything!

• **NOTE:** Although the above rhythm *looks* regular — close measurement (*with calipers*) reveals slight variation in the R-R interval. As previously stated (*on page 38*) — it is common for there to be at least *some* variation in R-R intervals when the underlying rhythm is sinus bradycardia. **Technically** — there should be *at least* **2-3 little boxes** (*0.08-0.12 second*) of variation in the R-R interval for a rhythm to qualify as "sinus arrhythmia".

⇒ *Bottom* **Line:** We would accept as the correct answer to the above rhythm strip *either* **sinus bradycardia** *or* **sinus bradycardia** *and* **arrhythmia**.

Practice **Tracing #9:**

 ➡ **PRACTICE** Tracing:

● Interpret the rhythm below using the **Ps,Qs,3R** **Approach**. The patient is *hemodynamically* stable.

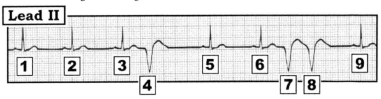

👉 **Answer to Tracing #9:** The **underlying** rhythm is **sinus** – as determined by the presence of a regular R-R interval at a rate of **70/minute** for the first 3 beats in the tracing. The QRS complex for these first 3 beats is narrow — and each QRS is preceded by an upright P wave with fixed PR interval.

• **Beat #4** occurs early. Its QRS is wide <u>and</u> this beat is *not* preceded by any P wave. This defines **beat #4** as a **PVC** (*Premature Ventricular Contraction*).

• Normal sinus rhythm resumes for beats #5 and 6.

• Two PVCs then occur in a row (*beat #7,8*). This is called a **ventricular couplet**. Sinus rhythm then resumes at the end of the tracing with beat #9.

• Full interpretation of the above rhythm strip would therefore be — **sinus rhythm _with_ PVCs** (*including a ventricular couplet*).

➡ *Clinical* **Note:**   The significance of PVCs depends on the clinical setting in which these beats occur. Many otherwise healthy individuals have at least *some* ventricular ectopy on 24 hours of monitoring — so the mere presence of PVCs on monitoring does not necessarily imply pathology.

• Have said this — the more frequent PVCs are, <u>and</u> the more repetitive forms (*2 or more PVCs in a row*) are seen — the more likely these beats are to be markers of concern. This is especially true when frequent and worrisome forms of PVCs occur in patients with *underlying* heart disease. *Clinical correlation* is everything! (*More on PVCs in Section 18*).

• As was the case for the rhythm on page 42 — It is impossible to assess the true "frequency" of PVCs from a *single-lead* rhythm strip.

Practice Tracing #10:

 ⇨ **PRACTICE** Tracing:

⬤ Interpret the rhythm below using the **Ps,Qs,3R Approach**. The patient is *hemodynamically* stable.

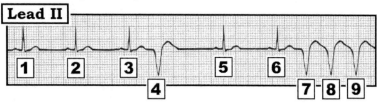

☞ **Answer to Tracing #10:** The rhythm strip shown above begins the same as did the rhythm on page 44. That is — the **underlying rhythm** is **sinus**; beat #4 is a **PVC**, which is followed by resumption of sinus rhythm for beats #5 and 6. Three PVCs then occur in a row.

- Several terms are used to describe the occurrence of 3 PVCs in a row. These include a **ventricular salvo** or **triplet**. Technically, the definition of **"VT"** (*Ventricular Tachycardia*) — is 3 PVCs in a row.
- <u>Clinically</u> — it is useful to classify VT as either being "sustained" or *"nonsustained"*, depending on whether (*and for how long*) VT persists. Be aware that the definition of **"sustained" VT** varies among experts, with most authorities requiring persistence of VT for *at least* 20-to-30 seconds <u>or</u> *long enough* to produce symptoms of hypotension or syncope.
- We would classify the 3-beat run seen at the end of the above tracing as **NSVT** (*NonSustained Ventricular Tachycardia*). That said — in reality, we have *no idea* of how long this run of VT lasts since the rhythm strip is cut off after beat #9 ...

⇨ *Clinical* **Note:** We emphasized on page 44 that the significance of PVCs depends on the clinical setting in which these beats occur.

- In general — PVCs are far less likely to be clinically significant when they occur in the absence of *underlying* heart disease. Even short runs of NSVT are unlikely to adversely affect outcome <u>IF</u> the patient in question does *not* have underlying heart disease. *Clinical correlation is everything!*

Practice Tracing #11:

 ➡ **PRACTICE** Tracing:

● Interpret the rhythm below using the **Ps,Qs,3R Approach**. The patient is *hemodynamically* stable.

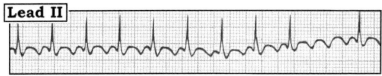

Lead II

📨 **Answer to Tracing #11:** Up until the end of the above tracing — the rhythm is regular at a rate just *under* 150/minute. The QRS looks to be narrow — although it is difficult to be certain about QRS duration without benefit of a 12-lead ECG obtained *during* tachycardia. The *KEY* clue to the etiology of this rhythm strip is seen at the end of the tracing where the rhythm slows. This is **AFlutter** (*Atrial Flutter*) — diagnosed by the presence of *regular* atrial activity at a rate *close* to 300/minute in a ***sawtooth*** **pattern**. There is 2:1 AV conduction early on — which slows at the end of the tracing to become 4:1 AV conduction.

• In our experience — AFlutter is *by far* the most commonly *overlooked* arrhythmia. It is easy to see why from the initial appearance of the above rhythm, in which the *rapid* rate makes it difficult to distinguish between the QRS complex, ST-T waves and *ongoing* flutter waves.

• The most common ventricular response to **untreated AFlutter** is with **2:1 AV conduction**. Because the atrial rate of flutter is almost always close to 300/minute (*250-350/min range*) — this means that the ventricular rate of a patient in AFlutter will most commonly be regular and **close** to **150/minute** (*140-160/min usual range*).

• The 2nd most common ventricular response to AFlutter is with **4:1 AV conduction**. This is seen at the end of the above rhythm strip.

➡ ***Clinical*** **Note:**   Were it not for brief slowing in the ventricular response toward the end of the above rhythm — we would <u>not</u> know for certain what the diagnosis is. All we could say is that the rhythm *appears to be* a **regular** SVT (*SupraVentricular Tachycardia*) at a rate *just under* 150/minute with *uncertain* atrial activity.

• We might *suspect* AFlutter (*because the rate is close to 150/minute,* <u>and</u> *there* <u>does</u> *seem to be suspicious atrial activity*) — but the true *sawtooth* pattern of flutter does *not* emerge until the relative pause at the end of the tracing.

• Full discussion of AFlutter (*including the approach to diagnosis and treatment*) is covered in Sections 13 and 14 (*esp. pp 147-158*).

Practice **Tracing #12:**

(?) ⇨ PRACTICE Tracing:

● Interpret the rhythm below using the **Ps,Qs,3R Approach**. The patient is *hemodynamically* stable.

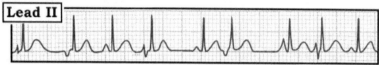

Lead II

☞ **Answer to Tracing #12:** The QRS complex is narrow. The rhythm is *irregularly* irregular. Despite this irregularity — this is *not* AFib because P waves <u>are</u> present. P waves are of *multiple* different shapes. The above rhythm is **MAT** (*Multifocal Atrial Tachycardia*).

• This tracing provides an excellent example of how working through the *Ps,Qs,3R Approach* facilitates deduction of the correct diagnosis.
• Next to AFlutter — MAT is (*in our experience*) the most commonly overlooked arrhythmia. Whereas P waves <u>are</u> well seen in the above rhythm — it would be easy to mistake the *irregular* irregularity of MAT for AFib if <u>only</u> a *single* monitoring lead with *less* clear P wave morphology was used. *12 leads are always better than one.*

⇨ ***Clinical* PEARL:** *Suspect* MAT *whenever* you encounter an irregularly *irregular* rhythm in a patient with *chronic/severe* pulmonary disease, as this is the most common clinical setting for this arrhythmia.

• The other clinical situation in which MAT may be seen is in severely ill patients with multisystem disease (*including electrolyte and acid-base disturbance, hypoxemia, septicemia, and other disorders*).
• ***Obtaining*** a **12-lead ECG** in such patients (*rather than depending on a single-lead rhythm strip*) should clarify whether an *irregularly* irregular rhythm is AFib or MAT.
• Full discussion of the management approach to AFib, MAT, and other SVT rhythms is covered in Sections 13 and 14 (*esp. pp 133-137*).

Section 03 – Unspecified Tachycardia (*pp 48-50*)

 # *O*verview of *U*nspecified *T*achycardia

● You are called to a code. The patient is in the rhythm shown below in **Figure 03-1**. *What to do next?*

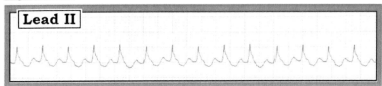

Figure 03-1: The patient is coding. We see *tachycardia* ...

☞ **The Very 1st Thing** to do when assessing a patient in tachycardia — is to assess the patient: *Is the patient hemodynamically stable?*

- IF the patient in *tachycardia* is **UnStable** — Treat the patient! It *no longer matters* what the specific rhythm diagnosis is — since **electricity** (*synchronized cardioversion* or *unsynchronized shock*) is **immediately** indicated (*See page 51 for HOW we define "stability"*).

- But IF the *tachycardic* patient is *hemodynamically* **STABLE** — then (*by definition*), there will be at least *some* time to more accurately assess what the rhythm is likely to be. Management options then depend on *which* of the following **3 possibilities** is present: i) *Stable* **VT**; ii) *Stable* **Narrow** **Tachycardia**; or iii) *Stable* **WCT** (*Wide-Complex Tachycardia*) of **uncertain** etiology.

NOTE: — The ACLS-PM *Tachycardia* Algorithm does *not* distinguish between stable tachycardia due to VT — vs tachycardia due to a WCT of *uncertain* etiology. We enhance this concept by *working through* the process of assessing the **unspecified** Tachycardia:
- The *initial* steps should take *no more* than seconds.
- *All* steps *need* to be followed for *each* Tachycardia!

Unspecified Tachycardia

 ➡ **Suggested** *Initial* **Approach:**

● **Check 1st for** a **Pulse!** This is because IF no pulse is present — the patient with *unspecified* wide tachycardia should be treated the *same* as VFib (ie, *with immediate unsynchronized shock* — *page 1*).
- On the other hand — IF a pulse is present — the *KEY* is to assess for **Hemodynamic** Stability (*Section 04 on page 51*).

- <u>Note:</u> IF the patient with Tachycardia *has* a pulse but is *not* **Stable** — then *immediate* treatment is needed. It *no longer matters* what the rhythm is since the patient needs to be *cardioverted* ASAP!

☞ <u>Remember:</u> The *fastest* way to convert a patient out of a *fast* rhythm is with *electricity* = **shock** (be this by *synchronized* cardioversion <u>or</u> defibrillation).

- **Cardioversion** (*Section 05 on page 53*) — Begin with 100-200 joules (*depending on symptom severity*) for the patient in need of *emergency* cardioversion. Increase energy as is needed. <u>IF</u> *unable* to cardiovert — then defibrillate.
- **Defibrillate** — Go straight to *unsynchronized* shock (*defibrillation*) if the rhythm is *polymorphic* VT/Torsades (*synchronized cardioversion will not work, since there is no consistent waveform to synch to ...*).

☞ IF the Patient is Stable:

If the patient with *unspecified* tachycardia is *initially* stable — then by definition, there is at least *some* time to proceed with further evaluation before beginning specific treatment. Hopefully you'll be able to determine the *type* of **Tachycardia**:

- Systematically **assess** the **5 Parameters**. That is: "*Watch Your Ps, Qs and 3Rs*" (*page 21*). Perhaps the *most* important of these 5 parameters when assessing the patient with *unspecified* tachycardia is determining <u>IF</u> the **QRS** *wide* <u>or</u> *narrow* ?

☞ Is the QRS Complex *Wide* <u>or</u> *Narrow* ?

IF the QRS complex is *truly* **narrow** in a patient with *stable* Tachycardia — then for practical purposes, the rhythm is **S**upra**V**entricular !

- Since the patient is stable — **Get** a **12-lead** to **confirm** that the **QRS** is *truly* **narrow** in <u>all</u> 12 leads.
- Our definition of **"WIDE"** — is *more* than **0.10 second** (ie, *more than half a large box in duration*). Once confirmed that the QRS is **normal duration** (≤0.10 second) in <u>all</u> 12 leads — Treat as per the **SVT Algorithm** (*pp 121-124*).

☞ IF the QRS Complex is *Wide* ...

The approach to *unspecified* tachycardia will be *different* **IF** *the* **QRS** *is* **WIDE**:

- Assess the patient. *Make sure the patient is stable!*
- Assess the ECG. *Get a* **12-lead**. Determine <u>IF</u> the rhythm is: **i)** *monomorphic* VT; **ii)** WCT of *uncertain* etiology; <u>or</u> **iii)** *Something* else (ie, *Torsades, polymorphic VT, WPW*).
- GO TO the **appropriate** Algorithm (*See Summary on page 50*).
- **IF** at *any* time the **patient** *becomes* **unstable** — *immediately* cardiovert <u>or</u> defibrillate.

Unspecified Tachycardia

 ⇒ *Summary*

● Bottom Line: — The **1st step** in management of *any* tachycardia — is to determine **IF** the ***patient* is stable?**

- Is there a pulse? If *not* — treat as VFib (*defibrillate*).
- IF a pulse is present but the patient is *not* stable (*as a direct result of the fast rate*) — Deliver electricity (*synchronized cardioversion* or *defibrillation*).

● But IF the patient in tachycardia is **Stable** — there is time to assess further. *Get a* **12-lead**. Begin targeted management based on your *best* guess as to what the rhythm is likely to be. *See **appropriate* algorithm**:

- **Hemodynamic Stability?** — *Section 04 on page 51.*
- *Synchronized* Cardioversion — *Section 05 on page 53.*
- *Using* Adenosine — *Section 06 on page 58.*
- ***Known* VT** — *Section 07 on page 63.*
- **WCTs of *Uncertain* Etiology** — *Section 08 on page 70.*
- *Polymorphic* VT/Torsades — *Section 11 on page 98.*
- *Very* Fast AFib with WPW — *Section 12 on page 104.*
- ***Narrow* Tachycardias** — *Section 13 on page 114.*
- AFib (*page 125*) – MAT (*page 133*) – PSVT (*page 138*)
  – AFlutter (*page 147*) – Sinus Tachycardia (*page 159*).

NOTE: IF at *any* time in the process the **patient *becomes* unstable** — *immediately* cardiovert or defibrillate.

☞ **A *Final* Word on Algorithms ...**

　　Algorithms provide guidance. They are excellent learning tools — and they help summarize the most common interventions for *most* situations. But — *"there is no one size that fits all"* — and the thinking clinician at the bedside will often need to consider additional measures.
- We *love* algorithms as a starting place.
- That said, sometimes — *"Ya just gotta be there"* (ie, *at the bedside of the patient ...*).

Section 04 – Is the Patient Stable? (*pp 51-52*)

 Is the P*atient* S*table?*

● **How to Assess:** *Is the Patient Stable?*
    Clinically, the *most* important parameter to assess in *any* patient with a cardiac arrhythmia — is whether the rhythm is **hemodynamically "significant"**. This holds true <u>regardless</u> of whether the rhythm in question is slow or fast. A rhythm is said to be *"hemodynamically"* significant — <u>IF</u> it **produces** **signs** or **symptoms** of concern as a *direct result* of the rate (*be the rate fast* <u>or</u> *slow*):

- **Signs** of **Concern** — include hypotension (ie, *systolic BP ≤80-90 mm Hg*); shock; heart failure/pulmonary edema; *and/or* acute infarction.
- **Symptoms** of **Concern** — include chest pain; shortness of breath; *and/or* impaired mental status.

☞ **KEY** *Clinical* **Points** — The definition of hemodynamic stability is *equally* applicable for *supraventricular* tachyarrhythmias — as it is for VT. That is, the patient with tachycardia who is **clearly symptomatic** (ie, *hypotensive; short of breath; confused*) is in need of *immediate* **synchronized** **cardioversion** — <u>regardless</u> of whether the rhythm is VT or SVT. In contrast — a trial of *medical* therapy is justified <u>IF</u> the patient is stable!

- Sometimes — ***"You just have to be there."*** For example, *despite* a systolic BP of 75 mm Hg — we would <u>*not*</u> necessarily cardiovert a patient with tachycardia who was otherwise tolerating the rhythm well (ie, *without chest pain, dyspnea, or confusion*). Some patients may *remain* stable for hours (or *even* days!) — *despite* being in *sustained* VT. **Treat the patient** — <u>*NOT*</u> the rhythm!

Is the Patient Stable?

 ⇨ ***Beyond-the-Textbook* ...**

● A *KEY* component to assessment is trying to determine <u>IF</u> it is the rate <u>or</u> the *rhythm* that is *causing* the patient to be unstable (<u>vs</u> *the underlying condition*).

- For **Tachycardia** — Consider the example of AIVR (*Accelerated IdioVentricular Rhythm*) at a rate of 110-120/minute. This rate is usually *not* fast enough to produce "instability". On the other hand — *loss* of the atrial "kick" in association with AIVR at ~110/minute in a patient with underlying ventricular dysfunction may clearly be enough to precipitate symptomatic hypotension.

- In general, **IF** the **rate of tachycardia** is *less* than **~150/minute** — it is *less* likely that hemodynamic instability is being caused by the rapid rate. That said, exceptions exist — as **VT** at **140/minute** in a patient with underlying heart disease may definitely precipitate hemodynamic compromise.

- For **Bradycardia** — A rate as slow as 30/minute will *not* necessarily cause symptoms. IF the situation is *not* acute — treatment with Atropine, Epinephrine or Dopamine may indeed cause more harm than good (*Careful observation may be all that is needed*). In contrast — other patients may be symptomatic with much less severe bradycardia (*if baseline low BP, ischemia or heart failure are present*).

Is the Patient Stable?

 ➡ *Bottom* ***Line***

⬤ There are **no** *"magic numbers"* for declaring hemodynamic "instability". Instead — this determination is a ***clinical*** **process** to be based on *ongoing* assessment of the patient by the clinician on-the-scene.

☞ A *special* rhythm to *be aware* of: — *AIVR* —

As a final note to this Section on *hemodynamic* stability — We comment on **AIVR** (*Accelerated* *Idio*Ventricular *Rhythm* = **Figure 04-1**).

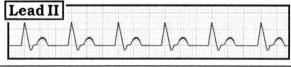

Figure 04-1: AIVR (*See text*).

⬤ We emphasize the following points about AIVR:
- The usual rate of an **idioventricular *ventricular* escape rhythm** is **20-40/minute** (*pp 190-192*). In contrast — the term **"VT"** (*Ventricular Tachycardia*) is usually reserved for ventricular rhythms *faster* than **130-140/minute**. Ventricular rhythms *in between* this range (*usually between ~60-120/minute*) are generally referred to as **"AIVR"** — since they are *"accelerated"* compared to the usual ventricular escape rate (*of 20-40/min*) — but *not quite as fast* as a VT rhythm likely to produce *hemodynamic* consequence.
- **AIVR** generally occurs in one of the following settings: **i)** as a rhythm during cardiac arrest; **ii)** in the monitoring phase of acute MI (*esp. with inferior MI*); *or* **iii)** as a *reperfusion* arrhythmia (*following thrombolytics, angioplasty, or spontaneous reperfusion*). The rhythm is often *transient* <u>and</u> treatment is usually *not* needed IF the patient is stable.
- **AIVR** is often an *"escape rhythm"* — that arises because *both* the SA and AV nodes are *not* functioning. IF treatment is needed (*because loss of atrial "kick" results in hypotension*) — Atropine is the drug of choice (*in hope of speeding up the SA node to resume its pacemaking function*). AIVR should *not* be shocked *nor* treated with Amiodarone/Procainamide — since doing so might result in asystole ...

Section 05 – *Synchronized* Cardioversion (*pp 53-57*)

 # Synchronized Cardioversion

● **Synchronized** Cardioversion (*as in* <u>Figure 05-1</u>) — entails delivery of the electrical discharge at a *specified* point in the cardiac cycle (*on R wave upstroke* <u>or</u> *S wave downslope*) — away from the *"vulnerable"* **period** (*which is near the end of the T wave*). Doing so makes cardioversion *safer* than unsynchronized shock (*defibrillation*).

• Cardioversion is especially effective in treatment of arrhythmias that depend on a *reentry* mechanism for their perpetuation. This includes (*among others*) atrial flutter; PSVT; ventricular tachycardia; <u>and</u> accessory pathway *reentry* tachycardias. Cardioversion is also very effective in terminating AFib.

• Synchronized electrical cardioversion works by producing a single, brief electrical discharge — that acts to terminate the arrhythmia by *interrupting* the reentrant circuit *and/or* altering conduction properties (*conduction velocity; refractoriness*) that led to perpetuation of the arrhythmia.

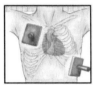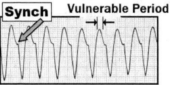

Figure 05-1: *Synchronized* cardioversion. The electrical impulse is *synchronized* to the QRS complex — so as to avoid delivery of the discharge during the "vulnerable" period. This *minimizes* the risk of precipitating VFib when energy is delivered.

Clarification of Terms:

☞ **KEY Clinical Points** — The term *"cardioversion"* may be the source of some confusion. This is because this term is commonly interchanged (*and mistakenly equated*) with two other terms: *defibrillation* <u>and</u> *countershock.*

• **Defibrillation** — is the process of passing an electrical current through the heart with express intent of completely depolarizing *all* myocardial cells. The electrical discharge that is delivered with defibrillation is *unsynchronized* — which means that it occurs at an entirely *random* point in the cardiac cycle.

• In contrast — use of the term **Cardioversion** implies that the electrical discharge has been timed (*synchronized*) to occur at a *designated* point in the cardiac cycle. Doing so not only facilitates conversion of certain tachyarrhythmias to sinus rhythm — but it also *minimizes* the chance that the electrical impulse will exacerbate the arrhythmia (*as may occur if the stimulus happens to be delivered during the vulnerable period*).

▶ NOTE: To avoid confusion about terminology (*as well as to clarify the mode of delivery of the electrical impulse*) — we frequently refer to the procedure as **"synchronized cardioversion"** (*rather than simply "cardioversion"*).

- Although use of the *combined* term *"synchronized cardioversion"* may seem redundant — it leaves *no doubt* as to how the operator is about to proceed.
- Use of the term *"synchronized"* cardioversion also helps to distinguish **electrical cardioversion** (*with delivery of a timed electrical discharge synchronized to a specific point in the cardiac cycle*) — from **medical cardioversion** (*in which a medication such as amiodarone or procainamide is given to a patient in AFib in hope of facilitating conversion to sinus rhythm <u>without</u> use of electricity*).
- The need for **synchronized** cardioversion may be **"emergent"** (*immediately needed because the patient is decompensating*) — <u>or</u> the procedure may be **"elective"** (*not immediately needed because the patient is hemodynamically stable*). There may be gradations of "urgency" in between (ie, *semi-elective*) — if the patient manifests symptoms from the arrhythmia but is not acutely decompensating.
- Finally — there may be **spontaneous conversion** (*rather than spontaneous "cardioversion"*) of the rhythm to normal when the tachyarrhythmia resolves on its own *without* any medical intervention.

⬤ The last 2 terms in need of clarification are **countershock** and its diminutive **"shock"**. Both of these terms are often freely interchanged with the term, **defibrillation**. We favor this free interchange, and unless otherwise specified — generally use these 3 terms synonymously to represent delivery of an *unsynchronized* electrical impulse to a patient in VFib.

☞ Selection of *Initial* Energy Levels

The clinical reality is that selection of initial energy levels for synchronized cardioversion is empiric. We suggest the following:

- **Atrial Flutter** — Use *low* energy first (*~50 joules*) — as flutter is usually *very* responsive to cardioversion.
- **Monomorphic VT/WCT** — Consider starting at 100-200 joules (*monophasic* <u>or</u> *biphasic* defibrillator — *depending on symptom severity*). Increase energy as needed.
- **AFib** — *Higher* energies are likely to be needed (*begin with 200 joules monophasic* <u>or</u> *~100-200 joules biphasic*).
- **Other Unstable SVT** — Consider 100-200 joules (*monophasic* <u>or</u> *biphasic*) — depending on symptom *severity* <u>and</u> the *likely* etiology of the rhythm.
- **Torsades/Polymorphic VT** — Defibrillate! (*Don't bother trying to synch, as doing so is unlikely to work and will delay the process*).

Synchronized Cardioversion

 ➡ *Beyond-the-Textbook* ...

● Although data for all situations are lacking — several points can be made regarding recommendations for how much energy to use:

- Various rhythms respond differently. In general — organized rhythms (*such as AFlutter, monomorphic VT*) tend to respond better (*to lower energies*) than less organized rhythms (*such as AFib*).
- Increase energy *as needed* <u>IF</u> patient *fails* to respond.
- **Certain SVT rhythms** (ie, *MAT; automatic atrial tach; junctional tach*) **are unlikely to respond** to synchronized cardioversion (*or if they do respond — the rhythm will usually recur*). Fortunately — it is *rare* that these rhythms require cardioversion (*Correcting the underlying disorder is key for these arrhythmias!*).

▶ NOTE: Whenever possible — **Sedate** the *conscious* patient <u>*prior*</u> to *synchronized* cardioversion (*and it almost always <u>will</u> be possible!*).

- Be sure to *continually* monitor the patient throughout the procedure.
- Obtain an ongoing *hard copy* of the rhythm just before, during, <u>and</u> immediately after delivery of the synchronized impulse — since a hard copy rhythm strip may be needed to detect subtle changes that may occur in the rhythm.

📡 Cardioversion: *If the Synch Discharge Won't Go Off* ...

Be Aware of common reasons why the defibrillator may not fire when attempting to cardiovert. These include:
- Synch mode not correctly on.
- Inability to synch on a particular QRS complex.
- Monitor gain set too low to sense.
- Personnel are unfamiliar with operating the device (*there are many different types of defibrillators in use — and each has its own particulars regarding activation and operation of synch mode*).

● IF for *any* reason you are *unable* to get the defibrillator to deliver a synchronized impulse — **Turn off** the **"synch" mode** and **defibrillate** the patient!
- It is usually *not* worthwhile spending extra time trying to figure out why the synch mode will not work in patient who is decompensating.
- Delivery of an *unsynchronized* discharge (*defibrillation*) — will almost always work as well as a synchronized one (*the increase in risk from unsynchronized discharge is minimal*).

📡 It is good to *anticipate* "the worst" that could happen during attempted cardioversion. This way you'll be prepared.
- IF delivery of a synchronized impulse precipitates VFib — then *immediately* defibrillate the patient. The "good news" — is that this

will usually be the *best* time to defibrillate (*since you are right there on-the-scene and can immediately shock after this witnessed VFib!*).
- It is rare that synchronized cardioversion will precipitate asystole. IF this occurs — Be aware that the patient will almost always respond to temporary pacing.

☞ Cardioversion: *ACLS Provider Manual Recommendations*

ACLS-PM (*Provider Manual*) recommends specific energy levels that differ slightly from the levels we suggest on page 54. Specifically — **ACLS-PM *recommends*** the following:
- *Narrow* Regular Tachycardia — 50-100 joules.
- Narrow *Irregular* Tachycardia — 120-200 joules biphasic (*200J monophasic*).
- *Wide* Regular Tachycardia — 100 joules.
- Wide *Irregular* Tachycardia — Defibrillate (*Don't synch!*).

▶ NOTE: Much *more* important than the details of how many joules to use for one's initial synchronized cardioversion attempt are the concepts involved!

- IF properly performed — **Synchronized cardioversion** offers a *safer* way to electrically convert a patient out of an *unstable* tachy-arrhythmia (*because it avoids the "vulnerable period" — and is therefore less likely to precipitate VFib*). Organized rhythms tend to respond better — but *regardless* of the starting energy level selected — You'll want to *increase* this amount if the patient fails to respond.
- IF in doubt — Defibrillation will almost always work.

☞ What about the *Precordial* Thump?

Use of the precordial thump dates back to 1920s, when the procedure was first used on a patient having Stokes-Adams attacks. A resurgence in use of the thump was seen in the 1970s with a serendipitous report of inadvertent passage by a transport ambulance over a parking lot speed bump surprisingly restoring sinus rhythm to a patient in cardiac arrest. The technique became popular and was routinely recommended during the early days of ACLS protocols.
- To **perform** a **precordial** thump — a sharp, quick blow is struck with the fleshy part of the fist (*hypothenar eminence*) from a distance of 8-12 inches above the chest — to the *midportion* of the sternum. The blow should be firm, but *not* so forceful as to break any ribs ...
- Mechanical energy generated by the thump has been shown to produce a low amplitude depolarization of *approximately* **2-5 joules**.
- The amount of electrical energy needed to defibrillate a patient in VFib increases *exponentially* after the first few moments following onset of VFib. The thought is that IF the thump generates ~2-5 joules of energy at an *early-enough-point* in the process — that this might be enough to convert VFib to sinus rhythm. The more time that passes

after onset of VFib — the *less* the chance that the thump will generate enough energy to be successful.

- A thump is <u>not</u> benign. Ribs may be broken — <u>and</u> if excessive in force, additional cardiac injury may occur. Although data are scarce — there are reports that delivery of a thump to a patient in VT at the *wrong* point (ie, *during the "vulnerable" period*) in the cardiac cycle may precipitate deterioration of VT to VFib. As opposed to application of *synchronized* cardioversion with a defibrillator — delivery of 2-5 joules via thump *cannot* be timed to the cardiac cycle.

● **BOTTOM Line** (*regarding the* **Thump**): Think of the precordial thump as a *"No-Lose"* **procedure**. It should *only* be considered in patients *without* a pulse (*if it is considered at all ... *).

- ACLS-PM *no longer* recommends use of the thump. IF a defibrillator is close by — it is far better to defibrillate asap rather than thump.
- We *might* consider a thump – <u>IF</u> we were quickly *on-the-scene* at a *pulseless* cardiac arrest in which *no* defibrillator was readily available. There is little to lose — <u>and</u> — a *promptly* delivered thump *might* work to convert VFib (*albeit realistic chance of success is admittedly small*).
- Do <u>not</u> use the thump if you feel a pulse! There IS *"something to lose"* in this situation (ie, *the pulse*). IF the rhythm is VT with a pulse — delivery of a precordial thump is statistically far more likely to precipitate deterioration to VFib than it is to convert the rhythm.

☞ **What about *Cough* Version for VFib?**

The technique for cough version is simple: As soon as the rhythm is noted — instruct the patient to, *"Cough hard, and keep coughing!"* Coughing should be continued at 1-to-3 second intervals — either until the arrhythmia is converted, <u>or</u> until the patient can be cardioverted.

- Impetus for advocating use of cough version resulted from observation in the cardiac catheterization laboratory that forceful and repetitive coughing (ie, *"cough CPR"*) — could sustain consciousness for surprisingly long periods of time (*of up to 90 seconds!*) in patients with pulseless VT, VFib or even asystole.
- Intrathoracic pressures of *more* than 100 mmHg are produced by such coughing — and are somehow able to generate adequate blood flow despite the presence of an otherwise *non-perfusing* rhythm. The mechanism for cough version remains unknown (*increased intrathoracic pressure* <u>vs</u> *autonomic nervous system activation* <u>vs</u> *conversion of mechanical energy from coughing into a few joules of electrical energy?*). What IS known — is that vigorous coughing occasionally converts malignant arrhythmias to normal sinus rhythm.
- Since original description of cough CPR by Criley et al in 1976 — instructing patients to cough at the onset of *nonperfusing* rhythms has been used in the cardiac catheterization laboratory. That said — the technique is still largely ignored by all too many other emergency care providers who rarely seem to invoke coughing in the conscious patient at the onset of a malignant arrhythmia.

Using **A***denosine*

● *Indications* for Adenosine

The ***primary*** **indication** for **Adenosine** has been tachyarrhythmias with a *reentry* mechanism — especially those involving at least a portion of the AV Node in the reentry circuit. Indications for Adenosine *have expanded!*

- **PSVT** — Adenosine is the drug of 1st choice for *emergency* treatment of **PSVT** (*>90% successful conversion rate*). That said — *longer-acting* drugs (ie, *diltiazem/verapamil, β-blockers*) may be needed to prevent PSVT recurrence (*pp 145-146*).
- ***"Chemical"*** **Valsalva** — in which Adenosine is given as a *diagnostic/therapeutic* trial for a *narrow* tachycardia of *uncertain* etiology (**Figure 06-1**). Presumably — Adenosine will convert the rhythm if it is PSVT. If not — it will hopefully *slow* the rhythm enough (*transiently*) to allow definitive diagnosis to be made (*like Valsalva ...*).
- **WCT** — ACLS-PM now recommends **Adenosine** as a drug of 1st choice for **regular *monomorphic* VT** or **WCT** of **uncertain etiology** (*See pags 60; 64; 73-74*).

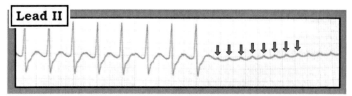

Figure 06-1: Chemical valsalva. Administration of Adenosine to this patient with a regular SVT at ~150/minute results in transient *diagnostic* slowing that reveals underlying flutter waves at 300/minute. (*The continuation of this rhythm strip is shown on page 59*).

☞ *Dosing* of Adenosine

Adenosine is administered **IV push** — giving the drug as rapidly as possible over 1-3 seconds (*so that it doesn't deteriorate in the IV tubing*). IV Adenosine half-life is *less* than 10 seconds!

- *Initially* give **6mg** by **IV push**. Follow each bolus with a fluid flush.
- IF *no response* after 1-2 minutes — give **12mg** by IV push (*for a total dose = 6+12=18mg*).
- ACLS-PM *no longer* recommends giving a second 12mg bolus if the patient has not responded.

▶ NOTE: Dosing protocols for use of Adenosine should *not* necessarily be *fixed* for all adults. Instead — it is well to be aware of occasional instances when *higher* or *lower* doses of the drug are indicated:

- **Lower Adenosine doses** (ie, *2-3mg initially*) — should be considered for older patients; those with renal failure; heart failure; shock; in transplant patients; if taking dipyridamole (*Persantine*) – and/or – when Adenosine is given by central IV line.
- **Higher Adenosine doses** — may be needed for patients taking theophylline (*or for those consuming large amounts of caffeine*) — since methylxanthines impede binding of adenosine at its receptor sites.

☞ *Adverse* Effects of Adenosine

Adenosine is *not* totally benign. Although the drug is usually fairly well tolerated — a series of adverse effects is common (*and to be expected*).

- **Adverse effects** may include: **i)** chest pain; **ii)** cough (*from transient bronchospasm*); **iii)** cutaneous vasodilation; **iv)** metallic taste; **v)** a sense of "impending doom"; and **vi)** transient bradycardia that may be marked (*and which may even cause a brief period of asystole*).
- The "good news" — is that *adverse* effects **most often resolve *within* 1 minute** — although this may be *very* alarming in the meantime IF the clinician is not aware of what to expect (Figure 06-2).

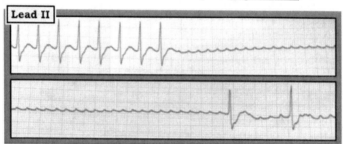

Figure 06-2: Chemical Valsalva (*continuation of the rhythm strip on page 58*). Administration of Adenosine was diagnostic of SVT etiology (*revealing underlying AFlutter at ~300/minute*). In so doing — a period of *over* 10 seconds ensued *without* a QRS complex. *Marked* bradycardia like this is *not* uncommon following Adenosine Fortunately — bradycardia almost always resolves *within* 30-60 seconds.

▶ NOTE: Some clinicians even *look away* for 20-30 seconds after giving Adenosine — so as not to be bothered by the transient marked rate slowing that so often is seen. While *not* suggesting you do this — it is well to be aware that *marked* rate slowing may *transiently* occur.

▶ FINAL Note: Adenosine may *shorten* the refractory period of *atrial* tissue — which could initiate AFib in a *predisposed* individual. As a result — Adenosine should be used with caution in patients with known WPW, given theoretic possibility of inducing AFib (*which could have significant consequence in a patient with accessory pathways*).

Using Adenosine

  ➡ *<u>Beyond</u>-the-Textbook ...*

⬤ Despite the above series of *adverse* effects — Adenosine remains an exceedingly useful agent in emergency cardiac care. It is usually well tolerated. Nevertheless, it is <u>not</u> completely benign – <u>and</u> – a balance must be reached between pros and cons of using this drug.

- It is a great drug for **SVT** (*of known or unknown etiology*).
- Adenosine **should <u>not</u> be used** for: **i)** *polymorphic* VT; **ii)** Torsades; <u>or</u> **iii)** WPW <u>with</u> *very rapid* AFib (*since Adenosine may precipitate deterioration to VFib if given for these rhythms*). Instead — *defibrillation* may be needed.
- ***EARLY* use** of **Adenosine** — may help greatly in evaluation/management of **stable** *monomorphic* **WCT**. We favor Adenosine: **i)** <u>IF</u> we think there is ***reasonable* chance** the **WCT** is ***supraventricular*** (*Adenosine will usually convert PSVT* – <u>and</u> – *it facilitates diagnosis of other SVTs by briefly slowing the rate*); <u>or</u> **ii)** <u>IF</u> we think the patient **might** have an ***adenosine-responsive* VT** (*See below*).
- <u>Admittedly</u> — there <u>are</u> times we ***empirically* try Adenosine** when we have *no idea* what the rhythm is (*VT* <u>vs</u> *SVT*). That said — we generally prefer <u>not</u> to use Adenosine when the clinical setting and 12-lead ECG suggest a *non-responsive* form of VT is likely. Sometimes — *"Ya just gotta be there"* to decide whether or not to try Adenosine.

▶ PEARL: Do <u>not</u> use Adenosine to treat SVT in a heart transplant patient (*much lower doses are needed due to Adenosine-hypersensitivity*). **Aminophylline** may reverse *adenosine-induced* extreme bradycardia (*See page 174*).

▶ *Final* PEARL: Adenosine should probably <u>not</u> be used to treat SVT by the IO route. Time for IO absorption may exceed the *less than* 10-second half-life of this drug (*probably better to use IV Diltiazem to treat SVT if only IO access is available*).

👉 **When to Suspect *Adenosine-Responsive* VT?**

A group of VT rhythms <u>do</u> respond to Adenosine! These ***adenosine-responsive* VTs** are most commonly *catecholamine-induced* <u>and</u> occur *during exercise* in younger adults <u>without</u> structural heart disease:

- Many of these VTs originate from the **RVOT** (*<u>R</u>ight <u>V</u>entricular <u>O</u>utflow <u>T</u>rack*) — though they can also arise from the LVOT, the hemifascicles, or elsewhere.
- We ***suspect* RVOT VT** — <u>IF</u> a young adult presents with an exercise-induced *regular* WCT showing LBBB in precordial leads and an *inferior* axis (<u>Figure 06-3</u>). That said — *adenosine-responsive* forms of VT can <u>not</u> always be predicted by their ECG appearance! This is the **rationale** for *empiric* **use** of **Adenosine** with a ***regular* WCT**.

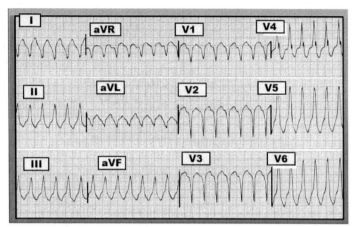

Figure 06-3: RVOT-VT. *Suspect* **RVOT VT** when a younger (*20-40 yo*) adult presents with an *exercise-induced* regular WCT showing a LBBB pattern in *precordial* leads – and – an *inferior* axis in the limb leads.

● The mechanism whereby Adenosine may work for certain forms of VT (*such as RVOT VT*) — is that initiation of these VTs is felt to be due to intracellular calcium overload (*which affects cellular depolarization thresholds*) with resultant "triggered activity" mediated by cyclic-AMP (*which Adenosine inhibits*).

• Mechanisms of *non-adenosine-responsive* forms of VT are generally ischemic, reentrant, or due to increased automaticity — *none* of which respond to Adenosine.

▶ NOTE: **Verapamil/Diltiazem** — may also terminate RVOT VT (*by a different mechanism that inhibits intracellular calcium channels*). That said — these 2 calcium blockers should *never* be used empirically for WCT rhythms (!!!) — because their *vasodilatory* and *negative* inotropic effects may precipitate deterioration to VFib.

• **Beta-Blockers** — may also at times terminate RVOT VT (*these drugs also lower cyclic-AMP levels*).

• *Vagal* **Manuevers** — may on occasion terminate RVOT VT (*such that the previous dictum saying response to a vagal maneuver rules out VT is no longer completely true*).

Using Adenosine for WCT/VT

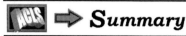 ➡ *Summary*

● A group of VT rhythms *do* respond to Adenosine. Overall — **this makes up *less* than 10% of all VT** — but true prevalence of *adenosine-responsive* VT depends on characteristics of the population being assessed (*healthy younger subjects* vs *older patients with ischemic heart disease...*).

- ***Polymorphic* VT** (*or polymorphic WCT*) — is unlikely to respond to Adenosine (*Adenosine is <u>not</u> recommended for this*).
- ***Ischemic*** and **reentrant VTs** (*as are commonly seen in older patients with coronary or structural heart disease*) — generally do <u>not</u> respond to Adenosine.
- ***Suspect*** an ***adenosine-responsive* form** of **VT** — when a regular *monomorphic* WCT is seen in a younger adult (*~20-40 years old*) <u>without</u> underlying heart disease — especially if the WCT was *precipitated* by exercise.
- **Most** (*>80-90%*) ***regular* WCTs** without clear sign of sinus-P-wave activity are ***due*** to **VT**. This figure goes up to >90-95% if the patient is older, has heart disease, and manifests certain morphologic features (*LIST #1 — See page 72*).

▶ **KEY Point:** In the past, it was thought that <u>IF</u> a WCT responded to Adenosine — that this "proved" the WCT was supraventricular. Given awareness that certain forms of VT may respond to Adenosine — We now appreciate that conversion of WCT to sinus rhythm with use of Adenosine does <u>not</u> prove anything regarding etiology of the arrhythmia.

 ⇨ *Bottom Line*

● IV Adenosine may be ***tried* early** on in the treatment algorithm of **monomorphic *stable* WCT**. Its use is *usually* safe in this situation — <u>and</u> the drug *may work* by converting the rhythm <u>IF</u> it is supraventricular <u>or</u> one of the uncommon forms of *adenosine-responsive VT*.

Known VT

● This Section deals with the approach to the patient who you *know* is in **sustained *monomorphic* VT** (*Ventricular Tachycardia*):

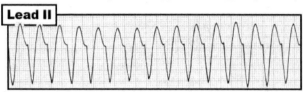
Lead II

Figure 07-1: Ventricular Tachycardia. This rhythm is further design- nated as **monomorphic VT** because QRS morphology (*outside of minor variation in amplitude*) does *not* change throughout the tracing.

- **Rhythm Description** — usually regular (or at least *fairly* regular) *wide*-QRS tachycardia *without* clear evidence of normal atrial activity.
- **Terminology** — The definition of *"sustained VT"* varies among experts. Most authorities require *persistence* of VT for *at least* 20-to-30 seconds *or* long enough to produce symptoms of hypotension or syncope. The term, **"NSVT"** (*Non-Sustained Ventricular Tachycardia*) is used to designate *shorter* runs of VT (*from 3 PVCs in a row — up to 15-20 seconds of VT*) that do *not* produce *hemodynamic* symptoms (*See Practice Tracing #10 on page 45*).

- **Bedside Pitfalls** — Do *not* depend on hemodynamic status to help with the differentiation between SVT and VT. Some patients remain awake and alert (*and normotensive*) for hours (*even days!*) — despite being in *sustained* VT!

☞ *Sustained* VT: *What to Do First?*

● The *KEY* to optimal management of VT lies with addressing these **3 Questions**: i) Is there a *Pulse?* — ii) Is the patient *Stable?* — and iii) Are you *certain* that the rhythm is *really* VT? (*See page 70*).

- IF there is **NO** *Pulse* — then *immediately* defibrillate. Treat **pulseless VT** the *same* as VFib (*page 1*).

But IF a **Pulse is present** during *sustained* VT — Assess the patient for *hemodynamic* stability (*page 51*).
- IF a pulse is present but the patient with VT is **unstable** — then *immediately* **cardiovert!**
- But IF the patient with *sustained* VT is **stable** — then there is at least *some* time for a trial of antiarrhythmic drugs (*See pp 64-69*).

▶ NOTE: If the rhythm is **polymorphic VT** (*in which QRS morphology varies throughout the tracing*) — the patient should be **defibrillated**.
• Many (*most*) patients in sustained *polymorphic* VT will be pulseless. Cardioversion is usually futile — because "synching" to a constantly changing QRST complex is not possible (*pp 98-99*). Acute treatment is with *unsynchronized* shock (*defibrillation*).

Sustained Monomorphic VT

 ➡ **Suggested *Initial* Approach:**

NOTE: The approach we propose below assumes: **i)** that we _know_ the rhythm is VT; _and_ **ii)** that the **VT *is* monomorphic** (*page 63*) — and _not_ polymorphic VT (*which should be immediately defibrillated*).
• It _also_ assumes: **iii)** that the patient **remains stable** throughout the process (*Shock is indicated IF the patient becomes unstable!*).

● **First Fix** the *"Fixables"* — Better than antiarrhythmic drugs is to *find* _and_ "*fix*" any potential *precipitating* causes of VT as soon as you can. These may include:
• Electrolyte disturbance **(***especially low Mg++ _or_ K+* **)**.
• Acidosis/Hypoglycemia.
• Hypoxemia.
• Shock (*from hypovolemia; blood loss; sepsis, etc.*).
• *Uncontrolled* ischemia/*acute* infarction/*acute* heart failure.
• Dig toxicity/Drug overdose.

 Use of Adenosine for *Sustained* VT

Strongly *consider* **Adenosine** as the **1st drug** you give (*page 58*) — especially IF an *adenosine-responsive* form of VT is likely (ie, *younger adult without underlying heart disease; exercise-induced VT*).
• Adenosine may also work when WCT/VT occurs in older patients with heart disease (*effective ~5-10% of the time*).
• Begin with **6mg** by **IV push**. IF no response in 1-2 minutes — Give **12mg** by IV push (*for a total dose = 6+12=18mg*).
• Side effects from Adenosine are usually short-lived (*due to the drug's ultra-short half-life — page 59*).
• Do _not_ use Adenosine for *polymorphic* VT or Torsades.
• NOTE: We do _not_ always start with Adenosine in all older patients with *ischemic* VT from *known* coronary disease.

Use of Amiodarone for *Sustained* VT

Amiodarone has become our preferred ***initial* agent** of choice (*after Adenosine*) for stable *sustained* VT:
• Give **150 mg IV** over 10 minutes. May repeat. IF the drug works — Consider maintenance **IV *infusion*** at **1 mg/ minute** (*See also pg 67*).

Use of Procainamide for *Sustained* VT

Procainamide is *also* recommended by ACLS-PM (*Provider Manual*) as a 1st-line drug of choice for *sustained* VT (*See also pg 67*):
- Give **100 mg IV** *slowly* over 5 minutes (*at ~20 mg/min*) — up to a loading dose of ~500-1,000 mg. May follow with **IV infusion** at **2 mg/minute** (*1-4 mg/minute range*).

Use of IV Magnesium for *Sustained* VT

Consider IV Magnesium for *non-responding* VT. Magnesium is the drug of choice for Torsades and when serum Magnesium levels are known to be low (*See also pg 68 for ACLS-PM Recs plus More on IV Mg++*).
- Give **1-2 gm IV** (*over 1-2 minutes*). May repeat (*especially IF serum Mg++ level is known to be low!*).
- *Higher* IV Mg++ doses may be needed with Torsades (*some cases have required up to 4-8gm IV*).

Use of IV Beta-Blockers for *Sustained* VT

IV β-Blockers are most likely to work IF excess *sympathetic* tone is *either* contributing to or is the cause of *sustained* VT (*See also pg 69*).
- **Metoprolol** — Give **5 mg IV** over ~2 minutes. May then repeat (*up to 15mg total*). May decrease dose and rate of administration depending on BP response.
- Many *other* IV β-blockers are available (*but the Metoprolol regimen is simple, and is commonly used*).

Use of Sotalol for *Sustained* VT

Sotalol is recommended by ACLS-PM as an additional option for *sustained* VT (*See also pg 67*). Do not use Sotalol if the QT is prolonged.
- Give **100 mg** (*1.5 mg/kg*) **IV** over 5 minutes.

Use of Lidocaine for *Sustained* VT

Lidocaine is now considered as a **3rd-line** option for *sustained* VT (*See also page 68*).
- Give **75-100 mg Lidocaine** (*~1.0-1.5 mg/kg*) as an *initial* **IV bolus**. At the same time begin Lidocaine **IV infusion** (*at **2 mg/minute***). May **repeat** the IV bolus (*giving ~**50-75 mg***) if needed in ~5 minutes.

Use of *Synchronized* Cardioversion for *Sustained* VT

There may well come a point during the above treatment process when **"it becomes time"** to get the patient out of *sustained* VT:
- At that point — **Cardiovert!** (*page 53*).

Sustained VT

  Beyond-the-Textbook ...

● ACLS-PM recommends IV antiarrhythmic infusion for **sustained stable monomorphic VT** — plus expert consultation. Our goal is to suggest an approach when expert consultation is *not* immediately available.

- **ACLS-PM** lists Procainamide — Amiodarone — and Sotalol (*but not Lidocaine*) as potential 1st-line antiarrhythmic options (*although Lido-caine is listed elsewhere as a potential alternative for monomorphic VT*). **ACLS-PM** does *not* make recommendation as to which antiar-rhythmic should be given in which sequence ...
- The **"good news"** — is that antiarrhythmic therapy may successfully convert *some* patients who are in stable *sustained* VT or WCT *without* need for electrical therapy.
- The **sobering clinical reality** — is that *none* of the antiarrhythmic agents are overly effective in such treatment (*and all of these drugs are associated with potential for adverse effects*). Many patients will simply *not* respond ...
- *Opinions* **vary** as to which drug should be given when. **Definitive data are lacking.** We provide *our* bias below — realizing that it may differ from other views ...
- *Potential* **problems** inherent **in any study** attempting randomized, prospective, double-blind assessment of the *relative* effectiveness of antiarrhythmic drugs are many: **i)** relative infrequency of *new-onset* stable sustained VT in an ED patient *not yet treated* with antiar-rhythmic drugs; **ii)** need for primary concern being welfare of the patient (*rather than implementation of strict study protocol*); **iii)** tendency toward use of *more* than a single treatment within the critical *initial* 20 minutes for studying this question; **iv)** subsequent *impossibility* of separating out potential *synergistic* detrimental effect when *more* than 1 antiarrhythmic drug is used; *and* **v)** tremendous *variation* among clinical and ECG characteristics of the case at hand. **BOTTOM LINE:** It may simply *not* be possible to "prove" (*or disprove*) the "superiority" of any particular drug for *sustained* VT ...

Antiarrhythmic Drugs for Sustained VT

 Clinical Pearls:

● We probably will *never* know which drug is "best" for **stable sustained monomorphic VT**. Clinical characteristics of the case at hand (*including personal preference and experience of the treating provider*) justify *several* potentially appropriate choices:

☞ **Adenosine** — Strongly consider Adenosine as your 1st drug for *most* patients in stable *monomorphic* VT (*See also pp 58; 64*).

- **Adenosine**'s duration of action is *very* short-lived (*allowing rapid use in most patients without lasting adverse effects*).

▶ **NOTE:** Effects (*beneficial* <u>and</u> *adverse*) of using *more* than one of the antiarrhythmic agents on pp 67-69 are *additive*.
  - Be aware that at <u>any</u> time — *electrical* therapy (*synchronized cardioversion* <u>or</u> *defibrillation*) may be needed <u>IF</u> the patient *becomes* unstable ...

☞ *More* on Amiodarone for *Sustained* VT

Amiodarone is in general **<u>our</u> preferred drug** for antiarrhythmic treatment of *sustained* VT. <u>Advantages</u> include: **i)** familiarity and ease of administration protocol; **ii)** ability to use in patients with heart failure; **iii)** low incidence of Torsades (*even though the QT may lengthen with use of this drug*); <u>and</u> **iv)** efficacy in treating a variety of rhythms (*may convert various SVTs including WPW with very rapid AFib*).
  - Watch BP; reduce IV infusion rate if/as needed.
  - <u>IF</u> effective — may continue as an **IV Amiodarone infusion** at **~1mg/minute** for up to 6 hours (*and 0.5 mg/min for 24-48 hours*).

☞ *More* on Procainamide for *Sustained* VT

Procainamide is preferred by many as their drug of choice for *sustained* VT. Efficacy appears *comparable* to Amiodarone for VT/ SVTs.
  - Give **20-50 mg/minute IV** until <u>either</u>: **i)** the arrhythmia is suppressed; **ii)** hypotension ensues; **iii)** QRS duration increases >50%; <u>or</u> **iv)** a max dose = 17mg/kg is given (*usual IV loading ~500-1,000 mg*).
  - May follow with **IV *maintenance* infusion** at **2mg/minute** (*1-4 mg/min range*).
  - *Potential* <u>Drawbacks</u> of Procainamide include: **i)** QT prolongation; **ii)** inadvisability with heart failure; **iii)** less clinician familiarity plus a more complicated administration protocol; <u>and</u> **iv)** greater tendency to develop hypotension, especially if *faster* infusion rates are used (*Our preference is to give 100 mg IV increments over ~5 min = ~20 mg/min*).

☞ *More* on Sotalol for *Sustained* VT

Although ACLS-PM conveys *comparable* priority for *initial* use of IV Sotalol — Procainamide — <u>and</u> Amiodarone in treating *sustained* VT — Sotalol is only recently approved for IV administration in the U.S..
  - <u>Advantages</u> — beta-blocker activity; efficacy also for SVT.
  - <u>Disadvantages</u> — *are* concerning to us. They include: **i)** lack of familiarity with emergency IV use by U.S. clinicians; <u>and</u> **ii)** significant QT prolongation with risk of precipitating Torsades. *Time will tell regarding use of this drug for VT and cardiac arrest.* For now — it is <u>not</u> one of our favored drugs for treating *sustained* VT.

☞ *More* on Lidocaine for *Sustained* VT

Lidocaine is **used much *less* often** at present than in the past. The primary reason for this is appreciation that ***other*** drugs (*Amiodarone; Procainamide*) — **are** clearly ***more* effective** for *sustained* VT.

- ACLS-PM *does* list Lidocaine as an alternative to Amiodarone for sustained *monomorphic* VT.
- Practically speaking — most patients will be cardioverted *before* consideration of Lidocaine is reached in the current VT treatment protocol.
- Advantages of Lidocaine that may merit its consideration on rare occasions include: **i)** purported efficacy in *ischemic-related* VT; **ii)** lack of significant QT prolongation; and **iii)** comfort/familiarity with use by clinicians trained in the era when Lidocaine was "standard" therapy. That said, the drug is *no longer* used much.
- Remember — *Lower* maintenance IV infusion rates (*of 0.5-1 mg/min*) should be used in older, lighter patients — especially if there is heart failure.

☞ *More* on IV Magnesium for *Sustained* VT

Realizing that **ACLS-PM** *only* recommends IV Magnesium for hypomagnesemia or Torsades — We feel there are **other indications** for **use** of **IV Magnesium** in the treatment of **VT:**

- While not nearly as effective for *polymorphic* VT as it is for **Torsades** — IV Magnesium *will* work for some cases. ECG distinction between **"polymorphic VT"** vs Torsades is sometimes equivocal (*it depends on whether the baseline QT is prolonged or not — which will not always be known at the time of the acute situation*). There would seem to be *no* downside to empiric trial of IV Mg++ for these patients (*page 99*).
- ***Empiric* Magnesium** (*given IV or PO*) may be useful on occasion in treatment of other arrhythmias (*including various SVTs and VT*).
- Most of the time — you will *not* be able to rule out the possibility of low *intramyocardial* Magnesium levels. This is because: **i)** no serum level may be available; **ii)** even if available — serum levels correlate poorly with intracellular (*and intramyocardial*) levels; and **iii)** cardiac arrest often precipitates flux and change in relative *intra-* vs *extra-cellular* K+ and Mg++ levels.
- The **"good" news** — Minimal side effects (*other than transient hypotension*) have been noted even when *very* large IV Magnesium doses are given. Reduce the rate (*or temporarily stop*) the infusion if BP drops (*adverse effects quickly resolve*).

☞ The **DOSE** of **IV Magnesium** to use varies — depending on the urgency of the situation:

- For *stable* VT or Torsades — Give **1-2 gm IV** over a period of **2-20 minutes** (*Give over 1-2 minutes for VFib*).
- For *less* urgent situations — 1-2 gm may be infused over 30-60 minutes (*or even slower*). May repeat as needed.

***More* on IV β-Blockers for *Sustained* VT**

ACLS-PM limits its recommendation for use of β-Blockers to *narrow-QRS* tachycardias. That said, there <u>are</u> times when **empiric use** of an IV β-Blocker may be lifesaving for VT/VFib <u>not</u> responding to any other therapy.

- Most cases of VT should <u>not</u> be treated with an IV β-Blocker (*although some patients may already be on this drug for acute MI or other indication*). Other agents (*Amiodarone, Procainamide*) are usually more effective for VT, and should be tried first.
- The time to **consider** *selective* use of an **IV β-Blocker** is for *sustained* VT when **increased sympathetic tone** is suspected as a contributing cause of the rhythm (ie, *anterior MI — especially if sinus tachycardia and hypertension preceded the onset of VT*).

When You KNOW the Rhythm is Sustained VT

  ⇒ *Bottom Line*

● This Section 07 **presupposes** that we KNOW the cardiac rhythm is **definitely VT** (*as it almost always will be when one has a regular WCT without sinus P waves*). That said — one can get fooled, so it is good to remain *open* to other possibilities … (*See Section 08 beginning on pg 70*).

- In the meantime — **Assume VT** <u>and</u> **treat** accordingly <u>until</u> proven otherwise (*As discussed in this Section 07 on pp 64-69*).

▶ NOTE: Do <u>**NOT**</u> use **IV Verapamil/Diltiazem** to *empirically* treat a WCT <u>unless</u> you are 100% *certain* that the rhythm is <u>not</u> VT – <u>and</u> – that the patient does <u>not</u> have WPW. This is because the *negative* inotropic and *vasodilatory* properties of these calcium blockers (*and their facilitating effect on accessory pathway conduction*) may precipitate *deterioration* to VFib if inadvertently given to a patient in either VT <u>or</u> very *fast* AFib <u>with</u> WPW.

- Finally — <u>IF</u> at <u>any</u> time during the process of treating *sustained* VT, the patient *becomes* hemodynamically unstable — **Be Ready** to stop giving drugs <u>and</u> **immediately cardiovert/shock** the patient!

 ⇒ *P.S.*

● Be sure the rhythm you have identified as "Known VT" **is <u>not</u> AIVR** (*page 52*). Ventricular rhythms are much *less* likely to cause hemodynamic instability at rates *below* 130-140/minute.
- Treatment with drugs (*Amiodarone/Procainamide*) <u>or</u> with cardioversion is rarely needed (*and may be harmful*) when the rhythm is **AIVR** at a ventricular rate *between* 60-110/minute.

Section 08 – WCTs of *Uncertain* Etiology (*pp 70-83*)

 # WCTs
of *Uncertain* *E*tiology

● You are called to a code. You see **Tachycardia** on the monitor (*Figure 08-1*). The patient is *hemodynamically* stable. *What to do next?*

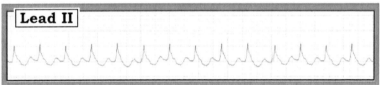

Figure 08-1: We see **tachycardia** – but the patient is stable.

☞ Assessing Tachycardia: *Initial Thoughts*

Since the patient in Figure 08-1 is stable — there is *at least* a moment of time to proceed with further evaluation:
• Optimal management will depend on determining the **specific type** of **tachycardia** — as per the assessment steps below. These steps should be accomplished *within* seconds!
• Some of these steps may overlap. The reality is that *definitive* rhythm diagnosis may *not* be possible at this time. That said — *as long as* the patient *remains* stable, we should be able to **narrow down diagnostic possibilities** and initiate appropriate treatment.

▶ NOTE: IF at *any* time during the process the **patient** *becomes* **unstable** — then *immediately* cardiovert *or* defibrillate.

Step #1: *Assessing Tachycardia*

☞ **Step #1:** *Is the QRS Wide or Narrow?*

● IF the QRS complex of a tachycardia is **narrow** (ie, *not more than* *0.10 second in any lead*) — then the rhythm is *almost* certain to be **supraventricular**.
• **SVTs** (*SupraVentricular Tachycardia*) — are *rarely* life-threatening. Treatment is *different* than for WCTs. This is why **ACLS-PM** highlights assessment of **QRS width** as an early *KEY* step for determining treatment!
• **Sometimes it will be obvious** that the QRS is wide! This is *not* the case for Figure 08-1 (*We think the QRS in Figure 08-1 is wide — but are not 100% certain from the single lead II that is shown here*).
• Given the importance of distinguishing between SVT vs VT — obtaining a **12-lead ECG** *during* **tachycardia** is an *invaluable* early

step in management of the stable tachycardia patient when *uncertain* about etiology.

▶ **Caveat:** Part of the QRS may lie on the baseline. When this happens, the QRS may *look* narrow in one lead — but be *very* wide in *other* leads (*Get a* **12-lead!**).

HOW to Define: *Is the QRS Complex Wide?*

Although ACLS-PM defines *"wide"* as ≥0.12 second — We favor using ***more*** than ***half*** a ***large* box** (≥*0.11 second*) as our definition. This is because the QRS of some VTs may only be 0.11 second in duration (*fascicular or outflow track VTs*).

• Practically speaking — it is often much *easier* to tell *at a glance* IF the QRS is *more* than half a large box or not — than to determine if the QRS is ≥0.12 second (*page 28*).

• Using ≥0.11 second to define "wide" will *not* overlook VT (*whereas requiring 0.12 second will miss some cases of outflow track or fascicular VT — especially if part of the QRS lies on the baseline in the lead[s] being monitored*).

Step #1A: *Assessing Tachycardia*

Step #1A: IF uncertain–*Get a 12-Lead!*

● There are *several* ways in which a **12-lead ECG** obtained ***during* tachycardia** may be helpful. These include:

• Determining *for sure* IF the QRS is wide or not (*Look in all 12 leads; Measure the widest QRS you see*). Remember — there may be distortion of QRS duration when using a portable ECG monitor/defibrillator (*due to time compression*) — so the only way to *truly* determine QRS width is by obtaining a 12-lead ECG *during* tachycardia.

• Assessing axis and QRS morphology *during* tachycardia.

• Looking in *all* 12 leads for signs of atrial activity.

• Getting a baseline *during* tachycardia may prove invaluable in management *after* conversion to sinus rhythm. The true etiology of the WCT will sometimes only be elucidated by *retrospective* comparison between the 12-lead ECG obtained *during* and *after* tachycardia.

▶ **Summary Point:** IF the **QRS** on 12-lead is **narrow** (*not more than half a large box*) — then the rhythm is an **SVT** (*Section 13 on page 114*).

• But **IF** the **QRS** is **Wide** — then by definition, you have a **WCT** (*Wide-Complex Tachycardia*). Go to STEP 2 (*page 72*):

Steps #2, 2A: _Assessing Tachycardia_

Step #2: _Is the WCT a Regular Rhythm?_
➡ **Step #2A:** _Is it a Monomorphic WCT?_

● Practically speaking — We assess **Steps 2** and **2A** together. Our reasons for doing so are the following:

- **Polymorphic WCT** (_in which QRS morphology during tachycardia changes_) — will often require defibrillation for conversion. These rhythms are typically irregular and include _polymorphic_ VT and Torsades de Pointes (_Section 11 on pp 98-103_).
- **Monomorphic WCT** (_in which the QRS during tachycardia stays the same_) — is often easier to treat. IF **no P waves** are seen and the rhythm is **irregularly irregular** — _Consider_ AFib.
- Keep in mind that _some_ VT rhythms may be _slightly_ irregular (_though not nearly as irregular as AFib!_).
- But **IF** the rhythm is a **regular** (_or almost regular_) **monomorphic WCT** _without_ clear evidence of normal sinus P waves — then the differential is as in **LIST #1** (_See Table 08-1 below_).

LIST #1: _Causes of a Regular WCT of Uncertain Etiology_

The common causes of a regular _monomorphic_ WCT rhythm _without_ clear sign of normal P wave activity are noted in **LIST #1** (_Table 08-1_).

Table 08-1: Presume VT until proven otherwise ...

LIST #1: Common Causes of a Monomorphic _Regular_ WCT of _Uncertain_ Etiology

1. **V**entricular **T**achycardia (_VT_)
2. VT (_esp. IF patient older/has heart disease_)
   Causes #3 _thru_ **8** – VT/VT/**VT** !!!
9. SVT with _pre-existing_ BBB
10. SVT with _aberrant_ conduction

Regarding **List #1** — We emphasize the following points:
- The reason for putting **VT** as the first 8 entities in LIST #1 is twofold: **i)** It is _by far_ the **most common cause** of a regular (_or almost regular_) WCT in adults when sinus P waves are lacking; and **ii)** It is **the most serious cause!**
- The **likelihood** that a **WCT** is **VT** goes up even more (_to at least 90%_) IF — **i)** the patient in question is **older** and **ii)** the patient has _underlying_ **heart disease** (_prior MI, cardiomyopathy, angina, heart failure_). This is true _regardless_ of whether the patient is alert — and _regardless_ of what the BP might be _during_ the tachycardia (_VT can be present even if systolic BP exceeds 180 mmHg!_).
- Availability of a **prior 12-lead ECG** during sinus rhythm may be invaluable for assessing the possibility of **preexisting** BBB.
- _See_ Section 19 (_pp 196-202_) — for _aberrant_ conduction considerations.

Step #3: *Assessing Tachycardia*

 Step #3: *Empirically Treat*
/Ongoing Diagnosis

● Optimal management of WCT rhythms depends on the type of WCT. You will *not* always know definitive diagnosis at the time you need to begin treatment:

- **Steps #1** and **#2** should *eliminate* most SVTs and *polymorphic* VT from consideration (*pages 70-72*).
- This leaves you with a **regular** (*or almost regular*) **monomorphic WCT** of **Uncertain** Etiology (*LIST #1*). *Presume* VT. Treat accordingly *until* proven otherwise.

▶ KEY Point: IF at *any* time the **patient** *becomes* **unstable** — then *immediately* cardiovert or defibrillate.

Unspecified WCT

 ➡ **Suggested** *Initial* **Approach:**

● Until such time that the clues discussed in *Beyond-the-Textbook* (*on page 74*) suggest a different diagnosis — it is most prudent to **presume** VT as the etiology of the WCT — and to **treat** accordingly. The "short answer" for our suggested *initial* treatment approach to *unspecified* WCT appears below (*pp 73-74*). More on the subject is found in Section 07 on treatment of *Known* VT (*pp 63-69*).

● **First Fix** the **"Fixables"** — Better than antiarrhythmic drugs is to *find* and *"fix"* any potential *precipitating* causes of VT as soon as you can. These may include:
- Electrolyte disturbance (*especially low Mg++ or K+*).
- Acidosis/Hypoglycemia.
- Hypoxemia.
- Shock (*from hypovolemia; blood loss; sepsis, etc.*).
- *Uncontrolled* ischemia/*acute* infarction/*acute* heart failure.
- Dig toxicity/Drug overdose.

 Use of Adenosine for WCT/*Presumed* VT

   Adenosine is usually well tolerated — and should be considered as the 1st drug that might be given.
- Adenosine will convert (*or at least slow down*) most *regular* SVT rhythms. It may convert 5-10% of VT rhythms.
- Begin with **6mg** by **IV push**. IF no response in 1-2 minutes — Give **12mg** by IV push (*page 58*).
- Side effects from Adenosine usually last <60-90 seconds (*page 59*).

- Do *not* use Adenosine for *polymorphic* VT or Torsades.
- Conversion of a WCT to sinus rhythm with use of Adenosine does *not* prove a supraventricular etiology!
- NOTE: We do *not* always start with Adenosine in all older patients with *ischemic* VT from *known* coronary disease (*as the drug is unlikely to convert ischemic-etiology VT*).

☞ Use of Amiodarone for WCT / *Presumed* VT

    Amiodarone is our preferred **initial agent** of choice (*after Adenosine*) for *stable* sustained *unspecified* WCT:

- Give **150 mg IV** over 10 minutes. May repeat. IF the drug works — Consider maintenance **IV infusion** at **1 mg/ minute** (*pp 64; 67*).
- Amiodarone may also treat *some* forms of SVT.

☞ Use of Procainamide for WCT / *Presumed* VT

    Procainamide is *also* recommended by ACLS-PM (*Provider Manual*) as a 1st-line drug of choice for *unspecified* WCT:

- The efficacy of Procainamide appears *comparable* to Amiodarone for VT and SVT rhythms.
- Give **20-50 mg/minute IV** until either: **i)** the arrhythmia is suppressed; **ii)** hypotension ensues; **iii)** QRS duration increases >50%; or **iv)** a maximum dose = 17mg/kg has been given (*usual IV loading ~500-1,000 mg*).
- May follow with **IV maintenance** infusion at **2mg/minute** (*1-4 mg/ min range*).
- *Potential* <u>Drawbacks</u> of Procainamide include: **i)** QT prolongation; **ii)** inadvisability with heart failure; **iii)** less clinician familiarity plus a more complicated administration protocol; <u>and</u> **iv)** greater tendency to develop hypotension, especially if *faster* infusion rates are used (*Our preference is to give 100 mg IV increments over ~5 min = ~20 mg/ min*).

☞ *Synchronized* Cardioversion for WCT / *Presumed* VT

    There may come a point during the treatment process when **"it becomes time"** to get the patient out of the *unspecified* WCT rhythm:

- At that point — **Cardiovert!** (*page 53*).

Diagnosing the Regular WCT

 ➡ ***Beyond-the-Textbook ...***

    ● Given that *optimal* management of **WCT rhythms** depends on **specific** diagnosis of the **type** of WCT — We conclude this section with insights for determining IF a **regular** (*or almost* regular) **monomorphic WCT** is likely to be VT (<u>vs</u> *SVT with aberrant conduction* <u>or</u> *preexisting BBB*). We emphasize the following points:

- A WCT rhythm is "guilty" (ie, *presumed VT*) <u>until</u> proven otherwise.

- As long as the patient *remains* stable — there is *little to lose* by *brief* attempt at refining your rhythm diagnosis. **Remain ready to cardiovert** at *any* time <u>IF</u> the patient begins to decompensate.
- IF unable to cardiovert — then *immediately* defibrillate.

▶ **NOTE:** No set of rules is "perfect" for interpreting WCT rhythms. Even the experts are *not* always certain. Our goal is merely to increase your odds of correct diagnosis by a *time-efficient* <u>and</u> *easy-to-remember* approach using those criteria we have found most helpful.
- We then devote Section 09 (*pp 84-96*) to a series of **Practice ECGs** that apply these principles.

WCT Diagnosis: *Using Statistics/Clinical Parameters*

One often forgets to recruit the wisdom inherent in the following statement: *Common things are common.* **Statistically** — VT is *by far* the most common cause of a *regular* WCT rhythm when sinus P waves are not clearly evident (*LIST #1 — on page 72*). Studies have shown that *at least* 80% of such *regular* WCT rhythms are VT.
- Is the patient *older* than 50-60 years old? Is there a history of *heart* disease? <u>IF</u> Yes — ***think* VT!** Statistical odds that a *regular* WCT without sinus P waves is VT attain *at least* 90% — <u>IF</u> the patient is older than ~50 years old *and* has underlying heart disease.
- Is there a *prior* history of VT? — *Telemetry* tracings showing PVCs or short VT runs? <u>IF</u> Yes — ***think* VT!**
- <u>OR</u> – Is the patient a *20-to-40* year old adult with *no* history of underlying heart disease who presents in a WCT *precipitated by* exercise or stress? <u>IF</u> Yes — then even if the WCT is VT, it is relatively *likely* to be an **adenosine-responsive form** of **VT** that will often be *well* tolerated (*pp 60-61*).

▶ **Remember:** — Even <u>IF</u> the patient is *asymptomatic* with BP>180 systolic for a *prolonged* period — this *in no way* rules out VT. *It simply means you have some time.*

- *Additional* steps in the diagnostic assessment of a *regular* WCT rhythm <u>require</u> a **12-lead ECG** obtained ***during*** the **WCT**.

WCT Diagnosis: *Prior 12-Lead During Sinus Rhythm?*

Some patients have *baseline* conduction defects (*baseline BBB; IVCD*). Availability of a 12-lead while the patient was in sinus rhythm allows **lead-to-lead** comparison *prior* <u>and</u> *during* the WCT to see if QRS morphology is the same.
- <u>IF</u> QRS morphology is *not* the same — ***think* VT!**
- Realistically — It will *not* be often that a prior ECG during sinus rhythm will be available (*or you may not have time to look at it with a WCT patient in front of you*).

☞ WCT Diagnosis: *Extreme Axis?* (*Simple Rule #1*)

We favor beginning our use of the 12-lead ECG obtained *during* the WCT rhythm with attention to **3 Simple Rules**. The 1st of these Rules relates to assessment of ***frontal* plane axis** *during* the WCT rhythm.

- The frontal plane axis may be approximated *at a glance* — simply from inspection (*and comparison*) of the net QRS deflection in leads I and aVF. **Lead I** is the *horizontal* lead — it is situated at zero degrees. **Lead aVF** is the *vertical* lead — it is situated at +90 degrees. If the *net* QRS deflection is positive in *both* leads I and aVF — then the mean QRS axis is normal (ie, *between zero and +90 degrees*).

- While details of axis calculation extend beyond the scope of this Section on ventricular tachycardia — the *"take-home"* **message** is that the presence of ***extreme* axis deviation** *during* a WCT rhythm is ***virtually* diagnostic** of **VT**.

- *Extreme* axis deviation is *easy* to recognize. The QRS complex will be *entirely* negative in *either* lead I *or* in lead aVF. This is the case for *both* **X** *and* **Y** in **Figure 08-2**. Awareness of this axis criterion *immediately* tells us that X and Y are *almost* certainly VT.

- **KEY Point:** The presence of mild or even *moderate* LAD or RAD (*Left or Right Axis Deviation*) does *not* assist in distinguishing between VT vs SVT. This is the case for **Z** in Figure 08-2 in which lead I is clearly positive, but lead aVF is not. Instead, we see a *slender* positive R wave in lead aVF — and a *wider* S wave. Whether some degree of left axis deviation is present in Z *(surface area of the negative S wave appears greater than surface area within the slender positive R wave)* — is not only uncertain, but unimportant. What counts is that **extreme axis deviation** is **not present** in **Z** (*because the net QRS deflection in lead aVF is not all negative*). This tells us *at a glance* that use of axis is *not* helpful in distinguishing between VT vs SVT for the rhythm in Z.

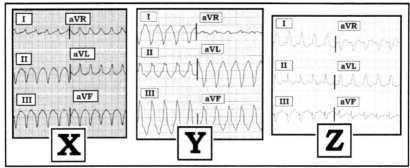

Figure 08-2: Use of **Axis** for WCT diagnosis. **Rhythm X** — shows *extreme* left axis (*QRS all negative in lead aVF*). This is VT. **Rhythm Y** — shows *extreme* right axis (*QRS all negative in lead I*). This is VT. **Rhythm Z** — clearly does *not* manifest extreme axis deviation, because the QRS complex in lead aVF is *not* all negative. Calculation of axis is of *no help* for distinguishing between VT vs SVT for Rhythm Z.

▶ **Bottom Line:** — We *LOVE* this **axis criterion** *during* **tachycardia.** When used as intended you'll find:

- *Calculation* of **axis** *during* WCT rhythms using **leads I** and **aVF** is easy. IF the QRS is *all* **negative** in either lead — then diagnosis of **VT** is *almost* **certain** (*X and Y in Figure 08-2*).
- Remember that anything other than *extreme* axis deviation is of <u>no use</u> in distinguishing between VT <u>vs</u> SVT.

☞ **WCT Diagnosis:** *Is Lead V6* <u>*all*</u> *Negative?* (*Simple Rule #2*)

We have found lead V6 to be the most helpful of the 12 leads to look at *during* a *regular* WCT rhythm. We ask: **Is Lead V6** <u>*all*</u> (*or almost all*) **Negative?**

- When the etiology of the rhythm is supraventricular — there will almost always be at least *some* positive activity traveling toward the left ventricle (*and therefore positive in lead V6*).
- IF ever the QRS in **lead V6** is <u>either</u> *all* **negative** (*or almost all negative*) as in <u>Figure 08-3</u> — then VT is *highly* likely (*See Figure 09-1 on page 84* and *Figure 09.4 on page 87*).
- Lead V6 is <u>only</u> helpful if it is negative … (*A positive R or RS in lead V6 is <u>not</u> helpful in ruling in or out VT*).

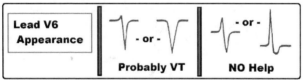

Figure 08-3: Using **QRS morphology** in **lead V6.** The presence of a QRS complex in lead V6 that is either all negative (*or almost all negative*) — is strongly suggestive of VT. This criterion is of *no help* if anything more than a tiny r wave is present in lead V6.

☞ **WCT Diagnosis:** *Is the QRS "Ugly"?* (*Simple Rule #3*)

Our 3rd *"Simple Rule"* is as follows: ***The "uglier" the QRS — the more* likely the rhythm is VT.** The reason for this clinical reality is that *aberrant* conduction almost always manifests some form of conduction defect (*RBBB; LBBB; LAHB; LPHB — or some combination thereof*) due to *relative* delay in the hemifascicles or bundle branches.

- In contrast — VT originates from a ventricular focus *outside* of the conduction system. As a result — VT is more likely to be wider and far <u>less</u> organized (*therefore "uglier"*) in its conduction pattern.

▶ **PEARL:** In our experience — Use of the **"3 SIMPLE Rules"** is easy and accurate for *recognizing* VT in the large majority of cases.
- **Rule #1** – Is axis deviation *extreme* during WCT? (*page 76*).
- **Rule #2** – Is lead V6 all (*or almost all*) negative? (*page 77*).
- **Rule #3** – Does the QRS look *"ugly"* during WCT? (*page 77*).

Diagnosing the Regular WCT

  ➡ **_Beyond-the-Core ..._**

⚫ What follows on pages 78-83 are a number of *Beyond-the-Core additional* ways to help distinguish *between* VT *vs* SVT:
- We emphasize that you do *not* have to remember all of these criteria! This is advanced (*beyond-the-core*) material for *experienced* providers with special interest in this fascinating area!

☞ *Is there an RS in any Precordial Lead?*

- IF there is *no* RS complex in *any* precordial lead (*V1-thru-V6*) — then **the rhythm** is **VT!** (*with >99% specificity*).
- Caveat: IF an RS complex is seen in ≥1 precordial lead — then this criterion is of *no* help (*because both SVT and VT rhythms may have an RS complex in no more than a single precordial lead*).

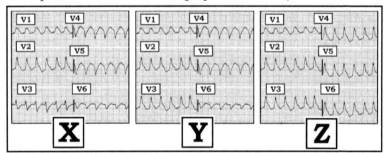

Figure 08-4: Is there an **RS** in *any Precordial* Lead? (*See text.*)

- *Both* **Y** and **Z** in Figure 08-4 are **VT** (*there is no RS complex in either*). In addition — the finding of **QRS concordance** in Z (*in this case global positivity*) is insensitive but 100% specific!
- In **X** — An RS complex is present in **lead V3** (*in the form of a small initial r wave and much deeper negative S wave*). We therefore can *not* rule out VT on the basis of this RS criterion. That said — We still think X is VT because of *other* criteria! (*'ugly' formless QRS, especially in lead V1; almost entirely negative QRS in lead V6*).

☞ *Is the R-to-S Nadir Delayed?*

IF an RS complex is present in *at least* one precordial lead, then the **rhythm** is **VT** (*with >99% specificity*) — IF the **R-to-S Nadir** (ie, *interval from the beginning of the R wave until the deepest portion of the S wave*) is ***delayed*** to **>0.10 second** (*100 msec*) – **Figure 08-5** (*pg 79*).
- Caveat: This criterion is *only* helpful for *ruling in* VT if ≥1 precordial lead clearly manifests an R-to-S nadir >0.10 second. It is of **no help** if you see an RS nadir that is *not* more than 0.10 second (*and the reality is that it is often difficult to be sure of RS nadir duration*).

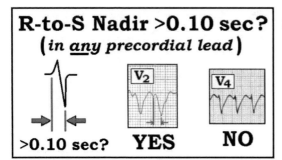

R-to-S Nadir >0.10 sec?
(in any precordial lead)

>0.10 sec?   YES   NO

Figure 08-5: Is the R-to-S Nadir >0.10 sec. in *any* **Precordial Lead?** If an RS complex *is* present in one or more precordial lead — then the rhythm is *almost* certainly VT if the *R-to-S* Nadir is *delayed* to >0.10 sec.

▶ **NOTE:** — The physiologic rationale for Figures 08-4 and 08-5 is that *supraventricular* activation should yield at least *some* change in the direction of ventricular activation with respect to the 6 precordial leads (*Fig. 08-4*) – and, that most of the time, *initial* ventricular activation will be slow (*>0.10 sec*) compared to significantly *faster* initial activation when the rhythm is supraventricular (*Fig. 08-5*).

☞ *Initial r or q ≥0.04 second in any Lead?*

Look in *all* 12 leads to see in which leads an *initial* r wave or q wave is present. IF an ***initial* r or q wave** is **≥0.04 sec** (*>1 small box*) in *any* lead — then the rhythm is *almost* certain to be **VT**.

• Caveat: This criterion is *only* helpful for *ruling in* VT if ≥1 lead clearly manifests an *initial* r or q wave ≥0.04 second. It is of *no help* if you do not see an initial r or q wave ≥0.04 second (*and the reality is that it is often difficult to be sure of q or r wave duration during WCT*).

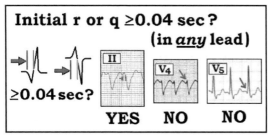

Initial r or q ≥0.04 sec?
(in any lead)

≥0.04 sec?   YES   NO   NO

Figure 08-6: Is the *initial* **r or q ≥0.04 sec** in *any* Lead? If an *initial* q or r wave is present and wide (*>0.04 sec*) in *any* lead – then the rhythm is *almost* certain to be VT.

▶ **NOTE:** — The physiologic rationale for Figure 08-6 is that initial conduction through myocardial tissue is *delayed* when the site of origin for a tachycardia is ventricular. In contrast — WCT rhythms of *supraventricular* etiology manifest more rapid *initial* conduction, because the impulse is *at least* in part transmitted over specialized conduction fibers.

☞ *Is there AV Dissociation?*

It is always good to look for potential ***confirmatory* criteria** when assessing WCT rhythms — since <u>IF</u> found, these virtually ***ensure*** the **diagnosis** of **VT**. Confirmatory criteria include: **i)** AV dissociation; <u>and</u> **ii)** Fusion beats.

- <u>Caveat:</u> Most WCT rhythms do <u>not</u> manifest either AV dissociation or fusion beats (*esp. when the rate of VT is >130/min*). Therefore, <u>not</u> seeing this proves nothing. But sometimes you'll get lucky! (<u>Fig. 08-7</u>).

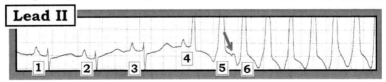

Figure 08-7: Use of AV Dissociation to prove VT (*arrow*). In addition — VT is proven because beat #4 is a *fusion* beat (*See text*).

- Beats #1,2,3 in <u>Figure 08-7</u> are sinus. The QRS then widens and dramatically changes in morphology. Although the beginning of this WCT is slightly irregular — We can ***prove*** this run is **VT** because: **i)** Beat #4 is a ***fusion* beat** (*short PR; QRS not overly wide <u>and</u> with QRS morphology intermediate between sinus beats and the other wide beats*); <u>plus</u> **ii)** there is **AV Dissociation**, at least for a brief period (*arrow highlighting an on-time P wave <u>not</u> related to neighboring QRS*).

▶ **NOTE:** — The easiest way to explain ***"fusion beats"*** is to contemplate what the QRS would look like <u>IF</u> beats #4 and #6 in Figure 08-7 had children? (ie, *with characteristics of both beats!*).

- The reason the PR interval preceding beat #4 is *shorter-than-normal* is that it only *partially* conducts to the ventricles until its path is interrupted by a *simultaneously* occurring ventricular beat.
- **PEARL:** You'll <u>need</u> **calipers** to look for AV Dissociation.

☞ *Large Monophasic R Wave in Lead aVR?*

With normal sinus rhythm — lead aVR manifests a predominantly *negative* QRS complex. This reflects the normal path of ventricular activation — which moves *away* from the right (*away from aVR*) — and toward the left ventricle. <u>IF</u> ever the **QRS** in **lead aVR** *<u>during</u>* WCT is ***entirely* positive** (*writing a large, monophasic R wave in aVR*) – then the rhythm is **VT** (*with virtual 100% specificity*)!

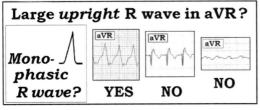

Figure 08-8: Is there a **large *monophasic* R** in **aVR?** If yes — then the rhythm is VT.

- Caveat: You will _not_ often see a monophasic R in aVR during WCT. But sometimes you'll get lucky! (_Figure 08-8_).

▶ **NOTE:** — The finding of a monophasic R wave in lead aVR _during_ WCT indicates that the electrical impulse _must_ _be_ **originating** from a site in the _**ventricular**_ **apex** and traveling upward toward the base (ie, _in the direction of lead aVR_). Therefore — a _quick_ look at **lead aVR** during WCT can _instantly_ tell you the rhythm is **VT** if you see a large monophasic R wave.

☞ _Does Lead V1 Suggest Aberrancy?_

   Much has been written about _aberrant_ conduction as a reason for QRS widening during WCT. For practical purposes — the _only_ QRS morphology with **high specificity** for **SVT** is the presence of _**typical**_ **RBBB** in lead V1. Thus, the presence of an **rsR' complex** (_with taller right 'rabbit ear'_ _and_ _S wave that descends_ _below_ _the baseline_) — **_strongly_** suggests a _**supraventricular**_ etiology (_H-1, H-2_ in Fig. 08-9).

- In contrast — _**any other**_ **QRS morphology** in lead V1 (_H-3,4,5,6 in_ Figure 08-9) **_favors_** **VT**.

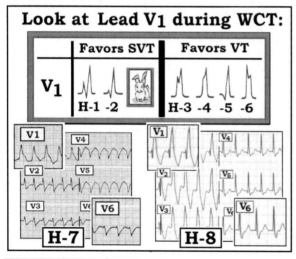

Figure 08-9: QRS morphology _**favoring**_ **aberrancy** in **V1** (_See text_).

▶ **CAVEAT:** — This criterion is strict. Only a _**typical**_ **RBBB** pattern in V1 (**H-1,H-2**) suggests aberrant conduction. _Any other_ QRS pattern in lead V1 suggests VT.

   We illustrate further in Figure 08-9 _diagnostic_ use of lead V1 QRS morphology characteristics in assessment of WCT rhythms:
- **Example H-7** — strongly _**suggests**_ **VT**. Lead V1 manifests a _mono-phasic_ R wave with taller _left_ rabbit ear (_resembles H-6, but without any notch_). Lead V6 in H-7 supports a diagnosis of VT because it is _predominantly_ negative.

- **Example H-8** — is *consistent* with a **supraventricular** **rhythm** (*either preexisting RBBB* – <u>or</u> – *aberrant conduction*). Lead V1 manifests an rSR' with taller *right* rabbit ear (*similar to H-2*).

▶ **NOTE:** — The reason for **aberrant** **conduction** is that there is *insufficient* time for a part of the ventricular conduction system to recover. This may be precipitated by <u>*either*</u> an *early* beat (*like a PAC*) — <u>or</u> — by tachycardia. Because the right bundle branch tends to have a *longer* refractory period than both the left bundle branch and the hemifascicles — a RBBB pattern is the most common form of aberrant conduction (*but LAHB or LPHB aberration, or any combination of patterns may also be seen*) — *See Section 19 beginning on page 196.*

🖎 *Is the Run of WCT <u>preceded</u> by a PAC ?*

The *best* way to *prove* aberrant conduction is <u>IF</u> you can find a **premature P wave** (*PAC*) preceding the run of WCT. This will often <u>*not*</u> be easy to do <u>BUT</u> you may occasionally see a tracing like <u>Figure 08-10</u>:

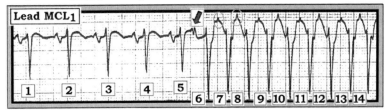

Figure 08-10: Beats #1-*thru*-5 in this **right-sided MCL-1 Lead** (*comparable to V1*) — are sinus conducted. There follows a 9-beat run of WCT (*beats #6-thru-14*). We <u>*know*</u> this is a run of **SVT** with **aberrant conduction** because of the PAC we see that *notches* the T wave *just prior* to the onset of the run (*arrow in Figure 08-10*). None of the other sinus beats (*#1-thru-4*) have this notch.

▶ *Beyond-the-Core* on **Figure 08-10:** — Although a *simultaneous* 12-lead ECG would be needed to know for sure — the similar *initial* r wave deflection with very *steep* S wave but *without* excessive QRS widening suggests an *incomplete* left bundle branch block form of *aberrant* conduction for beats #6-thru-14.

WCT Summary with Review of 3 Simple Rules

 ⇨ *Summary*

● *Despite* the length and complexity of this Section on WCT rhythms of *uncertain* etiology — the **"message"** is clear:
- **1st Priority:** — Is the patient stable? <u>IF</u> not — then immediately **shock** the patient! (*defibrillate or use synchronized cardioversion*).

- IF the patient **is Stable** — then *Apply* **Step #1** (*pp 70-71*) and **Step #2** (*page 72*) in your attempt at determining the diagnosis (*or at least narrowing your differential*).
- Application of the **3 *Simple* Rules** (*pp 76-77 — and summarized below* in Figure 08-11) will usually allow you to greatly increase your diagnostic certainty in *no more than* a few seconds.
- Begin *empiric* **treatment** based on your presumptive diagnosis as you continually refine your rhythm diagnosis as indicated in **Step #3** and in our *Suggested* **Approach** (*pp 73-74*).

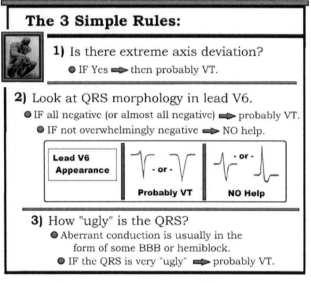

The 3 Simple Rules:

1) Is there extreme axis deviation?
- IF Yes ➡ then probably VT.

2) Look at QRS morphology in lead V6.
- IF all negative (or almost all negative) ➡ probably VT.
- IF not overwhelmingly negative ➡ NO help.

Lead V6 Appearance		
	Probably VT	NO Help

3) How "ugly" is the QRS?
- Aberrant conduction is usually in the form of some BBB or hemiblock.
- IF the QRS is very "ugly" ➡ probably VT.

Figure 08-11:
The 3 Simple Rules for assessing the 12-lead ECG of a WCT rhythm (*See text*).

▶ **NOTE:** — Although you may not be certain of the rhythm diagnosis at the beginning of this process (*you are after all, dealing with an "unspecified" WCT*) — the chances are great that with ongoing monitoring, treatment, and follow-up — that you'll arrive at the correct diagnosis.

- In any event — the *Suggested* **Approach** (*pp 73-74*) will be an appropriate course to follow.

☞ Now — **Test *yourself*** on our **WCT Practice Tracings** beginning on page 84.

Section 09 – WCT *Practice* Tracings (*pp 84-96*)

 # *WCT Practice*

● We reinforce the principles discussed in Section 08 (*pp 70-83*) with a series of **WCT** (*Wide-Complex Tachycardia*) *Practice* **Examples** ...
• Key concepts in *Rhythm Diagnosis* were discussed in Section 02 — in which we reviewed clinical application of the **Ps,Qs,3R Approach** (*page 21*). *Feel free to refer back to Sections 02 and 08 as needed.*

WCT *Practice* Tracing #1

 ➡ **PRACTICE Tracing:**

● Your patient is a 55-year-old man with CAD. His 12-lead ECG is shown below in **Figure 09-1**. The patient is *hemodynamically* stable with a BP =150/80.
• What should you do first?
• What is your diagnosis of the WCT rhythm in <u>Figure 09-1</u>?
• *How certain* are you of your rhythm diagnosis?

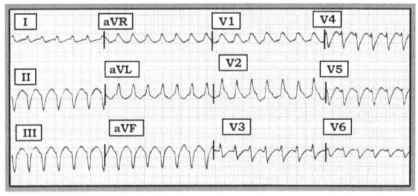

Figure 09-1: WCT Tracing #1. The patient is *hemodynamically* stable.

☞ **Answer to WCT Tracing #1:** As discussed in Section 03 on *Overview of Unspecified Tachycardia* — **the very 1st thing to do** is assess the patient for *hemodynamic* stability. This has been done — and we are told that the patient <u>is</u> **hemodynamically stable**.
• Since the patient is stable — there is *no need* to immediately cardiovert. Instead — there is *at least* a moment to **assess the rhythm**.
• The rhythm in <u>Figure 09-1</u> is a **regular** WCT *without* clear sign of atrial activity. Given that the patient is a 55-year-old man with *known* CAD — the **likelihood** of **VT** is already **at least 90%** <u>even</u> <u>without</u> looking further (*See List #1 on page 72*).

- As suggested by **Step #3** in Section 08 (*page 73*) — one could at this point *either* empirically treat the rhythm in Figure 09-1 as a **WCT** of **Unknown** Etiology (*pp 73-74*) – or – one could further assess the rhythm to see if we can **increase certainty** of our rhythm diagnosis.
- We emphasize that it would *not* be wrong to begin empiric treatment with *either* Adenosine, Amiodarone *and/or* Procainamide (*pp 73-74*). That said — We feel the treatment approach will be *far better* IF we can hone in on the rhythm diagnosis. It should take *no more* than *2-to-5 seconds* to assess the rhythm in Figure 09-1 by applying the **3 Simple Rules** (*pp 76-77*) — and this is the approach we favor.

▶ NOTE: IF at *any* time the **patient becomes unstable** — then *immediately* cardiovert or defibrillate.

☞ *Applying the 3 Simple Rules*

It should take no more than a few seconds to apply the **3 Simple rules** (Figure 09-2) to the rhythm in Figure 09-1:

The 3 Simple Rules:

1) Is there extreme axis deviation?
- IF Yes ➡ then probably VT.

2) Look at QRS morphology in lead V6.
- IF all negative (or almost all negative) ➡ probably VT.
- IF not overwhelmingly negative ➡ NO help.

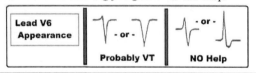

Lead V6 Appearance	⎞⎛ - or - ⎲	⎱⎰ - or - ⎱
	Probably VT	**NO Help**

3) How "ugly" is the QRS?
- Aberrant conduction is usually in the form of some BBB or hemiblock.
- IF the QRS is very "ugly" ➡ probably VT.

Figure 09-2:
The 3 Simple Rules for assessing the 12-lead ECG of a WCT rhythm (*See below*).

● Applying the 3 Simple Rules to Figure 09-1:

- **Rule #1: *Extreme Axis Deviation?*** — There is *extreme* LAD (*Left Axis Deviation*) in Figure 09-1 (*the QRS is entirely negative in the inferior leads*). This is virtually *never* seen with SVT ...
- **Rule #2: *Is Lead V6 Negative?*** — The QRS in lead V6 is *almost* entirely negative. This is rarely seen with SVT ...
- **Rule #3: *Is the QRS "Ugly"?*** — The QRS in Figure 09-1 is *extremely* wide (*almost 0.20 sec*) and formless. We say it is **"ugly"** because QRS

morphology does *not* resemble any form of BBB or hemiblock. This *strongly* favors VT.

☞ **Conclusion:** In *less* than 5 seconds — By the **3 *Simple* Rules** we have become 99% certain that the WCT in Figure 09-1 is VT.

• It would *not* have been wrong to start with **Adenosine**. That said — We would *promptly* switch to *other* treatments if Adenosine didn't work since the patient's age, history of CAD, and ECG appearance do *not* suggest an *adenosine-responsive* form of VT is likely (*pp 60-61*).

• Our preference after Adenosine would be Amiodarone — but *other* options are available (*pp 64-65*).

Regarding WCT Tracing #1

 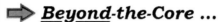 ⇨ ***Beyond*-the-Core ...**

● There are **no *"magic numbers"*** for declaring hemodynamic "instability". Instead — this determination is a ***clinical* process** to be based on *ongoing* assessment of the patient by the clinician on-the-scene.

▶ NOTE: We can actually be **100% *certain*** the WCT in Figure 09-1 is VT (*ventricular tachycardia*):

• There is a monophasic *upright* R wave in lead aVR. Although insensitive — this finding is highly specific for VT when found (*pp 80-81*).

QUESTION: Does the upright R wave in lead V1 of Figure 09-1 suggest RBBB or *aberrant* conduction?

• HINT: Feel free to review pages 81-82 *before* answering.

ANSWER: The very wide and formless (*very 'ugly'*) QRS in lead V1 does *not* in the least resemble either H-1 or H-2 in Figure 08-9 (*page 81*). If anything — QRS morphology in lead V1 of Figure 09-1 is strongly in favor of VT.

WCT *Practice* Tracing #2

 ➡ **PRACTICE Tracing:**

⬤ Your patient is a 50-year-old man with CAD and "heart awareness". His ECG is shown below. BP = 140/90 mmHg.
- Is the rhythm in <u>Figure 09-3</u> an SVT? *What should you do next?*

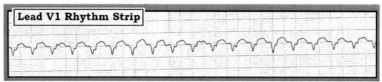

Figure 09-3: WCT Tracing #2. The patient is stable. *Is this SVT?*

☞ **Answer to WCT Tracing #2:** This patient seems to be stable (*BP=140/90*). The Lead V1 rhythm strip in <u>Figure 09-3</u> *appears* to show a regular *narrow* tachycardia at a rate just over 150/minute. The "good news" is that since the patient is stable — there <u>is</u> time to look further into what the rhythm might be!
- All we see is a *single* monitoring lead. Given that the patient is stable — We'd like to see **more leads** <u>before</u> proceeding. Therefore — *Get a* **12-lead ECG** <u>during</u> tachycardia!

▶ NOTE: IF at *any* time during the process the **patient *becomes* unstable** — then *immediately* cardiovert <u>or</u> defibrillate.

☞ ***Does Figure 09-3 belong in this WCT Section?***

The answer as to whether the rhythm in <u>Figure 09-3</u> "belongs" in this WCT *Practice* Section is forthcoming on seeing the **12-lead ECG** recorded at the *same* time as the lead V1 rhythm strip (<u>Figure 09-4</u>):

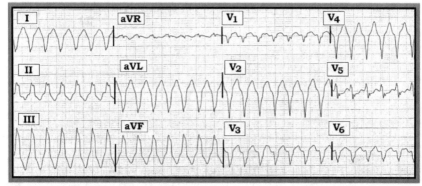

Figure 09-4: 12-lead ECG recorded at the *same* time as the lead V1 rhythm strip shown in <u>Figure 09-3</u>. The patient is stable (*BP=140/90*).

QUESTION: What is the rhythm in <u>Figure 09-3</u>: *VT or SVT?*
• What *degree of certainty* do you have about your rhythm diagnosis?
• <u>HINT:</u> What is the rhythm for the 12-lead ECG in <u>Figure 09.4</u> ?

ANSWER: Comparison of the *single-lead* V1 strip (*Figure 09-3*) with the *simultaneously* recorded **12-lead ECG** from this patient (<u>Figure 09-4</u>) illustrates the following KEY concept: ***"12 leads are <u>better</u> than 1".*** Part of the QRS may sometimes lie on the baseline in the *single* lead being monitored. For this reason — it is best *whenever possible* to always get a **12-lead ECG *<u>during</u>* tachycardia** to verify QRS width.

• It should now be *obvious* that the **QRS complex** in this case is **wide**! In fact — about the *only* lead in which the QRS looks to be narrow on the 12-lead tracing obtained *during* tachycardia is lead V1.
• We strongly suspect VT. Applying the **3 Simple Rules** to the 12-lead ECG shown in **Figure 09-4** allows us to *greatly* increase certainty of our rhythm diagnosis.

▶   <u>NOTE:</u> Although it would *not* be wrong to give Adenosine at this point — it should take *no more* than *2-to-5 seconds* to apply the **3 *Simple* Rules** (<u>Figure 09-5</u>).

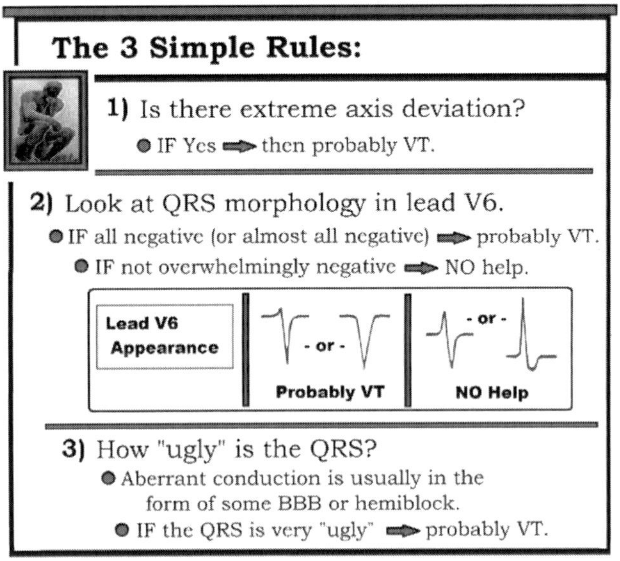

The 3 Simple Rules:

1) Is there extreme axis deviation?
   ● IF Yes ➡ then probably VT.

---

2) Look at QRS morphology in lead V6.
   ● IF all negative (or almost all negative) ➡ probably VT.
   ● IF not overwhelmingly negative ➡ NO help.

Lead V6 Appearance	⎰⎱ - or - ⎰⎱	⎰⎱ - or - ⎰⎱
	Probably VT	**NO Help**

3) How "ugly" is the QRS?
   ● Aberrant conduction is usually in the form of some BBB or hemiblock.
   ● IF the QRS is very "ugly" ➡ probably VT.

Figure 09-5:
The 3 Simple Rules for assessing the 12-lead ECG of a WCT rhythm (*pp 76-77; 83*).

●   Applying the 3 Simple Rules to Figure 09-4:

• **Rule #1: *Extreme Axis Deviation?*** — There <u>is</u> *extreme* RAD (*<u>R</u>ight <u>A</u>xis <u>D</u>eviation*) in <u>Figure 09-4</u> (*the QRS is entirely negative in lead I*). This is *not* seen with SVT.

- **Rule #2: _Is Lead V6 Negative?_** — The QRS in lead V6 _is_ entirely negative. This is virtually _never_ seen with SVT.
- **Rule #3: _Is the QRS "Ugly"?_** — The QRS in Figure 09-4 is _extremely_ wide (_almost 0.20 second_) and formless. We say it is **_"ugly"_** because QRS morphology does _not_ resemble any form of BBB or hemiblock. This _strongly_ favors VT.

▶ Conclusion: In _less_ than 5 seconds — We have become virtually **100% _certain_** the WCT in Figure 09-4 is **VT**.

- Although _acceptable_ to start with Adenosine — our preference would be to select Amiodarone first in view of virtual _certainty_ of _ischemic_ etiology VT (_given patient's age; history of CAD; ECG characteristics_) — and that this VT is unlikely to be _adenosine-responsive._
- _Other_ options for VT are available (_pp 64-65_).
- _Synchronized_ cardioversion may be needed <u>IF</u> the patient fails to respond to antiarrhythmic drugs.

Regarding WCT Tracing #2

 ➡ **_Beyond-the-Core_ ...**

● So certain are we at this point that diagnosis of the rhythm in Figure 09-4 is VT — that clinically, we would _not_ need to spend time looking further to confirm this. That said — for teaching purposes:
- The _blow-up_ of **Lead V5** from Figure 09-4 provides an excellent example of an RS complex in which the **_initial_ R** is **_clearly_ ≥0.04 second** — which virtually _ensures_ VT (_page 79_).

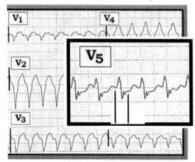

Figure 09-6: Blow-up of lead V5 from the 12-lead ECG previously shown in Figure 09-4. The very wide (_>0.04 second_) initial R wave in this lead virtually _confirms_ VT as the diagnosis (_page 79_).

▶ Final Point: The rationale for _routine_ incorporation of Adenosine at an _early_ point in VT management is that one can _not_ reliably identify all _adenosine-responsive_ cases on the basis of ECG characteristics.

- **_Adenosine-responsive_** forms of **VT** (_pp 60-61_) — are most likely to occur in _younger_ adults _without_ underlying heart disease. The ECG is more likely to manifest _minimal_ QRS widening _without_ bizarre morphology — and VT episodes are more likely to be precipitated by exercise (_or other causes of catecholamine release_). This is _not_ the case here.

WCT *Practice* Tracing #3

 ➡ **<u>PRACTICE</u> Tracing:**

🔴 Your patient is a 65-year-old woman with an exacerbation of heart failure. Her ECG is shown below. BP = 140/90 mmHg.
• Is the rhythm in <u>Figure 09-7</u> VT or SVT? *What should you do next?*

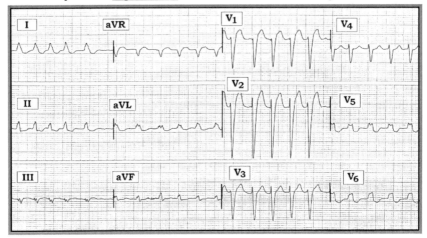

<u>Figure 09-7</u>: WCT Tracing #3. The patient is *hemodynamically* stable.

☞ **<u>Answer to WCT Tracing #3</u>:** Despite first glance impression that the rhythm in <u>Figure 09-7</u> appears to be regular — it is <u>not</u>. Fortunately, this patient is stable — so there <u>is</u> time to look further.
• **NOTE:** Use of ***calipers*** greatly facilitates assessing rhythm regularity.
• The *underlying* rhythm in <u>Figure 09-7</u> is *irregularly* irregular. No P waves are seen. We suspect this is **AFib (*Atrial Fibrillation*)** with a **fairly *rapid* ventricular response**.
• The **QRS complex** is ***wide***. Although VT is *usually* a fairly regular rhythm — it may at times be irregular. Thus, we can <u>not</u> with 100% certainty exclude the possibility of VT. That said — VT is rarely as *irregularly* irregular as is seen in <u>Figure 09-7</u>. We therefore ***suspect*** this patient has ***preexisting* LBBB** as the cause of QRS widening.

☞ *When You Don't Know for Sure What the Rhythm Is ...*

This case provides an excellent example of how one will <u>not</u> always know with 100% certainty what the rhythm is at the time treatment decisions need to be made.
• Assessment of **ECG features** in <u>Figure 09-7</u> is consistent with our presumption of a *supraventricular* etiology because: **i)** there is typical LBBB morphology (*upright monophasic QRS in leads I,V6; predominantly negative QRS in V1*); **ii)** the QRS is *not* overly wide; **iii)** there is

no extreme axis deviation; <u>and</u> **iv)** the downslope of the S waves in anterior leads is very steep (*unlike the delay often seen with VT*).

- It would be wonderful <u>IF</u> we had access to a **_prior_ ECG** on this patient. Evidence of LBBB in the past would confirm that the rhythm in <u>Figure 09-7</u> is AFib and *not* VT.

- Review of **_additional_ rhythm strips** on this patient might also help confirm the *irregularly* irregular nature of AFib (*vs VT that tends to regularize after a period of irregularity when the rhythm persists*).

- The "good news" — is that this patient is stable. Essential to management will be treatment of her heart failure. One would expect the rate of her presumed AFib to *slow* as her clinical condition improves.

▶ **Bottom Line:** We strongly suspect that the rhythm in <u>Figure 09-7</u> is AFib with *preexisting* LBBB. While remaining ready to cardiovert this patient IF at <u>any</u> time she were to decompensate — We would begin by treating her heart failure <u>and</u> cautiously use drugs to slow the rate of her presumed AFib (*See pp 130-132 in Section 14*).

Regarding WCT Tracing #3

  Beyond-the-Core ...

● The case scenario presented here is a common one. Progressive diastolic dysfunction from longstanding hypertension may predispose to *both* AFib <u>and</u> to development of LBBB. Sudden loss of the 'atrial kick' with onset of AFib may precipitate acute heart failure. Given minimal R-R interval variation when the rate of AFib is fast — the resultant ECG picture may mimic VT.

- It really helps to know if the patient has baseline LBBB.

- The best clues that the rhythm in <u>Figure 09-7</u> is **AFib** are: **i)** Awareness of the above common scenario; <u>and</u> **ii)** realization that the R-R interval *continually* changes.

PEARL: *Using Calipers ...*

Use of **_calipers_** may be *invaluable* to assist in assessing arrhythmias such as <u>Figure 09-7</u> — as well as for assessing AV blocks.

- **Calipers _instantly_ enhance your skills** in arrhythmia interpretation! They make obvious relationships between atrial activity and QRS complexes that would not otherwise be apparent. Detecting subtle variation in atrial or ventricular rate becomes easy.

- Using calipers conveys to others that YOU <u>know</u> what you are doing. All it takes is a *little* bit of practice to become facile in using calipers.

- Clearly — You will <u>not</u> have time to pull out calipers if your patient is "crashing" in front of you. That said, in such situations — a patient with hemodynamically *unstable* tachycardia (*where instability is due to the rapid rate*) should be immediately cardioverted or defibrillated <u>regardless</u> of whether the rhythm is regular or not.

WCT *Practice* Tracing #4

 ➡ **PRACTICE** Tracing:

⬤ Your patient is a previously healthy 30-year-old woman who presents with palpitations. Her ECG is shown below. BP=145/80.
• Is the rhythm in Figure 09-8 VT or SVT? *What should you do next?*

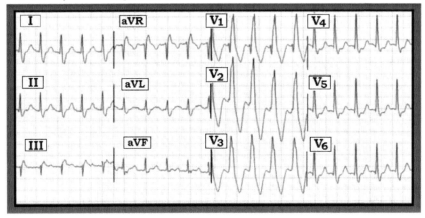

Figure 09-8: WCT Tracing #4. The patient is *hemodynamically* stable.

📖 **Answer to WCT Tracing #4:** A *regular* **WCT** at ~150/minute is seen in Figure 09-8. There is *no* clear sign of atrial activity. Although VT *always* needs to be presumed until proven otherwise (*LIST #1 on page 72*) — there are a number of reasons why we **strongly** **suspect** a **supraventricular** **etiology** in this case. Consider the following:

• The patient is young (*30 years old*) — she has been *previously* healthy – and – she is *hemodynamically* stable. While *none* of these features rules out the possibility of VT — they <u>do</u> make VT much *less* likely.

• Even if VT is present — the patient's age, *lack* of cardiac history, and hemodynamic status *increase* the likelihood of some type of fascicular VT <u>or</u> *adenosine-responsive* form of VT (*pp 60-61*). In *either* case — **trial** of **Adenosine** is the appropriate initial step.

• **QRS morphology** in Figure 09-8 — is *typical* **RBBB** (*rsR' with taller-right-rabbit-ear in V1; wide terminal S waves in I,V6*). This strongly suggests **PSVT** <u>*with*</u> QRS widening from ***RBBB* aberration**.

📖 *Approach to Management*

There would seem to be *no* downside from *initial* management of the rhythm in Figure 09-8 with **Adenosine** (*pp 58-62*) — since this drug stands *high* probability of converting the arrhythmia (*be the rhythm PSVT with aberrant conduction* <u>or</u> *some form of adenosine-responsive VT in this relatively young adult*).

- Application of a ***vagal* maneuver** (*See pp 118-120 in Section 13*) might also be tried (*even before Adenosine*). Vagal maneuvers often work for PSVT and on occasion, even for *adenosine-responsive* forms of VT and *fascicular* VT.
- Be ready to cardiovert IF at <u>any</u> time during the treatment process the patient decompensates.
- Obtaining a **post-conversion 12-lead ECG** would be very important in this case in the hope of determining <u>IF</u> there is *baseline* RBBB.
- An **Echo** should be done to assess for *underlying* structural heart disease – <u>and</u> – **referral** may be in order (*especially IF fascicular VT is suspected <u>or</u> if there is recurrence of WCT*).

Regarding WCT Tracing #4

 ⇨ ***Beyond-the-Core ...***

● In general — <u>neither</u> Verapamil <u>nor</u> Diltiazem should ever be given for a WCT rhythm unless one is 100% certain that the WCT is *not* VT. This is because the *vasodilating* and *negative* inotropic effects of these drugs is likely to precipitate deterioration of VT to VFib ...
- The above said — it is well to be aware that the special form of VT known as ***fascicular* VT** may respond (*and convert to sinus rhythm*) with use of Verapamil/Diltiazem. ECG recognition of fascicular VT may be subtle (*usually presents with a RBBB/LAHB pattern without P waves in a previously healthy younger adult*).

▶ **Bottom Line:** For the non-expert — it is probably best to <u>avoid</u> Verapamil/Diltiazem in the acute setting <u>unless</u> you are 100% certain that the WCT rhythm is <u>not</u> VT.

- Access to a **prior ECG** on this patient showing baseline RBBB of *identical* QRS morphology as during the WCT would confirm a supraventricular etiology. (<u>Unfortunately</u> — *Most of the time, <u>no</u> prior tracing will be available ...*).
- In 2013 — Certain forms of VT as well as many (*most*) reentry SVTs are potentially *curable* by ablation. **EP referral** may at some point be in order.

WCT *Practice* Tracing #5

  ⇨ <u>**PRACTICE**</u> **Tracing:**

⬤ Your patient is a 60-year-old man with "heart disease". His ECG is shown below. BP = 160/90 mmHg.
• Is the rhythm in <u>Figure 09-9</u> VT or SVT? *What should you do next?*

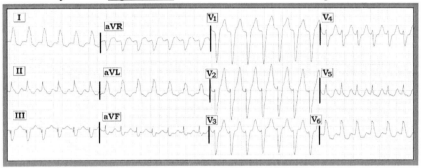

Figure 09-9: WCT Tracing #5. The patient is *hemodynamically* stable.

☞ **Answer to WCT Tracing #5:** A *regular* **WCT** is seen at a rate of ~160/minute. There is *no* clear evidence of atrial activity. The ***differential* diagnosis** is that as shown in **LIST #1** (*page 72*): = VT, VT, VT until *proven* otherwise.
• Given the patient's age <u>and</u> history of "heart disease" — *statistical* likelihood of VT is ~90% *without* going further.
• The above said — there IS a chance that the rhythm in <u>Figure 09-9</u> *could* be SVT (*with <u>either</u> aberrant conduction <u>or</u> preexisting BBB*).

☞ **Fig 09-9:** *Approach When Uncdertain of the Diagnosis*

The 12-lead tracing in <u>Figure 09-9</u> provides an excellent example of how to approach a **WCT Rhythm** when you do <u>not</u> know for sure what the diagnosis is (*discussed in detail in Section 08 on pages 70-83*):
• The patient is **stable** (ie, *there <u>is</u> time to look further*).
• The WCT is ***regular***. Therefore — this is <u>not</u> AFib (*Step #2 on page 72*).
• The QRS is **monomorphic** (*all QRS complexes in a given lead look the same*). Thus, this is <u>not</u> polymorphic VT/Torsades (*Step #2A — pg 72*).
• Assessment of **QRS morphology** is ***inconclusive***. That is — the '*3 Simple Rules*' do <u>not</u> suggest VT (*page 83*). Specifically — the **axis** *during* WCT is normal — **lead V6** is upright – <u>and</u> – the **QRS** is **<u>not</u> "ugly"**, but instead is perfectly consistent with LBBB.

▶ **KEY:** We <u>don't</u> know for sure what the rhythm in <u>Figure 09-9</u> is. Although our initial assessment does *not* point to a ventricular etiology — We still need to *assume* VT until *proven* otherwise. That said — the patient is stable <u>and</u> **Adenosine** is appropriate *initial* treatment (*pg 73*).

- **Failure of Adenosine** — to either temporarily *slow* the rate <u>or</u> convert the rhythm would support the premise that the rhythm in <u>Figure 09-9</u> is VT. At this point — We would then move on to **Amiodarone** (*or other VT dru*g).
- *Successful* conversion of the rhythm by Adenosine would support (*but <u>not</u> definitely prove*) a supraventricular etiology (*Summary on pp 61-62*).
- *Remain* ready to cardiovert — <u>IF</u> at <u>any</u> time the patient *becomes* hemodynamically unstable.
- Ask someone to search this patient's chart in the hope of finding a **prior 12-lead ECG** that might tell if this patient had *baseline* LBBB.

Regarding WCT Tracing #5

  ➡ ***Beyond-the-Core ...***

● This case highlights a number of important points:
- *Definitive* diagnosis of the rhythm in <u>Figure 09-9</u> is <u>not</u> needed to effectively treat the patient. Instead we follow the course laid out for WCT of *Uncertain* Etiology (*pp 73-74*).
- Use of the '3 Simple Rules' does <u>not</u> point toward VT in this case (*but these Rules still help as they make an SVT diagnosis more plausible*).
- Assessment of more *advanced* QRS morphologic features likewise fails to yield a definitive answer (*See Beyond-the-Textbook on pp 74-83*). That is — *at least* one rS complex is present in precordial leads (*seen here in V2,V3,V4*) <u>and</u> there is *no delay* in S wave downslope in V1,V2,V3. The initial r wave in lead V4 is *not* wide.
- The ECG shown in <u>Figure 09-9</u> is the 12-lead *during* tachycardia for the **lead II *rhythm* strip** previously shown in **Figure 03-1** (*page 48*) and in **Figure 08-1** (*page 70*). It is now obvious that the QRS complex is wide (*whereas QRS width was <u>not</u> certain in Figures 03-1 and 08-1*). "12 leads are *better* than one!"
- Use of the **12-lead *during* tachycardia** is also helpful in clarifying questions about atrial activity. For example — one might wonder <u>IF</u> the *upright* deflection midway between QRS complexes in lead II (*and in other leads*) could be a sinus P wave? (*arrows in* **Figure 09-10**).

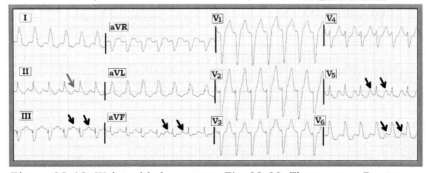

Figure 09-10: We've added arrows to <u>Fig. 09-09</u>. There are *no* P waves

▶ **NOTE:** While we <u>*cannot*</u> rule out the possibility that sinus P waves *might* be hiding within preceding T waves in <u>Figure 09-10</u> (*arrows*) — lack of "telltale" atrial notching defines this rhythm as a **monomorphic** *regular* **WCT** of **uncertain** **etiology** (*List #1 on page 72*). Ventricular tachycardia <u>*must*</u> be assumed until *proven* otherwise.

- Access to a **prior** **12-lead ECG** on this patient would favor SVT if LBBB with *identical* morphology was seen.
- <u>IF</u> the patient remained stable — Use of a **Lewis** **Lead** might be attempted looking for atrial activity (*page 97*).

Final **Point** !

The measures listed on pages 75-83 under '*Beyond-the-Core*' in Section 08 are just that = *advanced* <u>and</u> aimed for *experienced* providers desiring to know more.

- Appropriate management of <u>*all*</u> cases in this WCT *Practice Tracing* Section is possible <u>*without*</u> necessarily pursuing these advanced measures ...

Section 10 – Use of a Lewis Lead (*page 97*)

 # *Use of a Lewis Lead*

● Use of *special* lead systems may sometimes provide diagnostic insight in the search for atrial activity. By varying the anatomic landmarks used for electrode lead placement — a different electrical viewpoint is obtained, which may reveal atrial activity *not* previously visualized when using the 12 standard leads.

☞ *Application* of a *Lewis* Lead

Do the following to record a *Lewis* Lead (Figure 10-1):
• Place the **RA** (*Right Arm*) **electrode** on the *right* side of the sternum at the 2nd ICS (*InterCostal Space*).
• Place the **LA** (*Left Arm*) **electrode** on the *right* side of the sternum at the 4th ICS.
• Record the ECG. The *Lewis* Lead will now be seen in **Lead I**. Adjust calibration to 1mV=20mm (*which is twice normal size*) to facilitate visualization of atrial activity.

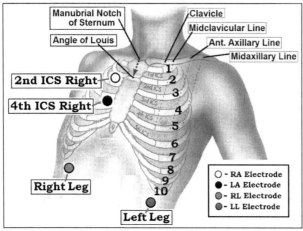

Figure 10-1:
Application of a
Lewis Lead
(*See text*).

▶ **NOTE:** Use of a *Lewis* Lead recording is an *advanced* intervention. It is *not* needed for appropriate evaluation and management in the overwhelming majority of cases. Nevertheless — this *extra* monitoring lead (*first described by Sir Thomas Lewis in 1931*) may at times help diagnose problematic **sustained WCT rhythms** of **uncertain** etiology.

• By facilitating detection of atrial activity — occult but *"telltale"* AV dissociation (*that is diagnostic of VT*) is much more easily recognized.
• By definition — the patient must be *stable* and in a *sustained* tachy-cardia for a Lewis Lead to be used.
• IF at *any* time the patient shows sign of decompensating — *STOP* monitoring and *immediately* cardiovert.

Section 11 – Polymorphic VT/Torsades (*pp 98-103*)

 Polymorphic VT/Torsades

● You are called to a code. The patient is in the **WCT** (<u>W</u>ide-<u>C</u>omplex <u>T</u>achycardia) rhythm shown in **Figure 11-1**.
• What is the rhythm? — *What to do next?*

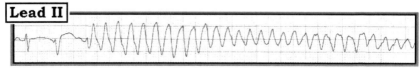

Figure 11-1: The patient is coding. There is a WCT rhythm. *What next?*

Figure 11-1: *What is the Rhythm?*

After an initial sinus beat — the rhythm in <u>Figure 11-1</u> dramatically changes. This is ***polymorphic* VT** — as defined by constantly *varying* QRS morphology *throughout* the rest of the tracing.

• ***Torsades de Pointes*** — is defined as ***polymorphic* VT** that occurs in association **with** a ***prolonged* QT** interval on baseline ECG. The very rapid *irregular* WCT seen in <u>Figure 11-1</u> manifests the shifting QRS polarity around the baseline (*"twisting of the points"*) that is characteristic of Torsades.

• The QT interval of the first sinus beat above appears to be prolonged. That said — it is extremely *difficult* to be certain where the "QT" ends in this this tracing. It simply will *not* always be possible to assess QT duration during *polymorphic* VT ...

Polymorphic VT/Torsades

➡ Suggested *Initial* Approach:

● The importance of distinguishing between *polymorphic* VT with <u>or</u> without QT prolongation lies with the likely cause(s) of the disorder <u>and</u> the response to treatment.

• The ***1st Thing* To Do** (*as always*) — is to check for a pulse. <u>IF</u> the rhythm in <u>Figure 11-1</u> is real — we would *not* expect the patient to be *hemodynamically* stable (*at least not for long ...*).

• **Defibrillation** (*as for VFib*) — is the acute treatment of choice for the patient with **persistent *polymorphic* VT**. Because (*by definition*) — the QRS complex *continually* varies during this *polymorphic* WCT — *synchronized* cardioversion will usually *not* be possible.

• Many episodes of Torsades will be relatively short and self-terminating — but *multiple* shocks may be needed given the tendency to recurrence <u>until</u> the precipitating cause(s) can be identified and corrected.

- **Magnesium Sulfate** — is the *drug* **of choice** for *polymorphic* VT. Give **1-2 gm IV** (*over 1-2 minutes*) — which can then be *repeated* 5-10 minutes later (*as much as* **4-8 gm** *of* **IV Mg++** *may be needed!*). Continuous **IV Mg++ infusion** (*at ~0.5-1gm/hour for up to 12-24 hours*) may help in preventing recurrence.
- IF there is **baseline QT prolongation** (*usually to a QTc ≥ 500msec*) — then the picture of *polymorphic* VT seen in Figure 11-1 is defined as ***Torsades* de Pointes**.

> ▶ **KEY Clinical Point:** *Regardless* of whether: **i)** the baseline QT is clearly prolonged; **ii)** the baseline QT is normal; or **iii)** You simply <u>can</u> <u>not</u> <u>tell</u> IF the baseline QT is normal or long — ***initial* treatment measures** (*defibrillation as needed; IV Mg++; find and fix potential causes*) are **the same!**

- ***Additional* Measures** — that on occasion <u>are</u> helpful in controlling episodes of *polymorphic* VT (*with* or *without long QT*): **i) Isoproterenol** infusion (*beginning at 2 mcg/min, and titrating upward as needed*); <u>and</u> **ii) overdrive** pacing. These measures are most likely to be useful for the *refractory* patient whose episodes are repeatedly *triggered* by **preceding bradycardia** (*which sets up conditions that prolong the QT of subsequent beats*). That said — IV Mg++; defibrillation when needed; <u>and</u> correcting precipitating causes should be tried first for the patient presenting with *polymorphic* VT.

Is the Baseline QT Interval Prolonged?

 ➡ ***Beyond-the-Core* ...**

● Full discussion of QT prolongation is beyond the scope of this book. Nevertheless, review of *key* principles may be helpful (**Figure 11-2**):
- The **QT interval** is the period that extends from the *beginning* of ventricular depolarization — <u>until</u> the *end* of ventricular repolarization.
- To **measure** the **baseline QT** on **12-lead ECG** — Select a lead where you can clearly see the *end* of the T wave. Use *that* lead in which the QT appears to be *longest* !
- ☞ **General Rule:** For practical purposes, the **QT** is **prolonged** — IF it clearly measures **more** than **half** the **R-R** interval.

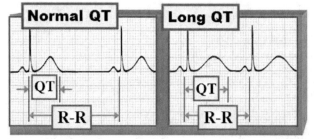

Figure 11-2: Normal <u>vs</u> long QT intervals. The QT should *not* be more than half the R-R interval (*See text*).

▶ **NOTE:** The **General Rule** on page 99 (*that the QT should not be more than half the R-R interval*) — works great when the rate is *less* than 80-90/minute. The Rule is *not* nearly as accurate when the heart rate is faster (*over 90-100/minute*).

• Clinically — You often will *not* have access to a *baseline* ECG on the patient you are treating. The underlying rhythm may not be sinus. The baseline QRS may be wide — in which case it becomes even more difficult to determine whether the QT is longer than it should be. **Bottom Line:** You will often *not* be able to determine IF the *baseline* QT of a coding patient is prolonged ...
• **'Rules of Thumb'** — Although the **corrected QT** (*QTc*) is *inversely* related to heart rate — a *measured* QT interval that *exceeds* 0.45 sec should be cause for concern.
• **IF** the **measured QT** is **>0.50 second** (*500 msec*) — it is *definitely* prolonged and worrisome (*increased risk of Torsades*).

☞ Measuring the QT: *Is the QT Prolonged in* <u>Figure 11-3</u> ?

Precise calculation of the QTc requires detailed tables specifying patient gender and heart rate. Fortunately — such precise calculation is not needed clinically. Instead — the **more-than-half** the **R-R-interval General Rule** works nicely in almost all cases — with the main caveat being *reduced* accuracy when heart rate exceeds 90-100/min. We illustrate clinical application of these principles in **Figure 11-3**. From this 12-lead tracing:
• *Which* lead(s) should be used to determine IF the QT is normal or prolonged?
• Which lead(s) should *not* be used to assess QT duration?
• What **clinical conditions** should be considered?

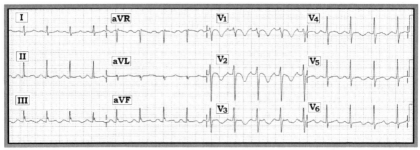

Figure 11-3: Assessment of QT duration from the 12-lead ECG. *Is the QT prolonged?* — What clinical conditions are suggested? (*See text*).

☞ Answer to Figure 11-3: *Is the QT Prolonged?*

As discussed — To determine IF the QT interval is prolonged, one should select a lead where you can clearly see the *end* of the T wave. One should use *that* lead in which the QT appears to be *longest*.
• Vertical **timelines** in **Figure 11-4** illustrate why we would *not* use leads such as lead I, II, aVR or aVL to determine if the QT is

prolonged. It is difficult to be certain where the QT interval ends in these leads (*and at most the QT is no more than half the R-R interval*).

- In contrast — the **QT interval** is *clearly* **prolonged** in *precordial* **leads V1** and **V2** (*despite uncertainty in* Figure 11-4 *about precisely where the T wave ends and the next P wave begins in these leads*).

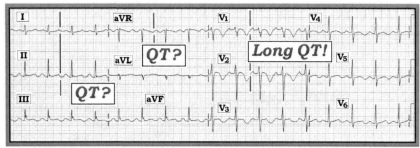

Figure 11-4: Vertical timelines have been added to Figure 11-3. The QT interval is clearly prolonged in precordial leads V1 and V2 (*See text*).

▶ **NOTE:** Despite the tachycardia in Figure 11-4 (*heart rate is slightly more than 100/minute*) — We can still comfortably state that the QT is prolonged because it is decisively *more* than half the R-R interval in *at least* certain leads (*such as V1,V2*).

- In addition to QT prolongation — the most remarkable ECG finding in Figure 11-4 is ST segment coving and **diffuse, *symmetric* precordial T wave inversion** that is marked in leads V1,V2,V3. This ECG picture should suggest the possibility of acute ischemia, ongoing infarction *and/or* pulmonary embolus.
- We add to the list of diagnostic considerations *any* of the *Common* Causes of QT prolongation:

☞ *Common* Causes of QT Prolongation

● To remember the common *causes* of QT prolongation: **Think "*Drugs – Lytes – CNS*"**. We list but a few of these below:

- **Drugs** — especially procainamide; sotalol; tricyclic antidepressants; older phenothiazines. (Note: *Although amiodarone lengthens the QT — the risk of Torsades is surprisingly low as a result of amiodarone use*).

- **"Lytes"** — *low* K+; *low* Mg++; *low* Ca++.

- **CNS** — *any* CNS catastrophe (*stroke; CNS bleed; coma; seizure; tumor; head trauma*). Acute CNS disorders may produce some of the most *bizarre* ECG changes imaginable — including *marked* ST elevation, depression, T wave inversion *and/or* extreme QT prolongation.

NOTE: Several *other* conditions (ie, *bundle branch block, infarction, ischemia*) may also prolong the QT. However, the presence of these **other conditions** will usually be obvious from inspection of the ECG.

▶ **KEY Clinical Point:** *Clinical correlation is essential!* Without it — it would be impossible to determine <u>IF</u> the *marked* QT prolongation seen in <u>Figure 11-4</u> was the result of ischemia, infarction, pulmonary embolus — <u>or</u> some drug effect, electrolyte disorder *and/or* acute CNS event.

☞ Polymorphic VT: *If the QT is Not Prolonged*

We *defined* the rhythm in <u>Figure 11-1</u> as **Torsades** IF the *baseline* QT was long. Alternatively known as **acquired LQTS** (<u>Long QT Syndrome</u>) — this disorder is most often due to *drug-induced* QT prolongation <u>and</u>/or electrolyte depletion (*low K+/Mg++*). As a result — primary efforts should be taken to: **i) *Stop*** all **meds** likely to contribute to QT prolongation; **ii) *Optimize*** serum **K+/Mg++ levels** (*IV Magnesium helps acutely with Torsades suppression even when serum Mg++ levels are normal*); <u>and</u> **iii)** Control whenever possible **other** factors that may contribute to QT prolongation (*page 101*).

- <u>IF</u> the **QT** is **not** prolonged — then the rhythm is simply referred to as polymorphic VT. **Initial** treatment is the **same** as for Torsades (*defibrillation as needed; IV Mg++*) — <u>BUT</u> the **response** to IV Mg++ is **not** nearly as good as it is when the QT is prolonged.
- Rather than being drug <u>or</u> electrolyte induced — **polymorphic VT** <u>with</u> a **normal QT** most often has an *ischemic* etiology (*less commonly due to Brugada syndrome or familial forms*). Efforts addressed at treating acute ischemia may therefore be helpful. IV Amiodarone <u>and</u>/or ß-blockers may reduce recurrence and should be considered if IV Mg++ is ineffective.

About Inherited LQTS

 ➡ *Beyond-the-Core ...*

● A rare **inherited form** of **LQTS** (<u>Long QT Syndrome</u>) exists — in which syncope/cardiac arrest from Torsades may occur. Onset is in childhood or adolescence, and there is usually a positive family history.

- Episodes typically occur during exercise or stress.
- Acute treatment (*of Torsades*) is similar as for the more common *acquired* form of LQTS (*pp 98-99*).
- Recurrence of Torsades episodes is common with inherited LQTS — so these patients should be promptly referred when discovered.
- *Adrenergic* modulation (*with beta-blockers*) <u>and</u> pacing (*to prevent precipitating bradycardia*) may be useful — but implantation of an **ICD** (*<u>I</u>mplantable <u>C</u>ardioverter-<u>D</u>efibrillator*) will often be needed.

On Recognizing and Treating Polymorphic VT

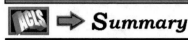 ⇒ **S*ummary***

● It is essential to *promptly* recognize *polymorphic* VT because of the *different* approach to treatment. *Varying* QRS morphology during this WCT rhythm usually makes such recognition easy (**Figure 11-5**):

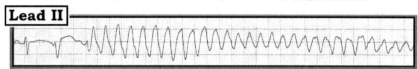

Figure 11-5: Polymorphic VT (*reproduced from* Figure 11-1 *on page 98*).

☞ **Summarized Treatment of *Polymorphic* VT:**

• Defibrillation is needed for persistent episodes (*it will usually not be possible to cardiovert given varying QRS morphologies that confound attempts to synchronize shock delivery to a specified point in the cardiac cycle*).

• **Magnesium Sulfate** is the *medical* treatment of choice. High doses (*up to 4-8 gm IV*) may need to be given. Magnesium is most likely to work IF the rhythm is **Torsades** and the baseline QT interval is prolonged — although realistically, you will not always be able to determine this. It is reasonable (*and appropriate*) to try IV Magnesium regardless of whether you know if the QT interval is prolonged ...

• Finding and fixing the **precipitating cause** of *polymorphic* VT/Torsades is key. ● Think *Drugs-Lytes-CNS.* Consider an acute *ischemic* etiology (*especially if the QT is not prolonged and the patient fails to respond to IV Magnesium*).

• *Avoid* drugs like Procainamide and Sotalol that lengthen the QT and predispose to Torsades.

• Amiodarone *also* lengthens the QT — but clinically, Amiodarone is surprisingly much *less* likely to precipitate Torsades.

• **Defibrillate** the patient *if/as* needed.

Fast Irregular VT
(VT <u>vs</u> AFib <u>vs</u> WPW)

▶ **NOTE:** The content in this Section 12 is *advanced*. It is *beyond-the-core* for the usual ACLS course given to *non-specialized* medical providers. We include this material for those wanting to know more.

● Your patient is *about* to code. The patient is in the **WCT** (*Wide-Complex Tachycardia*) rhythm shown in **Figure 12-1**.
• What is the rhythm? — *What to do next?*

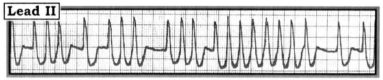

Figure 12-1: The patient is *about* to code ... (*See text*).

☞ **Figure 12-1: What is the Rhythm?**

The rhythm is rapid and *irregularly* irregular. *No* atrial activity is seen. Although the QRS is definitely widened — the gross irregularity of the rhythm makes VT (*Ventricular Tachycardia*) unlikely. This leaves **AFib** (*Atrial Fibrillation*) as the *probable* diagnosis.
• The rate of the rhythm is **much faster than** is **usually** seen in AFib (*the refractory period of the AV node usually limits AFib rate to <200 impulses/minute — whereas the rate in certain parts of* Figure 12-1 *is >250/minute!*).
• The rate is **too fast** for atrial impulses to be transmitted over the normal (*AV nodal*) conduction pathway. Therefore — **atrial impulses** must be **bypassing** the AV node (*We suspect the patient has WPW!*).

☞ **Why this is AFib with WPW and Not VT ...**

● **PEARL:** — The finding of AFib at an *exceedingly* rapid rate (*over ~220/minute*) — should *immediately* suggest the likelihood of **AP** (*Accessory Pathway*) **conduction** in a patient who has **WPW** (*Wolff-Parkinson-White*) **syndrome**.
• Two *additional* features in *favor* of Figure 12-1 being **WPW** rather than VT are: **i)** variation in QRS morphology (*not expected with mono-morphic VT — yet not nearly as erratic as polymorphic VT*); and **ii)** very *marked* change between some R-R intervals on the tracing (*some being extremely short with others being significantly longer*).

▶ **KEY Point:** The reason it is important to recognize WPW-associated arrhythmias is that acute treatment considerations of very *rapid*

AFib (*or AFlutter*) <u>with</u> WPW are very *different* than for other WCT rhythms. As a result — We first review ECG recognition before addressing treatment.

ECG Features of WPW

 ⇒ ***Beyond-the-Textbook ...***

⬤ WPW is a syndrome in which one or more accessory pathways exist that allow an *alternate* route for transmission of the electrical impulse from atria to ventricles.

- The **incidence** of **WPW** is **~2/1000** individuals in the general population (*just often enough that most emergency providers <u>will</u> see WPW from time to time!*).
- The **importance** of **WPW** is twofold: **i)** It is **"the great mimic"** — and may simulate other conditions (*such as ischemia/infarction, hypertrophy and/or conduction defects*) — <u>IF</u> it is not recognized; <u>and</u> **ii)** The presence of one or more accessory pathways **predisposes** the patient to a number of potentially important **cardiac arrhythmias**.

☞ **Recognition of WPW** is usually easy on a baseline 12-lead ECG when conduction *completely* utilizes the **AP** (<u>A</u>ccessory <u>P</u>athway). There are **3 ECG features** to look for (Figure 12-2):

- QRS widening.
- Delta waves.
- A *short* PR interval (*<0.12 second in lead II*).

Figure 12-2: With WPW — the electrical impulse will *bypass* the AV

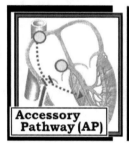

Accessory Pathway (AP)

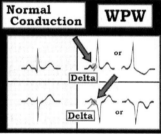

node. The AP is shown in this Figure to be passing along the *right* side of the heart — but the AP may pass on either side *and/or* pass in front or in back of the septum.

⬤ The **delta wave** is recognized as a distortion of the *initial* portion of the QRS complex. It is due to the fact that the electrical impulse *bypasses* the AV node — and arrives at the ventricles directly via conduction over the accessory pathway.

- Delta waves may be upright (*positive*) or downward (*negative*) — depending on where in the heart the AP is located (*arrows in* Figure 12-2). When delta waves are negative — they may simulate the Q wave of myocardial infarction.
- Even when conduction is entirely over the AP — delta waves will *not* always be seen in every lead. Moreover, delta waves may come and go

— since conduction over the AP may be intermittent. At times — conduction may *simultaneously* occur over both the normal and accessory pathway. When this happens — the ECG characteristics of WPW may be subtle because the contribution from conduction over the normal AV nodal pathway may predominate (*and thereby mask*) ECG features of pre-excitation.

● The reason the **PR interval** is ***short*** with WPW — is that the AV node is bypassed. With normal conduction in sinus rhythm — the electrical impulse *slows down* as it passes through the AV node on its way to the ventricles. As a result — most of the PR interval normally consists of the time it takes for the impulse to traverse the AV node. The electrical impulse arrives at the ventricles *sooner* with WPW because the relative *delay* that normally occurs when passing through the AV node is *avoided* by conduction over the AP.

• The **QRS *widens*** with **WPW** — because *after* the impulse arrives at the ventricles (*via conduction over the AP*) — it must then travel over *nonspecialized* myocardial tissue until such time that it attains whatever distal portion of the conduction system that has *not* yet depolarized. Thus the delta wave may extend for 0.04 second or more (*reflecting slow conduction over nonspecialized myocardial tissue*). When the delta wave is *added* to the rest of the QRS complex — the result is a *widened* complex.

▶ **NOTE:** All sorts of variations on the above theme (*that extend beyond-the-scope of this book*) are possible. The points to remember are the following.

• WPW is *not* common in the general population — but it <u>*does*</u> occur (*and you <u>will</u> see it*)!
• When a patient with WPW is conducting over their accessory pathway — you can ***diagnose*** **WPW** by ***recognition*** of the following **3 ECG features** in *at least* several of the 12 leads of an ECG: **i)** QRS widening; **ii)** a *delta* wave; <u>and</u> iii) a *short* PR interval (*Figure 12-2*).
• **Preexcitation (**ie, *WPW conduction over an AP* **)** — can be intermittent. There may be no indication on ECG that a patient has WPW if conduction is entirely (*or almost entirely*) over the normal AV nodal pathway at the time the tracing is recorded.

☞ **Figure 12.5-1: *WPW during Sinus Rhythm***

Emergency care providers will not always have the luxury of a baseline 12-lead ECG at the time a patient with *WPW-associated* tachycardia is initially seen. However, with luck — a ***baseline* 12-lead ECG** with ***telltale* features** of **WPW** may occasionally be found in the patient's chart — thereby *confirming* the diagnosis. We show such a tracing with overt WPW in **Figure 12-3**:

• Note in Figure 12-3 — that delta waves are <u>*not*</u> always prominent in every lead. One *cannot* diagnose LVH, ischemia or infarction from the tall inferior R waves, deep Q wave in lead aVL, or ST-T wave changes in V1,V2,V3 — since the patient has WPW.

- It should be apparent from **Figure 12-3** that the diagnosis of WPW could be *easily* overlooked <u>IF</u> one was not systematic in their approach. At *first* glance — the QRS complex does *not* look overly wide. That said — careful inspection of **lead II** clearly reveals a *short* PR interval with upward *delta* wave (*arrow in lead II of Figure 12-3*) — that when *added* to the remaining portion of the QRS results in *widening* of the QRS. Confirmation of WPW is forthcoming from recognition of delta waves in most other leads on the tracing.

- *Awareness* that the patient you are treating for an acute arrhythmia has WPW may be invaluable in *optimizing* management (*pp 110-112*).

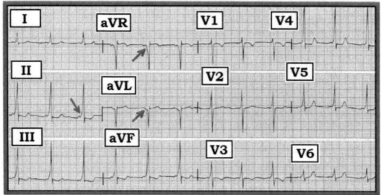

Figure 12-3: WPW during sinus rhythm. The PR interval is short (*best seen in lead II*) — and the QRS is prolonged (*best seen in leads II,III, aVF*). Delta waves are seen in most (*but not all*) leads on this 12-lead tracing (*there is no delta wave in lead V1 — and the delta wave is minimal in leads I and V2*). Delta waves are *positive* in most leads (ie, *arrow in lead II*) — but they are *negative* in leads aVR and aVL (*arrows*). On occasion — *negative* delta waves may simulate infarction.

☞ *SVT Pathways with WPW*

We have already emphasized how conduction of the sinus impulse in patients with WPW may be: **i)** via the normal (*AV nodal*) pathway; **ii)** down the AP; <u>or</u> **iii)** it may *alternate* between the two. The *same* 3 possibilities for conduction exist when a patient with WPW develops a supraventricular tachyarrhythmia (<u>Figure 12-4</u>):

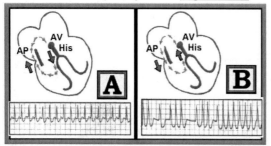

Figure 12-4: SVT pathways with WPW (*See text*).

It can therefore be seen from **Figure 12-4** (*pg 107*) — that conduction of the impulse from atria to ventricles during *WPW-associated* tachycardia may either be:
* **Orthodromic** (*Panel A in Fig. 12-4*) — in which the impulse goes down the *normal* AV nodal-His-Purkinje system — and back up the AP (*as commonly occurs with PSVT*) – <u>or</u> –
* **Antidromic** (*Panel B in Fig. 12-4*) — in which the impulse first goes down the AP — and then back up the normal pathway (*as commonly occurs with AFib or AFlutter — and only rarely with PSVT*).

▶ **NOTE:** Patients with WPW are prone to *supraventricular* tachyarrhythmias in which a **reentry circuit** is set up between the normal AV nodal pathway and the AP.

* Assuming there is no preexisting bundle branch block — Whether or not the QRS complex will be wide *during* the tachycardia in a patient with WPW will depend upon whether the reentrant pathway goes *up* <u>or</u> *down* the AP (*Figure 12-4*).

☞ PSVT with WPW: *When the QRS is Narrow*

With PSVT in WPW — the tachyarrhythmia is almost always **orthodromic** (*down the normal AV nodal-His-Purkinje system — and back up the AP* = **Panel A** in <u>Figure 12-4</u>).
* Because conduction goes *down* the normal AV nodal pathway — the **QRS is *narrow*** during the tachycardia. As a result — the usual **AV nodal blocking drugs** may be used effectively in treatment (*pg 121*).
* A delta wave will *not* be seen during the tachycardia. The presence of WPW may only be suspected in a patient with *narrow-complex* PSVT <u>IF</u> an ECG such as that seen in <u>Figure 12-3</u> (*pg 107*) is found in the medical chart or obtained following conversion of the tachycardia.
* PSVT is by far the most common tachyarrhythmia observed in patients with WPW. It is often well tolerated.
* *Beyond-the-Core:* A surprising number of patients with PSVT actually have one or more *concealed* accessory pathways. That is — a conduction pathway exists between atria and ventricles that *only* allows orthodromic (*but not antidromic*) conduction. Since forward conduction down the AP is not possible — a delta wave is *never* seen. However, ready availability of an AP reentry pathway may predispose such patients to frequent episodes of PSVT. While acute treatment considerations are similar to those for treatment of any other *narrow-complex* PSVT — awareness of this entity may lower one's threshold for EP referral after the episode if PSVT episodes are frequent *and/or* difficult to control with medication.
* *Way-Beyond-the-Core:* Taking the last *advanced* information bullet one step further — You may at times be able to *suspect* the presence of an AP in some WPW patients with *narrow* complex PSVT even without seeing a delta wave <u>IF</u> you see a *negative* P wave with *long* R-P interval reflecting *retrograde* conduction back to the atria during the reentrant cycle. When retrograde conduction is seen during

AVNRT in a patient *without* WPW — the RP is *very* short (*most often seen as a notch at the tail end of the QRS complex*) reflecting short distance travel within the AV node. The RP tends to be longer (*negative P usually seen midway within the ST segment*) for a patient in whom the reentry circuit runs down the AV node and back up an AP lying outside the AV node. Technically — this type of PSVT in a patient with accessory pathways is known as **AVRT** (*AtrioVentricular Reciprocating Tachycardia*). Distinction in the ECG picture *between* AVNRT vs AVRT (*when an AP is present)* is illustrated in Figure 14-16 (*See pp 141-144*).

▶ **Bottom Line:** Most of the time — PSVT in a patient with WPW will conduct with a *narrow* QRS complex (**Panel A** *in* Figure 12-4). Practically speaking — you do *not* have to worry in the immediate *acute* setting IF a patient with *narrow-complex* PSVT has WPW or not. Initial treatment measures are the same: Vagal maneuver — Adenosine *and/or* other AV nodal blocking agent (*Diltiazem, β-Blocker, etc.*).

☞ *Very Rapid AFib with WPW*

In contrast to the situation for PSVT with WPW — the occurrence of **AFib** in a patient with WPW *almost always* manifests a *wide* **QRS** during the tachycardia. This is because the direction of conduction for AFib with WPW is almost always **antidromic** (*first down the AP — and then back up the normal pathway* = **Panel B** *in* Figure 12-4 *on pg 107*).

- Because of the short RP (*Refractory Period*) of the accessory pathway — there may be 1:1 conduction of atrial impulses (*at times resulting in a ventricular response that may exceed 250/minute!*). As might be anticipated — these rapid rates are *not* always well tolerated (*may deteriorate to VFib*).
- It is recognition of the ECG picture of **exceedingly** rapid AFib (*over 220/minute in parts of the tracing*) in conjunction with **QRS widening** and **marked** variability in regularity of the tracing that clues the clinician into *almost certainty* of **AFib** **with** **WPW** as the diagnosis. This was the situation for the initial rhythm strip shown at the beginning of this Section (that we repeat below in **Figure 12-5**).
- We discuss management of *very rapid* AFib *with* WPW on pp 110-112.

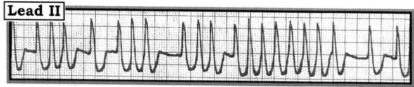

Figure 12-5: Same lead II rhythm strip previously shown on page 104. The patient is *about* to code. What is the rhythm? (*See text*).

AFlutter with WPW

With **AFlutter** in WPW — the tachyarrhythmia is also **antidromic** (*first down the AP — and then back up the normal pathway = as occurs in* **Panel B** *of* Figure 12-4 *on page 107*).
- As with AFib — the **QRS** is *wide* in **AFlutter** *with* **WPW**. There may be 1:1 AV conduction of atrial impulses (*so that the ventricular response may attain 250-300/minute*)!
- Very fast AFlutter with WPW is seen even *less often* than AFib (*but clinical manifestations and treatment are similar*).

PSVT with WPW: *When the QRS is Wide*

In *rare* instances — **PSVT** may be *antidromic* (ie, *travel first down the AP — and then back up the normal pathway = as occurs in* **Panel B** *of* Figure 12-4).
- In these rare instances — the **QRS** will be *wide* and the PSVT rhythm may be *indistinguishable* from VT.
- It may only be *after* conversion to sinus rhythm that "telltale" delta waves of WPW can be identified. Fortunately — the *vast* majority (~95%) of PSVT episodes with WPW are orthodromic (*with a narrow QRS complex*). **Synchronized** cardioversion will be the usual treatment of choice for episodes of a *regular* WCT (Wide-Complex Tachycardia) in which one suspects *antidromic* PSVT in a patient with WPW as the etiology.

Rapid AFib with WPW

 ➡️ **Suggested *Initial* Approach:**

● The importance of distinguishing between the very common form of *rapid* **AFib** (*Section 14 on pp 125-132*) – and – the relatively rare occurrence of **excessively rapid AFib** *with* **WPW** (Figure 12-5) lies with recommendations for treatment. Fortunately — distinctive ECG characteristics usually facilitate recognition.
- **Synchronized** Cardioversion — is the *acute* treatment of choice for the symptomatic patient who presents in **very rapid AFib** **with WPW**. That said — a significant number of patients who present with the rhythm in Figure 12-5 will be surprisingly stable *despite* attaining AFib rates of >220/minute. Therefore — a **trial** of **antiarrhythmic therapy** will often be warranted. Drug choices include: **i)** Procainamide; **ii)** Amiodarone; *and* **iii)** Ibutilide (*pp 110-112*).
- Remain ever ready to cardiovert for *any* sign of hemodynamic decompensation.
- IF for *any* reason you are unable to cardiovert (*as could happen when the rate is excessively fast*) — defibrillate.

Drugs for AFib/Flutter with WPW

 ➡ **Beyond-the-Core ...**

⬤ Controversy surrounds the use of antiarrhythmic agents for treatment of excessively *rapid* AFib (*or AFlutter*) with WPW. Prospective study of these rhythms is made **problematic** by: **i) rare occurrence** (*most emergency care providers see at most a handful of cases every few years*); **ii) life-threatening potential** (*mandating full attention to the case at hand rather than enrollment into a controlled prospective study*); and **iii)** difficulty sorting out cross-over treatments (*many patients being given more than a single agent and/or needing emergency cardioversion at an unpredictable point during the treatment process*).

Drug dosing is *not* consistent and details of study protocols in the small non-controlled trials that have been done are lacking — such that more questions remain than have been answered. What is known is the following:

• **AV Nodal Blocking Drugs** that are regularly used to treat the common form of rapid AFib are **contraindicated**. This includes Verapamil-Diltiazem-Digoxin — and *possibly* β-Blockers. By impeding conduction down the normal AV nodal pathway — *all* of these agents may inadvertently *facilitate* forward (*antidromic*) conduction of AFib impulses down the AP (*Accessory Pathway*), thereby *accelerating* the rapid AFib even more. This may precipitate deterioration to VFib ...

• Realizing that Adenosine is often used as a *diagnostic* measure during assessment of various WCT rhythms — it is best to **avoid Adenosine** whenever possible IF very rapid AFib *with* WPW is suspected (*since Adenosine may likewise accelerate AP conduction in a patient with WPW*). That said — the *ultra-short* half-life of Adenosine is much *less* likely to be deleterious compared to other AV nodal blocking drugs if it is inadvertently given.

☞ **WPW with Very *Rapid* AFib: *Drug of Choice?***

The **3 drugs** that have most commonly been recommended for antiarrhythmic treatment of **hemodynamically** stable very rapid AFib (*or AFlutter*) with WPW are **i) Procainamide**; **ii) Amiodarone**; and **iii) Ibutilide**. Each drug has its own set of advocates. Each (*at least theoretically*) slows forward (*antidromic*) conduction down the AP. To the best of our review of the current literature — no definitive case can be made at this time for use of one agent to the exclusion of the others for the reasons we state above.

▶ Bottom Line: Very *rapid* AFib *with* WPW is a medical emergency. **Synchronized cardioversion** is likely to be needed at some point in many (*most*) cases. Expert consultation is advised whenever possible. *Don't delay* cardioversion IF the patient at *any* time becomes unstable. In the meantime — IF it is YOU *on-the-scene* with a stable patient in very *rapid* AFib <u>with</u> WPW — You may consider medical treatment with one of the following:

- **Procainamide** — giving **20-50 mg/minute IV** until <u>either:</u> **i)** the arrhythmia is suppressed; **ii)** hypotension ensues; <u>or</u> **iii)** 17 mg/kg has been given (*~500-1,000mg is the usual IV loading dose*). Key to procainamide infusion is balancing the rapidity of IV infusion with the patient's blood pressure response (*slow the rate if hypotension occurs!*). Onset of action is relatively slow (*especially when starting at safer IV infusion rates ~20-30mg/minute*).
- **Amiodarone** — dosing as for VT (*giving ~**150 mg IV** over 10 minutes*). This dose may be repeated and followed by IV infusion of 1mg/minute for the next ~6 hours. Disadvantages include potential hypotension and potential for the AV nodal blocking properties of this drug to outweigh its beneficial effect on AP conduction.
- **Ibutilide** — giving **1mg IV** over 10 minutes (*use 0.01 mg/kg if patient weighs less than 60 kg*). May repeat 10 minutes later if no response. Although experience with Ibutilide for treating AFib with WPW is relatively limited — the drug acts fast (*average conversion time within 20 minutes*); appears to be effective; <u>and</u> is usually well tolerated in most patients. Although not yet listed in ACLS Guidelines — with time, cautious administration of this drug may become the agent of choice for very *rapid* AFib (*or AFlutter*) <u>with</u> WPW.

▶ *Clinical* <u>NOTE:</u> **After** the **acute tachycardia** **has resolved** — those patients with WPW who have had an episode of AFib or AFlutter should be **referred** to an **EP cardiologist** (*ablation of the "culprit AP" may cure this potentially life-threatening arrhythmia that is otherwise at high risk of recurring!*).

☞ By way of Review — Try your hand interpreting the *wide* tachycardia seen in **Figure 12-6** on page 113.

PRACTICE: *What is the Rhythm in Figure 12-6?*

 ⇨ **PRACTICE Tracing:**

● Imagine the 12-lead ECG in <u>Figure 12-6</u> was obtained in the ED (*Emergency Department*) from a *hemodynamically* stable young adult with *new-onset* palpitations.
- *What is the rhythm?* — What does this patient have?

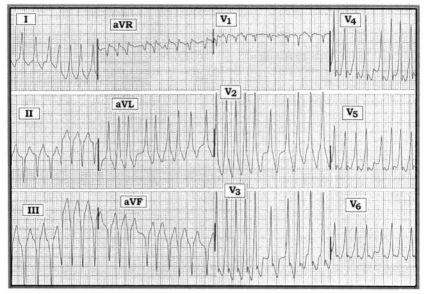

Figure 12-6: 12-lead ECG from a young adult with palpitations. What is the rhythm? (*See text*).

☞ **Answer to Figure 12-6:** The rhythm is an **irregularly *irregular*** **WCT** (<u>*Wide-Complex Tachycardia*</u>). No P waves are seen on any of the 12 leads — thus defining the rhythm as **AFib**. That said – the ***ventricular* response** is ***exceedingly* rapid** (*attaining a rate of nearly 300/minute in some parts of the tracing*). In addition — there is marked *variability* in rate of the ventricular response (*seen best in leads aVF and V3*).

- This 12-lead ECG is ***virtually* diagnostic** of **very rapid AFib** in a patient who has **WPW**. Treatment considerations are discussed on pages 110-112. The patient should be referred to an EP cardiologist after resolution of the acute tachycardia for consideration of an ablative procedure.

SVT of
Uncertain *E*tiology

● Your patient appears ill. You see **Tachycardia** on the monitor (*Figure 13-1*). BP = 120/80. The patient is *hemodynamically* stable.
- *What to do next?*

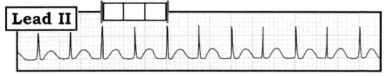

Figure 13-1: We see **tachycardia** — but the patient is stable.

☞ *Assessing* Figure 13-1: *Is the Rhythm an SVT?*

The "good news" about the rhythm shown in Figure 13-1 — is that the patient appears to be **hemodynamically** stable. Thus, there is a moment to assess the rhythm before determining need for treatment:
- By the **Ps,Qs & 3R Approach** (*page 21*) — We see a regular *narrow* tachycardia *without* identifiable P waves at a rate ~200/minute.
- That the **rate** of the *regular* SVT in Figure 13-1 is **~200/minute** can be easily calculated by the **every-other-beat** method (*page 33*). The R-R interval of *every-other-beat* is 3 large boxes. Therefore — *half* the rate = 300/3 = 100/min. This means that the *actual* rate = 100/min X 2 = 200/minute.
- The rhythm in **Figure 13-1** differs from Figure 03-1 at the beginning of the *Unspecified* Tachycardia section (*on page 48*) — in that the QRS complex clearly appears to be *narrow* in Figure 13-1. IF the **QRS** is **truly narrow** (ie, *NOT* more than half a large box in duration in *any* of the 12 leads — *page 28*) — then for practical purposes (*with ~99% accuracy*) — the **mechanism** of the rhythm will be **SupraVentricular** (ie, *the rhythm originates* at *or* above *the double dotted line in* Figure 13-2). Thus, the finding of a **narrow QRS** virtually defines a tachycardia as an **"SVT"** (*S*upra*V*entricular *T*achycardia).

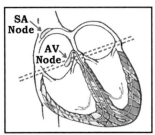

Figure 13-2: *Supraventricular* arrhythmias are defined as arising *at* or *above* the double-dotted line in Figure 13-2 = *at* or *above* the AV node. This means that *supraventricular* arrhythmias may arise from the SA node, AV node — or from somewhere in the atria (*See page 115*).

▶ **CAVEAT:** On occasion — the QRS complex of an SVT rhythm *may* be wide — IF there is either *preexisting* bundle branch block *or* aberrant conduction. This is the case for the supraventricular rhythm in **Figure 13-3** — in which a sinus mechanism is clearly present (*defined by an upright P with fixed PR preceding each QRS*) — despite the fact that the QRS complex is wide. The patient has *preexisting* BBB (*bundle branch block*).

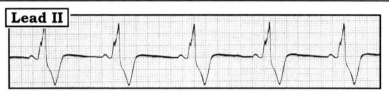

Figure 13-3: Sinus bradycardia and arrhythmia in a patient with *preexisting* bundle branch block. Despite QRS widening — the mechanism of the rhythm is sinus, as defined by the presence of an *upright* P with *fixed* PR interval preceding *each* QRS complex (*See text*).

▶ **SUMMARY:** We can therefore state the following regarding ECG assessment of tachycardia in an adult:

• IF the QRS complex during tachycardia is *clearly* narrow in *all* 12-leads — then we can say with ~99% accuracy that the rhythm is supraventricular. The rare exceptions to this rule are when the impulse arises from a part of the conduction system *below* the AV node (ie, *His or fascicular VT*).

• The converse to this rule is *not* true. That is, when the QRS complex during tachycardia is wide — we can *not* be certain of the etiology of the arrhythmia. Sections 08 and 09 emphasize how in the absence of sinus P waves — VT *must* be assumed until *proven* otherwise. That said — *wide-QRS* tachycardias may on occasion be supraventricular IF *either* preexisting BBB or *aberrant* conduction are present.

☞ *Differential* Diagnosis of SVT

⬤ The balance of this Section and the next address diagnosis and management of tachycardias that are *known* to be supraventricular (ie, *arising from at* or *above the double-dotted line in* Figure 13-2). For practical purposes — the principal entities included in the **differential diagnosis** of **SVT** consists of:

• Sinus Tachycardia
• AFib (*irregular*)
• AFlutter
• PSVT (*or AVNRT*)
• Junctional rhythms
• MAT (*irregular*)

| The list at the left is *not* all inclusive. Other entities (ie, *ectopic atrial tachycardia*) exist — although they are far *less* common and therefore *not* specifically addressed here. |

▶ **NOTE:** Certain types of VT may be misclassified as "supraventricular" — based on the fact that the QRS complex may not be overly wide. This is particularly true IF the VT site of origin is *within* the conduction system (ie, *fascicular VT*).

• The above said, in ~99% of cases — IF the QRS *during* tachycardia is narrow (*in all 12 leads*) — then the rhythm is supraventricular (*originating at* or above the double dotted line in Figure 13-2).

Key Points about SVT Rhythms

 ⇨ *KEY Points*

● We emphasize the following points about **SVT rhythms** such as that shown in Figure 13-1 (*page 114*) — in which the specific diagnosis is *uncertain* but the patient is *hemodynamically* stable.

• Since the patient is stable — Try to obtain a **12-lead ECG *during* tachycardia** as soon as possible. Doing so will: **i)** Verify that the QRS is *truly* narrow in *all* 12 leads; **ii)** Clarify if atrial activity is present in *any* leads; and **iii)** Provide a baseline ECG that may *retrospectively* assist in rhythm determination after conversion to sinus rhythm.

• **SVTs** (*SupraVentricular Tachycardia*) — are *rarely* life-threatening. Treatment is *different* than for WCTs. This is why **ACLS-PM** highlights assessment of **QRS width** as an early *KEY* step for determining treatment!

• Although ACLS-PM defines *"wide"* as ≥0.12 second — We favor **more** than **half** a **large box** (≥*0.11 sec.*) as our definition (*since the QRS of some VTs is only 0.11 second*).

• *Optimal* treatment — depends on the *type* of **SVT**. Rhythm diagnosis will be determined by: **i)** the heart rate; **ii)** the *regularity* of the rhythm; and **iii)** the presence (*and nature*) of atrial activity (*pp 116-118*). That said — **definitive** diagnosis is *not* always possible from a single rhythm strip. Fortunately — *definitive* diagnosis is **usually *not* necessary** to initiate treatment of most SVTs (*page 121*).

• **IF** at *any* time the **patient *becomes* unstable** — then *immediately* cardiovert or defibrillate.

Step #1A: Is the SVT an Irregular Rhythm?

 Step #1A: *Is the SVT Irregular?*

● Once you *verify* that the rhythm is supraventricular — Try to **define** the *type* of **SVT**. Assessing an SVT for *regularity* (*or lack thereof*) — is a *KEY* part of the process.

• IF the SVT is clearly *irregular* — Think *either* **AFib** (*if no P waves are present* — pp 125-132) — or **MAT** (*if multiple, different-looking* P waves *are seen* — pp 133-137).

● ***Other* forms** of ***irregular* SVTs** — are seen *less* often than AFib or MAT. The more common *other* forms include:
- Sinus rhythm with *frequent* PACs.
- Atrial Flutter with a *variable* ventricular response.
- A *regular* SVT that is <u>either</u> preceded <u>or</u> followed by a *brief* period of irregularity (*usually from PACs*).

▶ **Bottom Line:** *Think* **AFib** when you see an irregular *narrow-QRS* tachycardia without clear P waves.

- Lack of any P waves on a **12-lead tracing** *confirms* that the *irregularly* irregular rhythm is AFib.

Step 1B: *Is the SVT Regular?* (LIST #2)

☞ **Step #1B:** *Is the SVT Regular?*

● IF the rhythm is a **regular narrow QRS Tachycardia** <u>without</u> normal atrial activity (ie, *no clear upright P wave in lead II*) — then the principal entities to consider in ***differential* diagnosis** are those noted in **LIST #2:**

Table 13-1:
Common causes of a *regular* SVT when sinus P waves are *not* clearly evident.

LIST #2: Common Causes of a ***Regular* SVT**
(*<u>without</u>* sign of *normal* atrial activity)

1. **Sinus Tachycardia** — will rarely exceed a rate of 160-170/minute in an adult. (*Treat the underlying cause of Sinus Tach!*)
2. **Atrial Flutter** — most often has a ventricular rate *close* to 150/minute.
3. **PSVT** (*or AVNRT*).

☞ ***KEY* Points *about* LIST #2 (*Table 13-1*):**

We emphasize the following points about List #2:
- In our experience — one of the 3 entities noted in <u>List #2</u> will turn out to be the diagnosis for 90-95% of ***regular* SVT rhythms** when normal sinus P waves are not seen (*automatic atrial and junctional tachycardias are far less common — esp. if the patient is <u>not</u> digoxin-toxic*).
- **AFib** is ***not* included** in the differential for <u>List #2</u> (*because AFib is <u>not</u> a "regular" SVT rhythm!*).
- ***Junctional* Tachycardia** — most often occurs from digitalis toxicity. It is relatively *uncommon* outside of this setting (*it may be seen with acute MI; in very ill patients; and post-operatively*). The P wave in lead II is *negative* or *absent*, <u>and</u> the rate is usually *less* than 130/minute.
- ***Sinus* Tachycardia** — *rarely* exceeds **160-170/min** in adult patients (*may be >200/minute in children <u>or</u> >160/minute in adults during exercise*). This is <u>not</u> to say that you will never see sinus tachycardia in a non-exercising patient at a rate over 160-170/minute — <u>but</u>

rather to suggest that you consider *other* types of SVT rhythms when the rate is this fast.

- **Atrial** **Flutter** (*untreated*) — most often conducts at a ventricular rate *close* to **150/min** (*range ~140-160/min*). Be aware that <u>IF</u> the patient is on antiarrhythmic drugs — the rate of AFlutter may be *slower*.
- **PSVT** — is **likely** <u>IF</u> the **regular** SVT is **>170/minute** (*But the regular SVT rhythm could be <u>any</u> of the 3 possibilities in* <u>List #2</u> *if the rate is ≤160-170/minute*).

Step 2: *Which Regular SVT?*

☞ **Step #2:** *Which Regular SVT?*
— Working thru LIST #2 —

⬤ Let's revisit the rhythm we began this Section with in **Figure 13-4**. The patient was ill but *hemodynamically* stable with a BP = 120/80. Assume that a **12-lead ECG** *confirmed* that the QRS complex is *truly* narrow in *all* 12 leads.

- *Which* **regular** SVT is the most likely diagnosis?
- *Why* is this diagnosis most likely? – <u>and</u> – *What next?*

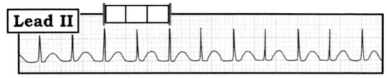

Figure 13-4: The patient is ill but *hemodynamically* stable. Which *regular* SVT rhythm from List #2 (*page 117*) is the *most* likely diagnosis?

☞ **Answer to Figure 13-4:** As discussed on page 114 — the rhythm in Figure 13-4 shows a regular *narrow* tachycardia <u>*without*</u> identifiable P waves at a rate ~200/minute.

- The differential diagnosis is as in **List #2** (*page 117*). That said — the **rate** of **~200/minute** makes sinus tachycardia <u>and</u> AFlutter both *highly* unlikely. By the process of elimination — the rhythm is *almost* certainly **PSVT**.
- <u>IF</u> the rate of the *regular* SVT in <u>Figure 13-4</u> would have been *less* than 170/minute — then we would <u>*not*</u> know which of the 3 entities in List #2 was the answer ...
- With regard to the question, *"What next?"* — One might at this point in this stable patient <u>either</u>: **i)** Try to confirm the diagnosis with use of a **vagal** *maneuver* (*See below*) — <u>and</u>/<u>or</u> **ii)** *Begin* treatment (*pg 120*).

Vagal Maneuvers: *To Diagnose/Treat SVT Rhythms*

☞ *Use of* **Vagal Maneuvers:**

⬤ *Vagal* maneuvers — are commonly used to *facilitate* ECG diagnosis – <u>and</u> – to treat certain arrhythmias. Vagal maneuvers produce a **tran-**

sient **increase** in ***parasympathetic* tone** (*thereby slowing AV conduction*). The maneuvers that are *most* often used are **carotid massage** (*CSM*) <u>and</u> **valsalva**.

☞ **C**arotid **S**inus **M**assage (*CSM*): — Always perform under **constant ECG monitoring**. Use the *right* carotid first. *Never* press on both carotids at the same time. Remember that the carotid sinus is located *high* in the neck at the angle of the jaw (*arrow in* <u>Figure 13-5</u>).
- Warn patient that the maneuver will be uncomfortable (*as very firm pressure sufficient to indent a tennis ball is needed*).
- Rub for <u>*no more*</u> than 3-5 seconds at a time.
- IF no response — may repeat CSM on the *left* side.
- *Don't* do CSM if patient has a carotid bruit (*you may dislodge a carotid plaque!*).

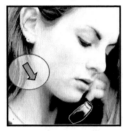

Figure 13-5: Carotid massage. Firm pressure is applied over the carotid sinus, which is located high in the neck at the angle of the jaw (*arrow*).

☞ ***Valsalva*** — Place patient in the *supine* position. Have patient forcibly exhale (*bear down*) against a closed glottis (*as it trying to go to the bathroom*) for up to 15 seconds at a time. IF properly performed — may be even *more* effective than CSM!
- Use of valsalva offers advantages over carotid massage of being safer (*no risk of dislodging a carotid plaque*) – <u>and</u> – of being a procedure that *selected* patients can be taught to do on their own.

▶ **NOTE:** There are *several* reasons for **constant ECG monitoring** during performance of any vagal procedure: **i)** Provides hard copy documentation of what was done; **ii)** Proves that you *only* pressed on the carotids for 3-5 seconds (*in the event that excessive bradycardia resulted*); <u>and</u> **iii)** Sometimes changes in the rhythm are subtle <u>and</u> are *only* evident *after* the procedure (*when the hard copy tracing is analyzed*).

☞ *Chemical* **Valsalva:** *Diagnostic Use of Adenosine*

The term, *"chemical Valsalva"* refers to use of **Adenosine** in management of an SVT rhythm of *uncertain* etiology. Given its rapid onset (*and rapid dissolution*) — the action of Adenosine is *similar* to application of a vagal maneuver. Thus, administration of Adenosine may convert PSVT <u>or</u> transiently *slow* the rate of other SVT rhythms — thereby allowing the diagnosis to be made (<u>**Figure 13-6**</u> — *page 120*).

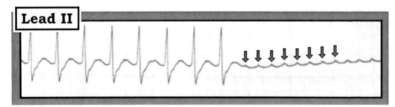

Figure 13-6: *Chemical* Valsalva. Administration of Adenosine to this patient with a regular SVT at ~150/minute results in transient *diagnostic* slowing that reveals underlying flutter waves at 300/minute. (*The continuation of this rhythm strip is shown in* Figure 13-7 — pg 122).

☞ *Usual* Response to *Vagal* Maneuvers

● Table 13.10-1 shows the usual response of various tachycardias to vagal maneuvers. A similar response would be expected with "chemical valsalva" (*from diagnostic/therapeutic use of Adenosine*):

Table 13-2:
Usual response to *vagal* maneuvers.

Usual Response to *Vagal* Maneuvers:
• **Sinus Tachycardia** — *gradual slowing* to CSM; *resumption* of tachycardia on *release* of pressure.
• **PSVT (or *AVNRT*)** — responds with *either* abrupt termination of PSVT (*and conversion to sinus rhythm*) – or – there is *no response* at all.
• **AFib or AFlutter** — CSM transiently *slows* the ventricular rate (*may facilitate rhythm diagnosis*).
• **Ventricular Tachycardia** — <u>no</u> response to CSM (*with rare exceptions of selected outflow track or fascicular VTs that surprisingly may respond ...*).

☞ Some ***Additional*** Points about *Vagal* Maneuvers:

• Like AV nodal blocking drugs (*such as verapamil-diltiazem-beta-blockers*) — a ***vagal* maneuver** would be expected to <u>either</u> abruptly **terminate** *AV-nodal-<u>dependent</u>* reentry arrhythmias (*such as PSVT*) — or have **no effect** at all.

• At times — ***reapplication*** of a ***vagal* maneuver** *after* administration of an AV nodal blocking drug (*such as diltiazem or a beta-blocker*) may work, whereas it did not work prior to giving the drug.

• For ***non-AV-nodal dependent* SVT rhythms** (*AFib/AFlutter — sinus tach — automatic atrial tachycardias*) — a ***vagal* maneuver** may transiently slow the rhythm <u>while</u> the maneuver is applied (*with resumption of tachycardia after CSM or valsalva is stopped*).

• *Avoid* vagal maneuvers with MAT (*which is clearly <u>not</u> an AV-nodal-dependent arrhythmia*).

Suggested Approach to SVT Rhythms

 ⇨ Suggested *Initial* Approach:

● What follows assumes you are relatively (*if not completely*) **certain** the tachycardia is an **SVT rhythm:**

- NOTE: IF at *any* time the patient *becomes* unstable — Treat electrically (*with cardioversion* or *defibrillation*).
- *As long as* **the patient** with an SVT **remains stable** — You have time to consider one or more of the actions below (*not necessarily in any particular sequence*).
- Actions below are divided between **diagnostic** and **therapeutic measures** (*as well as those that address both*).

☞ Get a **12-lead ECG** (*if you have not already done so*) — since *whatever* treatment you decide on will be *more* effective IF you can hone in on *specific* SVT diagnosis.
- *Verify* QRS width; look in all 12 leads for sign of atrial activity (*flutter waves; retrograde P waves; etc.*).

● **Fix** any *"Fixables"* that you can. Better than antiarrhythmic drugs is to *find* and *"fix"* any potential *precipitating* causes of the tachycardia as soon as you can. These may include:
- Electrolyte disturbance (*esp. low Mg++* or *K+*).
- Acidosis/Hypoglycemia.
- Hypoxemia.
- Shock (*from hypovolemia; blood loss; sepsis, etc.*).
- Uncontrolled ischemia/acute infarction.
- Acute heart failure.
- Dig toxicity/Drug overdose.

☞ *Consider* Use of a *Vagal* Maneuver

Whether or not to attempt a vagal maneuver at some (*usually early*) point in the diagnostic/therapeutic process depends on the comfort level, experience and preference of the treating clinician. Advantages of a vagal maneuver are that it may facilitate diagnosis, convert some cases of PSVT *and/or* augment the effect of drug treatment (*pp 118-120*).

☞ Use of Adenosine for SVT Rhythms

Consider *empiric* use of **Adenosine**. This drug is well tolerated by most patients. It will convert *most* PSVT – and – it usually produces transient *slowing* of other SVT rhythms (*which may be diagnostic*).
- *Adenosine* **DOSING:** Begin with **6mg** by **IV push.** IF no response in 1-2 minutes — Give **12 mg** by IV push.
- ACLS-PM *no longer* recommends giving a second 12mg bolus if the patient has not responded to the first two doses (*of 6mg +12mg*).

• ***Clinical* Note:** We now appreciate that conversion of tachycardia to sinus rhythm with Adenosine does <u>*not*</u> prove a *supraventricular* etiology. This is because ~5-10% of VT rhythms will respond to Adenosine — especially for VTs that occur in relatively *younger* adults *without* significant underlying heart disease when the QRS complex during VT is *not* overly wide (*pp 60-61*).

▶ **PEARL:** Dosing protocols for use of Adenosine should <u>*not*</u> necessarily be *fixed* for all adults. Instead — it is well to be aware of occasional instances when *higher* <u>or</u> *lower* doses of the drug are indicated.

• ***Lower* Adenosine doses** (ie, *2-3mg initially*) — should be considered for older patients; those with renal failure; heart failure; shock; in transplant patients; if taking dipyridamole (*Persantine*) – and/<u>or</u> – when Adenosine is given by central IV line.

• ***Higher* Adenosine doses** — may be needed for patients taking theophylline (*or for those consuming large amounts of caffeine*) — since methylxanthines impede binding of adenosine at its receptor sites.

☞ *Adverse* Effects of Adenosine

   Adenosine is <u>*not*</u> totally benign. Although the drug is usually fairly well tolerated — a series of adverse effects is common <u>and</u> *expected* !

• ***Adverse* effects** may include: **i)** chest pain; **ii)** cough (*from transient bronchospasm*); **iii)** cutaneous vasodilation; **iv)** metallic taste; **v)** a sense of "impending doom"; <u>and</u> **vi)** transient bradycardia that may be marked (*and which may even cause a brief period of asystole*).

• The "good news" — is that *adverse* effects **most often resolve <u>*within*</u> 1 minute** — although this may be *very* alarming in the meantime <u>IF</u> the clinician is not aware of what to expect (<u>Figure 13-7</u>).

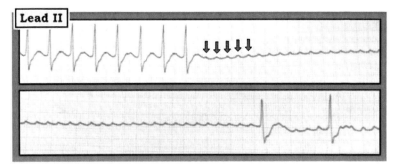

Figure 13-7: *Chemical* Valsalva (*continuation of Fig. 13-6 from pg 120*). Administration of Adenosine was *diagnostic* of the etiology of this *regular* SVT rhythm (*revealing underlying AFlutter at ~300/minute*). In so doing — a period of *over* 10 seconds ensued *without* a QRS complex. *Marked* bradycardia such as this is a *not uncommon* following Adenosine. Bradycardia almost always resolves *within* 30-60 seconds (*Adenosine half-life following IV administration is less than 10 seconds!*).

▶ **NOTE:** Some clinicians choose to *look away* for 20-30 seconds after giving Adenosine — so as not to be bothered by the transient marked rate slowing that so often is seen ...
- While *not* suggesting you do this — it is well to be aware that *marked rate slowing (as in* <u>Figure 13-7</u>*) may transiently* occur.

- ***Final* NOTE:** Adenosine may *shorten* the refractory period of *atrial* tissue — which could initiate AFib in a predisposed individual. As a result — Adenosine should be used with caution in patients with known WPW, given theoretic possibility of inducing AFib (*which could have significant consequence in a patient with accessory pathways*).

☞ Use of Diltiazem for SVT Rhythms

Consider *empiric* **use** of **IV Diltiazem**. Once you have established that the tachycardia is an SVT — treatment by IV Diltiazem **bolus** <u>and</u> **infusion** may be *invaluable* for rate slowing/conversion/maintenance of effect.

- ***Never*** use Verapamil/Diltiazem to treat a **WCT** (*wide QRS tachycardia*) — <u>unless</u> you are 100% certain of a *supraventricular* etiology. This is because the *negative* inotropic and *vasodilatory* effect of these drugs may facilitate *deterioration* of VT to lethal VFib.
- That said — Calcium blockers (*Verapamil/Diltiazem*) may convert *some* forms of **outflow-track** or **fascicular** *VT* (*pp 92-93*). Use of these drugs for this purpose is an *advanced* topic (<u>not</u> *recommended here in the acute setting*).
- Verapamil and Diltiazem have similar antiarrhythmic effects. **We *favor* Diltiazem** — because of greater physician familiarity with this drug plus longterm established use of a formulation for IV infusion.

● **DOSING:** — Begin with **15-20mg IV Diltiazem** (*0.25 mg/kg*) as an *initial* IV bolus; give over a 2 minute period.
- <u>IF</u> no response in 15 minutes — may give a 2nd IV bolus of **~25mg** (*0.35 mg/kg*).
- Use *lower* bolus **doses** (*given slower*) for lighter, older, or frail patients (ie, *10-15 mg over 3-4 minutes*).

- **Diltiazem <u>IV INFUSION</u> Rate:** Begin at **10mg/hour**. Titrate dose as needed (*usual range ~5-15 mg/hour*).

- <u>IF</u> *extreme* bradycardia is produced after giving Diltiazem — may treat with **Calcium** Chloride (*250-500mg by slow IV over 5-10 minutes; may repeat*) – <u>or</u> – with **IV Glucagon** (*5-10mg IV; may repeat in 3-5 minutes*).
- Many **oral forms** exist using Diltiazem (*range ~90-360 mg/day*) – <u>or</u> – Verapamil (*range ~120-480mg/day*).

☞ **Use of Beta-Blockers for SVT Rhythms**

Consider a **Beta-Blocker**. Clinically — β-blockers may exert *similar* AV-nodal *blocking* effects as Verapamil/Diltiazem (*albeit by a slightly different mechanism*).

- **Beta-blockers** tend to be most effective treating arrhythmias influenced by excess **sympathetic tone** (ie, *stress; anxiety; underlying sinus tachycardia; post-operative state*).
- Acutely — *many* emergency care providers favor use of IV Diltiazem for *initial* treatment of SVTs (*perhaps because of its ease of use* — page 123). That said — a case can be made for use of a Beta-blocker instead.
- The two agents (*β-blocker + Diltiazem*) can be used together for *synergistic* effect on AV conduction — which may be very helpful in *selected* SVT rhythms.

▶ ***KEY* Point:** Do *not* give an IV β-blocker together with IV Diltiazem/Verapamil (*because excessive bradycardia or even asystole may result*). However — You *can* give IV Diltiazem to a patient already taking an *oral* beta-blocker (*or add oral β-blocker after IV Diltiazem*).

● **Esmolol** (*Brevibloc*): — Give an initial **IV loading dose** (*of 250-500 mcg/kg*) over a 1-minute period. Follow this with a 4-minute infusion at 25-50 mcg/kg/minute.

- IF desired response is *not* obtained — titrate the rate of infusion upward (*by 25-50 mcg/kg/minute*) at 5-10 minute intervals (*up to 200 mcg/kg/minute*). Watch hypotension.

Other IV β-blockers exist (*there are many oral forms*):

- **IV Metoprolol** — Give 5 mg IV over 5 minutes; may repeat.
- **PO Metoprolol** — Begin with 25mg PO Bid (*increasing as needed up to 100 mg Bid*).
- **PO Atenolol** — Begin with 25-50 mg PO daily (*up to 100-200 mg/day*).

Section 14 – SVT *Practice* Tracings (*pp 125-162*)

 SVT *Practice*

● We reinforce principles discussed in Section 13 (*pp 114-124*) with a series of **SVT** (*SupraVentricular Tachycardia*) ***Practice* Examples** ...
• Basic concepts in *Rhythm Diagnosis* were discussed in Section 02 — in which we reviewed clinical application of the **Ps,Qs,3R Approach** (*page 21*). *Feel free to refer back to Sections 02 and 13 as needed.*

SVT *Practice* Tracing #1 (*AFib* — pp 125-132)

 ➡ PRACTICE Tracing:

● The patient is a *hemodynamically* stable adult who presents to the ED with the rhythm strip shown below. The **QRS** is *confirmed* to be **narrow** on 12-lead ECG.
• *What* is the Rhythm?
• Clinically – *What* should you do next?

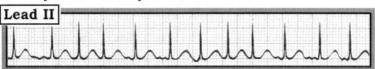

Figure 14-1: The patient is stable. What is the rhythm? *What next?*

☞ **Answer to SVT Tracing #1:** The rhythm in Figure 14-1 is rapid and *irregularly* irregular *without* P waves. The QRS is narrow. This is **AFib** (*Atrial Fibrillation*) — shown here with a **rapid ventricular response**.
• AFib is an *irregularly* irregular rhythm *lacking* P waves. Undulations in the baseline (*from the fibrillating atria*) are sometimes seen (*Note fine **"fib waves"** in parts of Figure 14-1*).

KEY Points: *ECG Diagnosis of AFib*

 ECG Diagnosis:

When "fib waves" are absent — the diagnosis of AFib is more difficult to make. In such cases — it is the *irregular* irregularity in the _absence_ of P waves in any of the 12 leads that by default leads to the diagnosis of AFib.
• Whenever in doubt about the rhythm diagnosis of a hemodynamically stable patient — ***Get a 12 lead!*** This is particularly true when contemplating the possibility of AFib (**Figure 14-2**).

- As will be seen with discussion of the *next* Practice Tracing (*on page 133*) — use of a **12-lead ECG** will often be essential for ruling out the possibility that an irregular rhythm might be MAT (*Multifocal Atrial Tachycardia*).

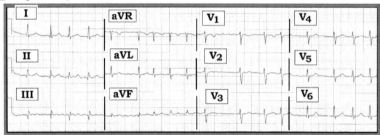

Figure 14-2: 12-lead ECG from a patient in AFib with a *relatively* rapid ventricular response. Although it almost looks like P waves are present in lead II — close inspection of other leads reveals that this is *not* the case. Fib waves *are* evident in leads III, aVF and V1. It is the *absence* of P waves and overall *irregularity* of this rhythm that *confirms* the diagnosis of AFib. This tracing provides an excellent example of how *all* 12 leads will sometimes be needed to be sure that the diagnosis is AFib.

☞ AFib: *Defining the Ventricular Response*

Depending on the rate — the ***ventricular* response** of **AFib** is said to be: **i) rapid** (*if the rate averages over 120/minute — as in* Figure 14-1 *on page 125 —* and *also for* **Tracing A** *below in* Figure 14-3); **ii) controlled** (*rate ~70-110/minute — as in* **Tracing B** *below*); or **iii) slow** (*rate less than 50-60/minute as in* **Tracing C** *below*).

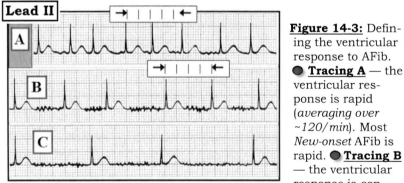

Figure 14-3: Defining the ventricular response to AFib. ● **Tracing A** — the ventricular response is rapid (*averaging over ~120/min*). Most *New-onset* AFib is rapid. ● **Tracing B** — the ventricular response is controlled (*between 70-110/minute*). Attaining rate control is one of the principal goals of treating *new-onset* AFib. ● **Tracing C** — the ventricular response is slow (*less than 50-60/minute*). New-onset *slow* AFib is unusual — and should suggest a *different* set of diagnostic considerations (*pp 127-128*). **NOTE:** There are *"fib waves"* that are coarse in B; fine in C; and barely detectable in A.

▶ **NOTE:** Far better than simply saying the rhythm is "AFib" — is to clarify to your colleague that AFib is conducting with either a rapid, controlled, or slow ventricular response. Most *new-onset* AFib presents with a **rapid** (*or at least relatively rapid*) **ventricular response**.

- Since by definition the rate of AFib varies from beat-to-beat — a period of monitoring may be needed to optimally define rapidity of the ventricular response.

☞ *Rapid* AFib: *Distinction from PSVT*

When AFib is rapid — the irregularity in the rhythm may be subtle. As a result — AFib may sometimes *simulate* PSVT (<u>Figure 14-4</u>).

- Close inspection of the rhythm (*including measurement with calipers*) may be needed to detect the irregular *irregularity* of rapid AFib.

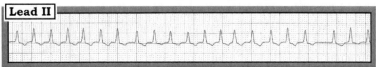

Figure 14-4: Rapid AFib. It is easy to see how the initial part of this tracing might be mistaken for PSVT. It is not until the end of this rhythm strip that its irregularity becomes readily apparent. That said — measurement with **calipers** of the initial portion of this rhythm strip *confirms* that the irregular irregularity <u>is</u> in fact present throughout.

KEY *Clinical* Points: *Regarding AFib*

☞ **KEY** *Clinical* **Points:**

● **AFib** — is the most common *sustained* cardiac arrhythmia (*far more common than AFlutter*). The frequency of AFib continues to increase as the population ages (*seen in up to ~10% of patients over 80 years old*).

- The most *common* ventricular response to *new-onset* AFib is rapid (*Tracing A in* <u>Figure 14-3</u>). **KEY** *Clinical* **Priorities** are to: **i)** *Find* the **cause** of **AFib**; **ii)** *Fix* the **cause** of AFib (*if possible*); **iii)** *Slow* the rate; **iv)** *Convert* the rhythm; <u>and</u> **v)** *Prevent* **thromboembolism**.

- The reason we suggest *considering* these 5 clinical priorities in the **sequence** we list them — is that <u>IF</u> you can *"find and fix"* the cause of *new-onset* AFib — then you may as a result slow the rate, convert the rhythm <u>and</u> reduce the chance of stroke (ie, <u>IF</u> *the cause of AFib is heart failure – then diuresis may facilitate conversion*).

☞ New-Onset *Slow* AFib

It is unusual for *new-onset* AFib to present with a **slow ventricular response** (*average rate less than 50-60/minute*). When this is seen

(*Tracing C in* <u>Figure 14-6</u> *on page 126*) — it should prompt a *different* set of diagnostic considerations. These include:

- Use of **rate-slowing drugs** (*digoxin; β-blockers; verapamil/diltiazem; amiodarone; sotalol; clonidine; various herbal preparations*). Ask about all pills that the patient is taking — including herbal preparations (*you may need to look up specific preparations to find out which ones may be rate slowing*). Be sure to also enquire about glaucoma eye drops (*β-blocker eye drops are in part systemically absorbed — and may sometimes produce significant rate-slowing*).
- **Acute ischemic heart disease** (*from ischemia/infarction; acute coronary syndrome*). Recent infarction may present with *slow* AFib *without* any history of chest pain.
- **Hypothyroidism** (*an uncommon but important and very treatable cause of new-onset slow AFib*).
- **SSS** (*Sick Sinus Syndrome*) — which can *only* be diagnosed after drugs, ischemia, and hypothyroidism have all been ruled out. Almost by definition — a patient older than 60-70 years old who presents with new-onset *slow* AFib, but who is <u>not</u> on any rate-slowing drugs — has *no* acute or recent ischemia — <u>and</u> has *normal* thyroid function — will have SSS.

☞ AFib *Clinical* Points: *Common Causes of AFib*

⬤ There are many *potential* causes of AFib. The 3 *most* common are:
- Heart failure/cardiomyopathy.
- Acute ischemic heart disease (*acute MI/acute coronary syndrome*).
- Hypertension (*especially when longstanding*).

Among the many other potential causes of AFib are the following:
- Valvular heart disease.
- Hyper/hypothyroidism;
- Drugs (*cocaine, sympathomimetics*).
- Pulmonary embolus / Hypoxemia
- Other *significant* medical illness
- Sick sinus syndrome.
- Finally — **"Lone" AFib** (*See below*).

☞ What is *"Lone"* AFib ?

The term, "lone" AFib — is applied to those patients who develop AFib <u>despite</u> having an *otherwise* "normal" heart. This occurs in approximately 10-20% of patients with AFib, although the *true* incidence really depends on one's definition of *'lone'* AFib <u>and</u> patient characteristics of the population studied.

- The precise **definition** of **"lone AFib"** varies among experts. The definition we prefer is: AFib in a patient *not more* than 50-60 years old who has *no* underlying heart disease (*not even hypertension*) — <u>and</u> *no* thyroid disease or diabetes. A **normal** Echocardiogram <u>and</u> **normal *thyroid* function** studies are essential to our definition.

- Our reasons for preferring this definition for *"lone AFib"* — is that it selects out a **low-risk group** for **thromboembolism** (*stroke*). This greatly simplifies discussion on the need for chronic anticoagulation. The risk for stroke in patients with *true* "lone AFib" is well *under* 1%/year — which is significantly *less* than the ~5%/year risk for other *nonvalvular* AFib patients. Patients with *true* "lone AFib" can probably be treated with **aspirin *alone***. While risk for stroke might be further reduced by longterm anticoagulation (*with either Coumadin or other new anticoagulants*) — potential for harm from longterm anticoagulation probably counters any potential for benefit by stroke reduction in this already very *low-risk* group. Therefore — comparable outcome is attained by aspirin alone ...

- The reason for ***limiting* age** to between 50-60 years old in our definition of "lone AFib" — is that risk of thromboembolism increases dramatically as patients get older. Marked increase in stroke risk especially begins at 60-65 years of age — such that even in the absence of underlying heart disease, adults over 60-65 years old with chronic AFib clearly benefit from longterm anticoagulation. Dropping the age range for our "lone AFib" definition to under 60 *minimizes* any increase in stroke risk from age alone.

- The reason for ***excluding* patients with **hypertension** from our low-risk group — is that longstanding BP (*blood pressure*) elevation results in structural and functional change in the heart. This is the entity of ***"diastolic dysfunction"***. As a result of chronic BP elevation — the LV (*left ventricle*) becomes thicker and stiffer (*less compliant*). A thicker and stiffer LV does not fill nearly as well in diastole as a normal-sized compliant LV. This produces an increase in LA (*left atrial*) pressure, and ultimately in LA size — as passive diastolic LV filling that normally occurs *early* in diastole (*as soon as the mitral valve opens*) is impeded.

- Instead of the normal 5-10% contribution of the ***"atrial kick"*** to cardiac output — in patients with *longstanding* hypertension, increased LV filling pressures *delay* LV filling during diastole. It is only *late* in diastole with atrial contraction (*at the time of the atrial kick*) that LA pressures finally rise enough to complete diastolic LV filling. The "atrial kick" may contribute as much as 30-40% to cardiac output in patients with diastolic dysfunction from chronic hypertension. This explains why such patients with chronic hypertension may *rapidly* decompensate if they suddenly *lose* their atrial kick due to development of *new-onset* AFib.

- ***Diastolic* dysfunction** is easy to diagnose on **Echo**. One sees *concentric* hypertrophy (*comparably increased septal and LV posterior walls*) with LA dilatation <u>and</u> echo parameters indicative of delayed filling (*reduced E-to-A ratio*). LV function (*contractility*) is often preserved until late in the course. The problem is <u>not</u> with contraction. Instead — the problem is with LV *diastolic* filling that is impeded by LV thickening and stiffening from longstanding increased afterload of chronic hypertension.

Medical *Work-Up* of *New-Onset* AFib

The medical work-up of *new-onset* AFib is easy to remember <u>IF</u> one considers the list of likely *precipitating* causes of AFib. Thus, the workup should *at least* include:

- **12-lead ECG** — to *verify* the diagnosis of AFib <u>vs</u> MAT <u>or</u> PACs (*and to rule out acute MI/ischemia*).
- CBC — to rule out blood loss/anemia.
- Chem profile — to assess electrolytes (*K+/Mg++*).
- TSH — looking for hyper/hypothyroidism.
- **Chest X-Ray** — pulmonary disease? / Heart failure?
- O2 Sat — hypoxemia as a *contributing* factor?
- **ECHO** — as the best *noninvasive* test to identify an underlying *cause* of AFib. Echo may also help **predict** the **likelihood** of **successful cardioversion** (*less likely if the LA is overly large and greater than 45mm on Echo*). Finally, **stroke is *less* likely** — <u>IF</u> the LA is: **i)** *not* enlarged <u>and</u> **ii)** if LV function is normal (*information that may be helpful in cases when decision to anticoagulate is not clearcut*).

AFib: *Treatment Priorities*

 ➡ *Treatment* Priorities:

⬤ The overwhelming majority (~98-99%) of patients who present in AFib are *hemodynamically* stable. Given that most of the time the ventricular response of **new-onset** AFib will be **rapid** — the initial **treatment priority** will be to **slow** the **rate** (<u>Figure 14-5</u>).

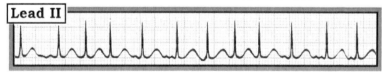

Figure 14-5: Repeat of the rhythm strip shown on page 125. Most of the time — *new-onset* AFib will be *rapid* <u>and</u> the patient will be *hemodynamically* stable. Slowing the rate is the *initial* treatment priority.

⬤ Initial *Rate-Slowing* of *Rapid* AFib:

Initial rate-slowing of *new-onset* rapid AFib is most commonly done in an ED setting with **IV Diltiazem** (*bolus and infusion — page 123*):
- **Diltiazem** — Give **~15-20 mg IV bolus**. IF no response — May follow in 15 minutes with a 2nd bolus (*of ~25mg IV*).
- May then start **IV infusion** at **10 mg/hour** to *maintain* rate control (*usual range ~5-15mg/hour range*).
- Alternatively — an **IV β-blocker** could be used *instead* of IV Diltiazem (*page 124*) — especially if increased *sympathetic* tone is a likely *contributing* cause of AFib.

- Be sure to **replace Mg++** and **K+** (*depletion of one or both of these electrolytes may exacerbate the arrhythmia*).
- Digoxin — is much *less* commonly used in 2013 than in the past (*though it may still help on occasion as a supplemental agent for AFib with acute heart failure*).

Clinical Perspective: *Is Acute Cardioversion Needed?*

 Clinical **Perspective:**

⬤ **Up to 50%** of *all* patients with **new-onset** AFib will **convert** to sinus rhythm **within 24 hours** (*even if no treatment is given*). A greater percentage will convert if treated (*especially* IF *the cause of AFib is found and corrected*).

- The above clinical reality provides a rationale for *not* reflexively trying to cardiovert all patients with *new-onset* AFib within the first few hours of their presentation *unless* the patient is: **i)** *very* symptomatic; or **ii)** *unstable* hemodynamically (*since many of these patients will be in sinus rhythm on their own within the next 24 hours ...*).
- *The need to emergently cardiovert new AFib is rare!* As stated — the overwhelming majority (>98-99%) of patients with *new-onset* rapid AFib are *hemodynamically* stable. This means there is usually time to attempt "finding *and* fixing" the precipitating cause – and – slowing the rate (*which can usually be done with medication*).

▶ **NOTE:** The issue in the ED is *not* whether *synchronized* cardioversion of *new-onset* AFib can be done (*because ED physicians are clearly capable of cardioverting*) — but rather whether or not it *should* be done, and, if so — for *which* patients. There are pros and cons on *both* sides of this debate that extend *beyond* the scope of the book.

- The above said — IF you do need to *emergently* cardiovert AFib (ie, *as might occur with new-onset rapid AFib and a large acute MI*) — realize that *higher* energy levels may be needed (*pp 54-56*).
- *Medical* **conversion** of **AFib** — is usually accomplished with agents such as Amiodarone – Sotalol – Flecainide – Propafenone – Ibutilide. This topic (*as well as the topic of elective electrical cardioversion in the ED* or *during the hospital stay*) extends beyond the scope of this book. Clinically — medical conversion of *new* AFib (*using drugs*) need *not* be started within the first few hours. There is almost always some time to allow for the effects of rate control and treatment of underlying (*potentially precipitating*) causes.
- PEARL: — Although *not* necessarily the most effective agent for *medical* conversion of AFib — **IV Amiodarone** conveys the *advantages* of: **i)** additional *AV-nodal-rate-slowing* effect (*if still needed for acute rate control*); and **ii)** the drug helps maintain sinus rhythm.
- *KEY* **Point:** — *Not* all patients with AFib should be converted to sinus rhythm. The *best* chance to achieve successful conversion and maintenance of sinus rhythm is with the **1st AFib episode** (*before atrial remodeling becomes established*). Realistically — it will *not* be

possible to convert many patients with *longstanding* AFib. In many cases (ie, *when it is unlikely that sinus rhythm can be maintained*) — it may be better <u>not</u> to try.

• **EP (**<u>E</u>lectro<u>P</u>hysiology**) Referral** — Recent years have seen amazing developments in the field of EP cardiology. Ablation of the initiating AFib focus has resulted in "cure" of a surprising number of even chronic AFib patients. In 2013 — the *problematic* AFib patient should be considered for EP referral.

☞ Anticoagulation of Patients with AFib

The risk of stroke in patients with *chronic* AFib is clearly reduced by longterm anticoagulation (*~60-70% reduction in stroke risk*). Use of Coumadin or *one* of the newer anticoagulants for patients with nonvalvular AFib is clearly more effective than use of aspirin alone. As a result — *virtually* all patients with *persistent* AFib should be anticoagulated <u>unless</u>: **i)** there is reason not to anticoagulate; <u>or</u> **ii)** the patient has *"lone AFib"* <u>and</u> is therefore *very low* risk of stroke (*in which case aspirin alone may be adequate — pp 128-129*).

• It is therefore important (*as soon as you are able*) to address the issue of anticoagulation in patients with new-onset AFib — although acute *rate-control* measures should be initiated first.

• Because of potential risk for stroke — *elective* synchronized cardioversion in the ED is <u>not</u> advised <u>unless</u>: **i)** the patient is *adequately* anticoagulated; <u>or</u> **ii)** one is relatively certain that AFib onset is *less* than 24-48 hours old (*risk of post-cardioversion stroke increases greatly in AFib of longer duration*).

SVT *Practice* Tracing #2 (*MAT*— pp 133-137)

➡ PRACTICE Tracing:

● The patient is a *hemodynamically* stable adult who presents to the ED with the rhythm shown in Figure 14-6. The **QRS** is *confirmed* to be **narrow** on 12-lead ECG.
• *What* is the Rhythm? Clinically — *What* should you do next?

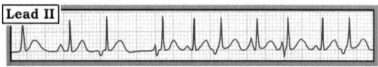

Lead II

Figure 14-6: Why is this *irregular* rhythm *not* AFib?

 Answer to SVT Tracing #2: The rhythm in Figure 14-6 is rapid and *irregularly* irregular. The QRS is narrow. That said, this is **not AFib** — because there *are* P waves. Instead — the rhythm is **MAT** (*Multifocal Atrial Tachycardia*).
• **MAT** — is characterized by the features inherent in its name: there are **multiple** forms of **atrial** activity at a rapid (**tachycardia**) rate. Note constantly varying shape of P waves in Figure 14-6.

KEY Points: *ECG Diagnosis of MAT*

ECG Diagnosis:

● In our experience — **MAT** is the 2nd most **commonly overlooked** cardiac arrhythmia (*next to AFlutter*). MAT is easy to overlook — because the overwhelming majority of sustained *irregular* SVT rhythms seen will turn out to be AFib (*Atrial Fibrillation*).
• MAT is *not* AFib.

The *best* way to *avoid* overlooking **MAT** is to *think* of this diagnosis *whenever* you see an irregularly *irregular* rhythm in *either* of the **2 common *clinical* settings** in which **MAT** is likely to occur:
• *Clinical* Setting #1: **Pulmonary** disease (*COPD; longterm asthma, pulmonary hypertension*);
• *Clinical* Setting #2: **Acutely ill** patients (ie, *with sepsis; shock; electrolyte and/or acid-base disorders*).

▶ **PEARL:** Be sure to *always* obtain a **12-lead ECG** (*and to search for P waves in all 12 leads*) — whenever you are contemplating the diagnosis of MAT. The *multiple* P wave morphologies characteristic of MAT will *not* always be appreciated if only a *single* monitoring lead is used (*See* **Figure 14-7** *on page 134*).

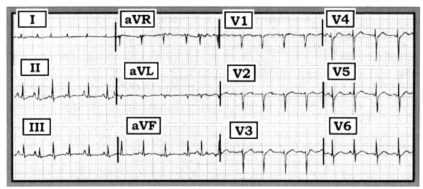

Figure 14-7: 12-lead ECG from a patient with longstanding *pulmonary* disease and MAT. Multiple and varied P wave morphology is obvious in lead II. That said — it is easy to see how this irregular rhythm might be mistaken for AFib IF monitoring was performed from a *single* lead in which P waves are *not* readily seen. Thus, there is no indication that the rhythm is MAT from inspection of leads I; V1,V2,V3 — and the inferior leads are really the only place where *beat-to-beat* change in P wave morphology is readily apparent.

☞ MAT vs Sinus Tachycardia with *Multiple* PACs

Rather than a discrete entity — it is best to think of AFib and MAT as **two ends** of a **spectrum**. On the one hand is **AFib** — in which there are *no* P waves at all in any of the 12 ECG leads. The atria are fibrillating (*usually at ~400-600/min*) — and, as a result produce **"fib wave"** **oscillations** of varying size (*usually quite small*) in random fashion.

- **MAT** — is at the *other* end of the spectrum. P waves *are* present — but they are completely *random* in their appearance and *varied* in morphology (*consistent with our understanding that these P waves arise from multiple irritable atrial foci*). Another name that was previously used for MAT (*chaotic atrial mechanism*) is wonderfully descriptive of the ongoing pathology.

● The rhythm in **Figure 14-8** illustrates middle ground. We interpret this *irregular* SVT rhythm as **Sinus** Tachycardia with *multiple* **PACs.**

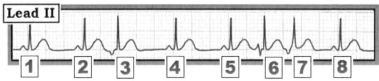

Figure 14-8: Sinus tachycardia with PACs. This irregular SVT rhythm is *not* MAT because underlying sinus rhythm is present (*See text*).

☞ **Interpretation of Figure 14-8:** As opposed to MAT (*in which the P wave erratically and continually changes from beat-to-beat*) — with

***Sinus* Tach _and_ PACs** — there _is_ an *underlying* sinus rhythm with *intermittent* periods of the *same* sinus P wave appearing *consecutively* for at least a few beats in a row.

- Note similar P wave morphology (*and similar PR interval*) for beats #1,2,4,5, and 8 in Figure 14-8. These are the P waves of the **underlying sinus rhythm** in this tracing.

- The *irregularity* in Figure 14-8 is produced by the **multiple PACs** that are present (*beats #3,6,7*). Note variation in P wave morphology for these PACs. That said — clear indication of *underlying* sinus rhythm suggests that the rhythm in Figure 14-8 is _not_ MAT.

- Realize that **Figure 14-8** represents no more than a *"snapshot"* of what is occurring clinically. This is merely a **4-second rhythm strip**. True appreciation for the real degree of variation in rate and P wave morphology can only be determined by a longer period of monitoring.

⬤ Many possibilities exist for "middle ground" *irregular* SVT rhythms that are *neither* AFib *nor* strict definition of MAT. For example — rhythms otherwise suggestive of being "MAT" are not always "tachycardic". Moreover — the point of transition between sinus rhythm with multiple *different-shaped* PACs into "MAT" is often elusive.

- Most of the time — it will be obvious when the rhythm is sinus tachycardia with PACs. That said — it may at times be difficult (*impossible*) to distinguish between **MAT** vs *Sinus* Tach _with_ PACs.

- The "good news" — is that clinically it does _not_ matter which of the two are present. This is because *clinical* implications of MAT vs Sinus Tach *with* multiple PACs are the same when _either_ rhythm is seen in a patient with one of the clinical settings *predisposing* to MAT (*page 133*). In either case — priority rests with identifying and treating the underlying disorder (*page 136*).

▶ ***Final* Caveat:** — MAT is **_not_** a **wandering pacemaker** (*in which there is gradual shift in P wave morphology* — *rather than a different-looking P wave from one beat to the next*). Wandering pacemaker is often a *normal* variant. MAT is *anything but* a "normal" variant (*See below*).

🖙 Wandering Pacer: *Different from MAT*

⬤ Wandering atrial pacemaker is often confused with MAT. The two entities are _not_ the same. As opposed to erratic *beat-to-beat* change in P wave morphology (*as occurs with MAT*) — there is **gradual change** with wandering pacer over a period of several beats as the site of the atrial pacemaker shifts to two or more additional sites in the atria. We illustrate this with the example of ***wandering* atrial pacemaker** shown on the top of the *next* page (Figure 14-9 — *on page 136*):

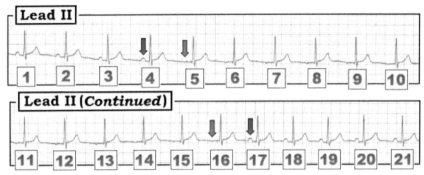

Figure 14-9: Wandering pacemaker. There is *gradual* change in P wave morphology as the site of the atrial pacemaker changes. Initially the P wave in lead II is an upright sinus complex (*1st arrow preceding* **beat #4**) — with *gradual* change to an isoelectric P wave (*2nd arrow that precedes* **beat #5**) — followed followed by eventual *resumption* of sinus rhythm with **beat #17** toward the end of the bottom tracing. Note that there is minimal change in heart rate throughout the rhythm strip.

▶ *Beyond-the-Core:* It should be apparent from <u>Figure 14-9</u> that a more *extensive* period of monitoring would really be needed to definitively diagnose "wandering pacemaker". <u>Technically</u> — Figure 14-9 does <u>not</u> qualify, because only two different atrial sites are seen. Nevertheless, we use this illustration because it highlights *gradual* **change** from one P wave morphology (*upright for beats #1,2,3,4 and #17,18,19,20,21*) to another (*isoelectric P wave for beats #5-thru-16*).

Wandering Pacemaker is *Often* a *Normal* Variant
⬤ Wandering pacemaker is often a *normal* variant rhythm (*pp 26-27*) — especially when it occurs in otherwise healthy individuals *without* underlying heart disease.
• In contrast — Patients with MAT almost invariably have significant comorbid conditions (*especially pulmonary disease and/or multisystem problems*).
• MAT and wandering pacer represent two ends of a spectrum. In a sense — MAT is simply a "wandering pacemaker" with a *rapid* rate <u>and</u> *beat-to-beat* change in P wave morphology. Clinical judgement (*with awareness of the patient's medical history*) will therefore be needed for assessment of *middle-ground* cases in which the rate is slower and P wave variation is intermediate between the two forms.

▶ **PEARL:** Wandering pacemaker is *easy* to overlook! The best way to avoid doing so is to **routinely** scrutinize a **long** lead II **rhythm strip** to ensure that P wave morphology and the PR interval are not subtly changing.

MAT: *Treatment Priorities*

 ➡ *Treatment* Priorities:

⬤ While treatment and clinical course are similar for MAT vs sinus rhythm with *multiple* PACs — It is important to distinguish these rhythms from AFib, which acts in a very different manner:

- AFib is by far more common. **MAT** almost always occurs in one of the **2** *clinical* **settings** discussed on page 133 (*pulmonary disease or acutely ill patients from multisystem disease*).
- The principal treatment priority of MAT is to identify and **correct** the **underlying** **disorder** (ie, *correct hypoxemia; sepsis; shock; low K+/Mg++; etc.*). IF this can be done — MAT will often resolve.
- *Drug* **treatment** will **usually** **_not_** be **needed** to slow the rate of MAT (*because the rate is typically not excessively fast — and the rhythm is usually fairly well tolerated*).
- IF medication is needed to slow the rate — Our preference is to use **IV Diltiazem** (*page 123*).
- Beta-blockers may be equally effective — but caution is advised if there is underlying *pulmonary* disease (*with bronchospasm that may be exacerbated by Beta–blockers*).
- Be sure to *optimize* **serum K+/Mg++** levels!
- *Avoid* Digoxin (*strong tendency for patients with MAT to develop digoxin toxicity*).

SVT *Practice* Tracing #3 (*PSVT* — pp 138-146)

➡ **PRACTICE** Tracing:

● The patient is a *hemodynamically* stable adult who presents to the ED with the rhythm shown below in Figure 14-10. The **QRS** is *confirmed* to be **narrow** on 12-lead ECG.

• *What* is the Rhythm? Clinically — *What* should you do next?

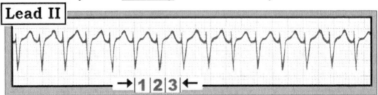

Figure 14-10: What is this rhythm likely to be? — *What next?*

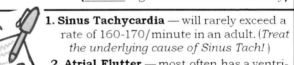 **Answer to SVT Tracing #3:** The rhythm in Figure 14-10 is rapid and regular. We are told that a **12-lead ECG *confirms* QRS narrowing** in all leads. The rate is just *under* 200/minute. No P waves are seen. We have therefore described a **regular** SVT *without* clear sign of normal atrial activity. This description should prompt consideration of the **3 entities** on **LIST #2** (Table 14-1 — *previously seen on page 117*):

▶ **NOTE:** Because the rate of the *regular* SVT in Figure 14-10 is very rapid (*well over 160/minute*) — **PSVT** (*Paroxysmal Supra-Ventricular Tachycardia*) is clearly the most *likely* diagnosis.

Table 14-1: Common causes of a *regular* SVT when sinus P waves are *not* clearly evident.

LIST #2: Common Causes of a **Regular** SVT
(*without* sign of *normal* atrial activity)

1. **Sinus Tachycardia** — will rarely exceed a rate of 160-170/minute in an adult. (*Treat the underlying cause of Sinus Tach!*)
2. **Atrial Flutter** — most often has a ventricular rate *close* to 150/minute.
3. **PSVT** (*or AVNRT*).

KEY Points: *ECG Diagnosis of PSVT*

📖 **ECG Diagnosis:**

● As discussed on page 117 — our purpose in developing **LIST #2** is that in our experience, one of the 3 entities on this list will turn out to be the diagnosis for 90-95% of **regular SVT rhythms** when normal sinus P waves are not seen (*automatic atrial and junctional tachycardias are far less common — especially if the patient is not digoxin-toxic*).

☞ Regarding the 3 entities in **List #2** (*page 138*) — Calculation of the ***rate*** of the *regular* SVT rhythm may greatly assist in determining the specific etiology.

> ▶ **PEARL:** Use of the ***Every-other-Beat* Method** (*page 33*) — facilitates calculation of heart rate when the rhythm is regular and the rate is fast. **Pick a QRS** that ***begins*** on a ***heavy* line** (*as does the S wave for the 6th beat in* Figure 14-10). **Measure** the **R-R interval** for ***every-other-beat*** — which is just *over* 3 large boxes. Thus, ***half*** the rate in Figure 14-10 is just *under* 100/minute — which means the ***actual*** rate is a bit ***below*** **200/minute** (*we estimate ~190/minute*).

☞ The rhythm in **Figure 14-10** provides an excellent example of how to ***narrow* down** one's differential diagnosis for the SVT rhythms:
- The fact that this **SVT** rhythm is ***regular*** — essentially *rules out* AFib and MAT as possibilities. This leaves us with the **3 most common causes** of a ***regular*** SVT to contemplate: **i)** Sinus tachycardia; **ii)** Atrial flutter; and **iii)** PSVT (*Table 14-1 on page 138*).
- Children may attain sinus tachycardia rates of 200/minute or more. A young adult (*in their 20s or 30s*) may attain sinus tachycardia rates of ~180/minute or more during vigorous exercise (ie, *running a 100-yard dash*). Outside of these two situations — it is *unlikely* for a patient presenting for medical attention to have sinus tachycardia at rates over 160-170/minute. It is also highly *unlikely* for AFlutter to present with a rate of 190/minute (*which is too slow in an untreated patient for AFlutter with 1:1 AV conduction — and too fast for AFlutter with 2:1 AV conduction*). This is why **PSVT** is *almost certainly* the diagnosis of the rhythm in Figure 14-10.

☞ The *Regular* SVT: *When the Rate is Close to 150/min*

● IF the rate of the *regular* SVT is *slower* than that in Figure 14-10 (*say, closer to 150-160/minute*) — then we would *not* be able to distinguish between the 3 entities in List #2. This is the case for the *regular* SVT rhythm shown below in **Figure 14-11**:

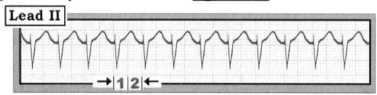

Figure 14-11: Regular SVT *without* sign of normal sinus P waves. Because the rate of this ***regular*** SVT is **~150/minute** — *Any* of the 3 entities in List #2 (*page 138*) might be present. Although we suspect PSVT (*since we see neither sinus P waves nor indication of flutter waves*) — there is *no way* to be certain of the diagnosis from this *single* monitoring lead. Other means (ie, *drugs, a vagal maneuver*) will be needed to determine which of the 3 entities in List #2 is present (*See text*).

KEY *Clinical* Points: *Regarding PSVT*

 KEY *Clinical* **Points:**

PSVT is a regular *supraventricular* tachycardia that most often occurs at a **rate** of **between** **150-to-240/minute**. Atrial activity is usually *not* evident — although *subtle* notching or a negative deflection (*representing retrograde atrial activity*) may at times be seen at the end of the QRS. Mechanistically — **PSVT** is a **reentry tachycardia** that almost always involves the AV node (*ergo the other name for this rhythm* = **AVNRT** = <u>A</u>V <u>N</u>odal <u>R</u>eentry <u>T</u>achycardia).

- The impulse *continues* to circulate *within* the AV node <u>until</u> the reentry pathway is either *interrupted* (ie, *by AV nodal blocking drugs* <u>or</u> *a vagal maneuver*) — or until it *spontaneously* stops (<u>Figure 14-12</u>).

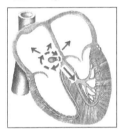

Figure 14-12: The *mechanism* of PSVT (*AVNRT*) is **AV nodal reentry**. As suggested in this figure, *each* time the impulse completes the reentry circuit — *retrograde* conduction (*back to the atria*) as well as *forward* conduction to the ventricles (*through the His-Purkinje system*) occurs. This *retrograde* conduction back to the atria can sometimes be seen on the ECG during tachycardia (*See text*).

PSVT: *The Clinical Importance of Reentry*

Awareness of reentry as the mechanism in PSVT is important diagnostically and therapeutically. It means that the arrhythmia is likely to be *self-perpetuating* <u>unless</u>/<u>until</u> *something* happens to interrupt the cycle.

- Think of 50 young children holding hands and running around in a circle. If someone sticks out their foot to trip one of the children — it is likely that *all* of the children will fall down... So it is with reentry. Interruption of the cycle for the briefest of moments (*by an AV-nodal-blocking drug or a vagal maneuver*) may be all that it takes to *break* the cycle and convert the rhythm.

PSVT: *Use of a Vagal Maneuver*

Use of a *vagal* maneuver may be helpful diagnostically <u>and</u> therapeutically in management of the SVT rhythms. Consider **Figure 14-13** (*on page 141*) — which is *continuation* of the rhythm strip shown in <u>Figure 14-10</u> on page 138 at the start of this section.

- What happens to the *regular* SVT in the beginning of <u>Figure 14-13</u> **after** the **arrow** when **CSM** (*Carotid Sinus Massage*) was applied?
- Is this an *expected* response?
- <u>HINT:</u> Feel free to refer back to <u>Table 13-2</u> (*page 120*) — regarding the usual response of SVT rhythms to vagal maneuvers.

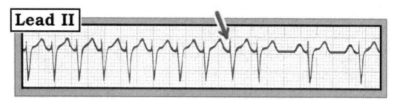

Figure 14-13: What happens *after* CSM (*arrow*)? Is this an expected response? (*See text*).

☞ **ANSWER to Figure 14-13:** PSVT typically responds to vagal maneuvers with *either* abrupt conversion to sinus rhythm – or – there is *no* response at all …

- *Abrupt* conversion to sinus rhythm is seen in Figure 14-13 shortly after CSM is applied (*Note sinus P waves after the arrow*).
- Do not be alarmed if several ventricular beats are initially seen right after a vagal maneuver. This almost always rapidly resolves.
- Realize that a vagal maneuver will *not* always work for PSVT. It is not uncommon for *nothing* to happen — in which case trial of an AV nodal *rate-slowing* drug may be in order (*page 145*).
- Sometimes *reapplication* of a vagal maneuver *after* administration of *rate-slowing* medication may be effective, whereas the vagal maneuver had no effect prior to giving the drug.

Beyond-the-Core: **Recognizing *Retrograde* P Waves with PSVT**

⇨ *Beyond-the-Core …*

● As a more *advanced* facet of this topic — Consider the situation in Figure 14-14. This 12-lead ECG was obtained from a *hemodynamically stable* patient with "palpitations". A **regular SVT rhythm** at ~150/min is seen. Normal sinus P waves are absent (ie, *there is no upright P wave preceding each QRS in lead II*). Instead — **retrograde atrial conduction** indicative of reentry is present. *Do you see the retrograde P waves?*
- *Which* leads in **Figure 14-14** manifest *retrograde* atrial activity *during* the tachycardia? — How does this help you clinically?

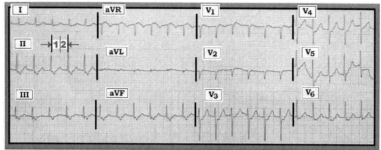

Figure 14-14: Regular SVT at ~150/minute. Which leads manifest *retrograde* P waves *during* the tachycardia? (*See text*).

☞ **ANSWER to Figure 14-14:** As illustrated previously in discussion of the rhythm in Figure 14-11 (*page 139*) — the differential diagnosis of a ***regular*** SVT at ~150/min ***without*** normal ***sinus*** P waves includes the 3 entities in **List #2** (*page 138*): **i)** Sinus tachycardia; **ii)** Atrial flutter; <u>and</u> **iii)** PSVT. When no atrial activity at all is seen (*as was the case in Figure 14-11*) — then the rhythm could be *any* of these 3 entities.

• ***Retrograde* P waves** <u>are</u> seen in *many* leads in Fig. 14-14. We highlight some of these *retrograde* P waves by **arrows** in **Figure 14-15**. Specifically — **negative *retrograde* P waves** are clearly seen in *each* of the inferior leads (*II,III,aVF*). Negative *retrograde* P waves account for angulation in the ST segment just prior to ascent of the T wave in lead V3 (*arrow in V3*) — and probably also in V4,V5,V6. In addition — **positive *retrograde* P waves** are clearly seen in leads aVR and V1 (*arrows in these leads*), and possibly also in aVL and V2.

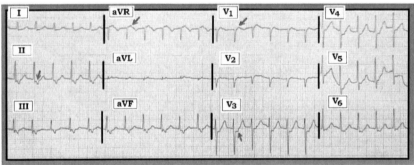

Figure 14-15: Arrows highlight *retrograde* atrial activity that was present in Figure 14-14 (*page 141*). Retrograde P waves are seen in virtually all leads in this tracing, except perhaps for lead I (*See text*).

☞ **Clinically** — the importance of recognizing retrograde atrial activity is twofold:
• It solidifies the diagnosis of ***reentry*** as the mechanism for the *regular* SVT rhythm in Figure 14-14. Knowing that P waves come *after* the QRS complex (*not before*) — <u>and</u> knowing there is only *one* P wave for each QRS *rules out* sinus tachycardia and AFlutter — therefore ***confirming*** PSVT as the diagnosis.
• Awareness of reentry as the mechanism for this *regular* SVT rhythm facilitates *decision-making* for management (*page 145*).

Way Beyond-the-Core:

☞ **Distinction *between* AVNRT *vs* AVRT**

Up until now — we have preferentially used the term, **"PSVT"** (<u>P</u>aroxysmal <u>S</u>upra<u>V</u>entricular <u>T</u>achycardia) to designate *regular* SVT rhythms with *reentry* as their underlying mechanism. The word ***"paroxysmal"*** was chosen because of the common *sudden* onset of these tachycardias (*often precipitated by a PAC, PJC, or PVC occurring at just the right moment in the cardiac cycle to initiate a circuit of self-perpetuating reentry in or around the AV node*). This reentry was schematically illustrated in <u>Figure 14-12</u> (*page 140*).

- A more accurate terminology distinguishes between **AVNRT** (*AV Nodal Reentry Tachycardia*) — in which the reentry circuit is contained within (*or just next to*) the AV node — <u>vs</u> **AVRT** (*AtrioVentricular Reciprocating Tachycardia*) — in which the reentry circuit extends further away *outside* of the AV nodal area to the vicinity of the atrioventricular valvular rings over an **AP** (*Accessory Pathway*).
- We have already discussed AVRT in Section 12 (*pp 107-109*) under the various SVT pathways in patients with WPW. The "good news" — is that most of the time it does <u>*not*</u> matter clinically in the *acute* situation whether the *true* mechanism of PSVT is **AVNRT** (*reentry over a small circuit within the AV node in a patient who does not have WPW*) – <u>vs</u> – **AVRT** (*reentry that extends outside the AV node involving a longer circuit that travels over an AP in a patient who has WPW*). This is because *initial* treatment measures are the same for AVNRT <u>and</u> AVRT when the QRS complex is narrow.
- ***Longterm* management** of the patient with **AVRT *may* differ** from that for AVNRT in certain regards. Patients with AVRT have an accessory pathway. There is therefore potential for sudden onset of *very rapid* supraventricular rates <u>IF</u> these patients develop atrial fibrillation or flutter (*pp 109-110*). In addition — patients with WPW who develop PSVT (*AVRT*) may occasionally manifest QRS widening with this supraventricular tachycardia IF conduction is antidromic (*first down the AP*) instead of orthodromic (*down the AV nodal-His-Purkinje system — then retrograde up the AP*). As discussed in Section 12 (*page 110*) — On those rare occasions when this happens, the QRS will be wide and the PSVT rhythm may be indistinguishable from VT. ● **Bottom** <u>**Line**</u>**:** Suspecting the presence of a *concealed* AP in a patient who presents with PSVT may *lower* one's threshold for **referral to** an **EP** cardiologist. **Ablation** of the AP is usually curative.

☞ We contrast the *usual* ECG picture of ***narrow-complex* AVNRT** <u>vs</u> **AVRT** in **<u>Figure 14-16</u>** shown below:

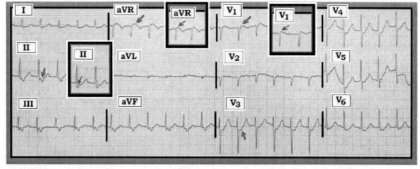

<u>Figure 14-16:</u> Comparison of *retrograde* R-P' intervals (*See text*).

● **QUESTIONS** regarding <u>Figure 14-16</u> (*on page 143*):
  • What is the *difference* in the **R-P' interval** for the arrows *within* the inserts in leads II,aVR,V1 — compared to the R-P' interval for the arrows *outside* the inserts in these leads?
  • <u>Clinically</u> — In which case would you suspect AVNRT as the mechanism? — In which case would you suspect AVRT?

☞ **ANSWER to Figure 14-16:** The **R-P' interval** (ie, *retrograde distance between the QRS complex and the retrograde P wave that follows*) — is clearly ***shorter*** for the P waves *within* the inserts:
  • PSVT due to **AVNRT** typically has a very *short* R-P' interval (*arrows within the inserts*). This is because the reentry circuit is contained either *within* or right *next to* the AV node. As a result — there is *less* distance for the impulse to travel during the reentry cycle. This is by far the most common situation for PSVT — in which *retrograde* atrial activity is either completely hidden within the QRS complex during tachycardia, or at most notches the most terminal aspect of the QRS (*as it does for the arrows within the inserts in Figure 14-16*).
  • In contrast — ***narrow-complex* AVRT** in a patient with WPW is more likely to manifest a *longer* R-P' interval (*arrows outside the inserts in Figure 14-16, as previously shown in* <u>Figure 14-15</u>). This is due to the *longer* distance the impulse must travel from the AV node to the AP during the reentry cycle.
  • **Clinical** *"Take-Home"* **Points:** Although the various mechanisms of AVNRT and AVRT rhythms are complex (*clearly extending Beyond-the-Core for many ACLS providers*) — Recognition of **retrograde** atrial **activity** during *narrow-complex* PSVT rhythms is <u>not</u> difficult once you become aware of what to look for. **Figure 14-16** compares the two common situations. In either case — recognition of retrograde P waves during PSVT **confirms** **reentry** (*and rules out sinus tachycardia and atrial flutter*) as the mechanism for the tachycardia. This facilitates initial clinical decision-making in treatment (*page 145*).
  • ***Beyond-the-Core:*** Recognition that the R-P' interval during PSVT is *longer* than expected (*extending to the middle of the ST segment*) suggests there may be a *concealed* AP (<u>Figure 14-15</u>). Our threshold for EP referral of such patients is lower.

▶ **PEARL:** It is good practice to *always* obtain a **12-lead ECG** <u>after</u> conversion of PSVT to sinus rhythm. Doing so sometimes facilitates *retrospective* detection of "telltale" *retrograde* atrial activity that may not have been readily apparent during tachycardia (*by carefully comparing the terminal portion of the QRS complex and ST-T wave during* <u>and</u> *after the tachycardia*).

  • **FINAL Note:** Other types of reentry supraventricular tachycardias exist (*beyond the scope of this book*). These include sophisticated *fast-slow* AVNRT, in which the retrograde P wave is negative in lead II with a *very long* R-P' interval. Suffice it to say that initial treatment measures as discussed on page 145 are usually effective in the acute situation.

PSVT: *Acute Treatment Priorities*

 ⇨ *Treatment* Priorities:

⬤ Although PSVT may occur in any population — it is often seen in otherwise *healthy* individuals. Patients with **PSVT** will *almost* **always** be *hemodynamically* **stable** (*exceptions include older patients with significant underlying heart disease and persistent PSVT*). As a result — *medical* **treatment** will *usually* be **effective** in the acute situation. Electrical cardioversion is only *rarely* necessary.

- Consider initial use of a *vagal* **maneuver** if no contraindications (ie, *Do not do carotid massage in an older patient in whom a carotid bruit is heard*). Some patients with PSVT are highly responsive to vagal maneuvers (*pp 118-121*).
- **Adenosine** — is a *drug of choice* for **PSVT** (*and* for SVT *of uncertain etiology that occurs in an ED or hospital setting*). Give **6mg IV** by rapid **IV push** (*over 1-3 seconds!*) — followed by a fluid flush. IF no response is seen after 1-2 minutes — a **2nd dose** (*of 12mg*) may be given. (*See also pp 121-123*).
- The *half-life* of **Adenosine** is *very* **short** (*less than 10 seconds*) — so PSVT may recur. As a result — consider the need for starting the patient on a *longer-acting* drug.
- *Other* **options** for treatment of PSVT include **Diltiazem** (*IV bolus and/or drip*) — or Verapamil — or a **β-blocker** (*IV or PO*). Selection of one of these agents may be made for PSVT or SVT of *uncertain* etiology that *either* occurs in- or out of the hospital. Oral forms of these drugs are used for PSVT that occurs in an ambulatory setting (*pp 123-124*).
- Use of an **anxiolytic** (ie, *a benzodiazepine*) — will often be helpful as an adjunct. In addition to attenuating anxiety that so often accompanies this highly symptomatic arrhythmia — anxiolytics may *reduce* sympathetic tone (*thereby slowing conduction down over a portion of the reentrant pathway*).
- Once the patient has been converted to sinus rhythm — *Minimize* or *eliminate* **potential precipitants** (ie, *caffeine; alcohol; cocaine; amphetamines; OTC sympathomimetic drugs including cough-cold preparations and diet pills — as well as psychological stress*).

PSVT: *Longterm Treatment Considerations*

Many patients with PSVT will experience recurrence of this arrhythmia. In some — episodes are infrequent. In others — PSVT may recur often. This brings up the issue of longterm management. Although complete discussion of this topic extends beyond the scope of this book — several basic concepts regarding longterm treatment issues can be stated:

- Identification and elimination of *precipitating* **factors** may sometimes be all that is necessary. The most common "culprit" is caffeine

— but *other* potential precipitants include *over-the-counter* sympatho-mimetics (*including cough-cold preparations and diet pills*), ampheta-mines, alcohol, cocaine, and psychologic stress.

- In general — PSVT is <u>not</u> a life-threatening arrhythmia. As a result — longterm treatment is *not* necessarily needed, especially in patient who only have infrequent episodes.

- In patients who continue to have frequent PSVT recurrence *despite* attempts at addressing potential precipitating factors — **daily use** of an **AV nodal blocking drug** (*diltiazem, verapamil, a β-blocker*) may be indicated. The dose required to minimize episodes may be titrated for each individual patient.

▶ **PEARL:** Surprisingly — no more than a very *low* dose of a beta-blocker may be all that is needed to prevent PSVT recurrence in patients for whom sympathetic tone plays a prominent causative role.

- **NOTE:** Maintenance therapy <u>need not</u> be daily in those patients who only have **intermittent episodes** every few months. Instead, in selected *appropriate* cases — such patients may be able to stay at home and take a **single dose** of an AV nodal blocking drug <u>plus</u> a benzodiazepine at the *onset* of an episode (*thereby often avoiding the need to go to the ED*).

SVT *Practice* Tracing #4 (*AFlutter* — pp 147-158)

 ⇨ **PRACTICE** Tracing:

● The patient is a *hemodynamically* stable adult who presents to the ED with the rhythm shown in Figure 14-17. The **QRS** is *confirmed* to be **narrow** on 12-lead ECG.
• *What* is the Rhythm? Clinically — *What* should you do next?

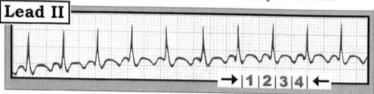

Figure 14-17: The patient is stable. What is the rhythm? *What next?*

☞ **Answer to SVT Tracing #4:** The rhythm in Figure 14-17 is rapid and regular. We are told that a **12-lead ECG *confirms* QRS narrowing** in *all* leads. The rate is *close to* 150/minute. Normal atrial activity is *not* seen (*the small, rounded upright deflection preceding each QRS has a PR interval that appears too short for normal conduction*). We have therefore described a **regular SVT** at ~**150/minute** *without* sign of normal atrial activity. This description should prompt consideration of the **3 entities** to consider in the differential diagnosis of a **regular SVT** (Table 14-2 — *previously seen on pages 117 and 138*):

▶ **NOTE:** Although *normal* atrial activity is *not* present in Figure 14-17 — it is likely that *some* form of atrial activity *is* present (*be this the upright rounded deflection preceding each QRS with short PR – or – the negative deflection midway between each QRS*).

Table 14-2: Common causes of a *regular* SVT when sinus P waves are *not* clearly evident.

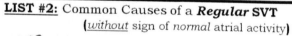
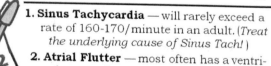

LIST #2: Common Causes of a *Regular* SVT (*without* sign of *normal* atrial activity)

1. **Sinus Tachycardia** — will rarely exceed a rate of 160-170/minute in an adult. (*Treat the underlying cause of Sinus Tach!*)
2. **Atrial Flutter** — most often has a ventricular rate *close* to 150/minute.
3. **PSVT** (*or AVNRT*).

☞ Regarding the **differential** diagnosis for a *regular* SVT rhythm without normal sinus P waves (*such as that seen in* Figure 14-17) — We can state the following:
• Overall *regularity* of the rhythm *rules out* AFib/MAT.
• The **3 most common causes** of a **regular SVT** to consider are: **i)** Sinus tachycardia; **ii)** Atrial flutter; *and* **iii)** PSVT. The **rate** of ~**150/minute** that is seen in Figure 14-17 could be consistent with

any of these 3 diagnoses. That said — a rate of ~150/minute for a _regular_ SVT of _uncertain_ etiology should suggest AFlutter as our first consideration to rule out (_See subsection on ECG Diagnosis below_).

▶ **PEARL:** Obtaining a **12-lead ECG** _and/or_ use of a **_vagal_ maneuver** may be invaluable for determining what the diagnosis is.

KEY Points: _ECG Diagnosis of AFlutter_

ECG Diagnosis:

● _Definitive_ diagnosis of the rhythm in <u>Figure 14-17</u> is simply <u>_not_</u> possible from the _single-lead_ tracing we are given. That said — We _strongly_ suspect **Atrial Flutter** until proven otherwise:

- In our experience — **AFlutter** is by far the **most commonly overlooked rhythm diagnosis**. It is _easy_ to overlook — because flutter waves are <u>_not_</u> always evident in all leads. **Always <u>suspect</u> AFlutter** (_until proven otherwise_) — <u>whenever</u> there is a **_regular_ SVT at ~150/minute** <u>_without_</u> normal atrial activity. This is precisely what we see in <u>Figure 14-17</u>.
- The diagnosis can be confirmed with a **_vagal_ maneuver** (_pp 118-120_).

▶ **NOTE:** Initiation of treatment for SVT rhythms in the hemodynamically _stable_ patient need <u>_not_</u> necessarily await definitive diagnosis. Depending on the clinical situation — one may (_or may not_) hold off on starting treatment until "the answer" is known.

AFlutter: _Diagnostic Use of a Vagal Maneuver_

Figure 14-18 shows the effect of **CSM** (_<u>C</u>arotid <u>S</u>inus <u>M</u>assage_) on the rhythm in Figure 14-17 (_page 147_).
- _What_ happens _after_ carotid massage (_CSM_) is applied?

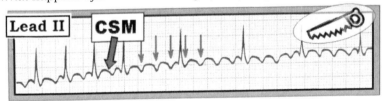

Figure 14-18: What happens _after_ CSM (_large arrow_) ?

Answer to Figure 14-18: Application of CSM _slows_ the ventricular response of the _regular_ SVT rhythm in <u>Figure 14-17</u>. As seen in <u>Figure 14-18</u> — this _facilitates_ recognition of **regular _sawtooth_ atrial activity** at **~300/minute** (_regular small arrows occurring each large box = 300/minute_).

• Thus, application of a vagal maneuver (*CSM*) as seen in Figure 14-18 **confirms** the **diagnosis** of **AFlutter** (*the only rhythm that produces regular atrial activity at ~300/minute is AFlutter*).

▶ **NOTE:** Following carotid massage — we count 4 *negative* deflections within *each* R-R interval. Application of CSM in Figure 14-18 has therefore *reduced* the ratio of AV conduction of AFlutter from 2:1 to 4:1.

KEY *Clinical* Points: *Regarding AFlutter*

 KEY *Clinical* Points:

⬤ Atrial flutter is characterized by a special pattern of *regular* atrial activity that in adults *almost* always (*and almost magically*) occurs at a rate of **~300/minute** (*250-to-350/min = usual range*). AFlutter typically manifests a **sawtooth** appearance that is usually best seen in the *inferior* leads (*and in lead V1*). At times, flutter waves may be *very* subtle — and only seen in a handful of leads.

• The **most common** ventricular response to AFlutter (*by far!*) — is with **2:1 AV conduction**. As a result, the ventricular rate with **untreated AFlutter** will usually be *close* to **150/minute** (*300/2 =150/minute*). NOTE: The atrial rate may be *less* than 250-300/minute — IF the patient is *already taking* certain antiarrhythmic drugs.

• The next most common ventricular response to AFlutter is **4:1 AV conduction** (*atrial rate ~300/minute; ventricular rate ~75/minute*).

• Occasionally — AFlutter may manifest a **variable** (*irregular*) **ventricular response**. In such cases — there will be an irregularly *irregular* ventricular response resembling AFib (*except for the presence of regularly occurring sawtooth flutter waves*).

• **Odd** conduction ratios (*1:1; 3:1; 5:1*) are **uncommon** for AFlutter (*with the exception being the patient with WPW who is prone to 1:1 AV conduction*).

▶ **Semantic Point:** It is best *not* to say that the example of AFlutter in Figure 14-17 represents "2:1 AV block". The term "block" implies pathology. Rather than being a bad thing that only 1 out of every 2 flutter impulses arriving at the AV node is conducted — it is indeed very fortunate that an intrinsic AV nodal refractory period exists that normally *prevents* 1:1 AV conduction from occurring. Thus, **2:1 AV conduction** with **AFlutter** is *"physiologic"* (*it is beneficial because it prevents an excessively fast ventricular rate*).

AFlutter: *Appearance on a 12-Lead Tracing*

It is helpful to become comfortable with several aspects regarding the recognition of AFlutter on 12-lead ECG (**Figure 14-19** — *page 150*).

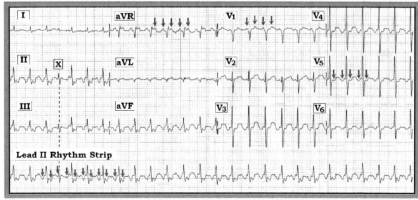

Figure 14-19: Atrial flutter on 12-lead ECG (*See text*).

📌 **Figure 14-19: *AFlutter* on 12-Lead** — Note in <u>Figure 14-19</u> that the rhythm is a *regular* SVT (*narrow-complex tachycardia*) at a rate of ~150/min. AFlutter should be assumed <u>until</u> proven otherwise (*pg 148*).
- Typically with AFlutter — flutter waves will be best seen in the 3 inferior leads (*II,III,aVF*). This is the case in <u>Figure 14-19</u>.
- We <u>know</u> the rhythm in figure 14-19 is <u>not</u> sinus. This is because there is *no* upright P wave with fixed PR interval preceding the QRS in lead II. Instead — there is a negative deflection preceding each QRS in lead II (*if not 2 negative deflections within each R-R interval*).
- Always look for a **long lead II rhythm strip** when contemplating the diagnosis of AFlutter. This is seen at the bottom of the tracing in <u>Figure 14-19</u>. Regularly occurring **arrows** mark out **negative atrial activity** at an approximate rate = **300/minute**. The only arrhythmia that produces regular atrial activity at ~300/minute is **AFlutter**.
- Use of **calipers** tremendously facilitates the diagnostic process. There is no easier way to identify if baseline deflections are regularly occurring or not.
- Flutter waves are <u>not</u> always seen in all leads on a 12-lead tracing. This is why we *meticulously* search *each* of the 12 leads for clues to underlying atrial activity. In <u>Figure 14-19</u> — **arrows** highlight flutter waves in several additional leads where they are seen. Note that flutter waves will often manifest *positive* deflections in leads aVR and V1 (*as they do here*). There is no indication of AFlutter in leads I or V2 of this tracing.
- Assessment of ST-T wave morphology is made more difficult when the underlying rhythm is AFlutter. This is because *sawtooth* flutter activity may *mask* underlying ST-T wave changes.
- <u>*Beyond-the-Core:*</u> There is actually slight irregularity in the early part of the rhythm in <u>Figure 14-19</u> (*See* **beat X** *in lead II*). Despite slightly *earlier-than-expected* occurrence of this QRS complex — note how regular flutter activity (*arrows*) nevertheless continues in the long lead II rhythm strip. Whether beat X represents fusion from a PVC or

aberrant conduction from *transient* change in AV conduction ratio to 3:2 Wenckebach within the AV node is unimportant. What counts is persistence of *underlying* flutter activity that <u>*proves*</u> AFlutter as the diagnosis.

☞ AFlutter: *Variable Conduction*

Although AFlutter most often manifests either 2:1 or 4:1 AV conduction — it may also commonly present with a **variable ventricular response**. When this happens — the ventricular response will resemble that of AFib in being *irregularly* irregular (<u>Figure 14-20</u>).
• The diagnosis of AFlutter is made by recognition of regular *sawtooth* atrial activity at a rate *close* to 300/minute.

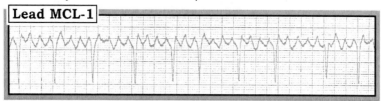

Figure 14-20: AFlutter with a *variable* ventricular response. The ventricular response is *irregularly* irregular and resembles AFib — but regular *sawtooth* atrial activity at a rate *close* to 300/minute identifies the rhythm as AFlutter.

☞ AFlutter: *Unusual 3:1 AV Conduction*

Odd conduction ratios are distinctly uncommon for AFlutter. Most non-cardiologist providers only rarely encounter AFlutter with 1:1 or 3:1 AV conduction. Higher level odd ratios are even rarer.
• <u>Figure 14-21</u> shows an example of **AFlutter** with **3:1 AV conduction**. The ventricular response in this tracing is regular at a rate of ~85/minute. There are 3 flutter waves for each QRS (*therefore an atrial rate of 85 X 3=255/minute*).

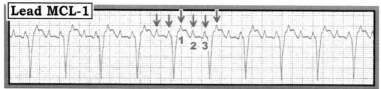

Figure 14-21: Atrial flutter with 3:1 AV conduction.

☞ There will usually be "something else" going on medically with the patient when you encounter AFlutter with an *odd* conduction ratio. Many such patients will be receiving one or more antiarrhythmic drugs (*that may slow the flutter rate and affect AV conduction ratio*).
• **AFlutter <u>with</u> 1:1 AV conduction** (*ventricular rate close to 300/min*) — should lead one to inquire <u>IF</u> the tracing is from a child who may

have congenital heart disease *and/or* a patient of any age with WPW (*page 110*). ● **BOTTOM Line:** You will probably only *rarely* see AFlutter with an odd conduction ratio, if at all …

▶ *Beyond-the-Core:* As opposed to the situation for AFlutter with a *variable* ventricular response (<u>Figure 14-20</u>) — in which the distance between the flutter wave immediately preceding each QRS and the QRS complex itself varies — there <u>is</u> a constant *flutter-to-QRS* distance before each QRS complex in <u>Figure 14-21</u>. This confirms that there <u>is</u> conduction of one out of every 3 flutter waves in this tracing!
• Interestingly — it is *not* the flutter wave closest to the QRS that conducts. Instead, "bombardment" of the AV node by 255 flutter waves each minute results in relative *refractoriness* of the AV node to forward conduction (*the flutter wave that conducts each third impulse to the ventricles in* <u>Figure 14-21</u> *is probably either #1 or #2 — but not #3*).

☞ AFlutter: *Is it AFlutter or Atrial Tach with Block?*

In the days when Digoxin was regularly used for treatment of heart failure and atrial fibrillation — **atrial tachycardia** <u>***with***</u> **block** (*previously known as PAT = <u>P</u>aroxysmal <u>A</u>trial <u>T</u>achycardia with block*) was commonly seen as a manifestation of **digoxin toxicity**. So characteristic was atrial tachycardia with block of Digoxin toxicity — that patients taking Digoxin were *presumed* to be toxic <u>IF</u> this arrhythmia was seen <u>*regardless*</u> of what the serum digoxin level was.
• Given that AFlutter is one of the few arrhythmias *not* attributable to digoxin toxicity — much attention used to be focused on distinguishing between atrial tachycardia with block <u>vs</u> AFlutter. If the arrhythmia was deemed "PAT with block" — then Digoxin was *withheld* for presumed toxicity. If on the other hand, the rhythm was felt to represent AFlutter with 2:1 AV conduction — then *additional* Digoxin was often recommended in hope of slowing down the ventricular response.

☞ While the above described approach to management has long ago been rendered obsolete by numerous advancements in treatment of supraventricular tachyarrhythmias (*as well greatly reduced use of Digoxin, such that digoxin toxicity is seen far less often than it used to be*) — it is nevertheless insightful to draw upon this historical perspective in interpreting the rhythm shown in <u>Figure 14-22</u>:

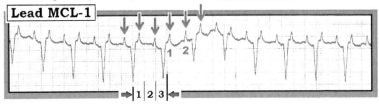

Figure 14-22: Is this rhythm AFlutter <u>or</u> atrial tachycardia with block? Clinically — *Does it matter* which one it is? (*See text*).

☞ **Answer to Figure 14-22:** The tracing in this *right-sided* MCL-1 lead shows a *regular* SVT rhythm at a ventricular rate of ~115/minute. Two P waves are seen to occur within each R-R interval. The P-P interval is regular at a rate of ~230/minute (ie, *115 X 2 = 230/minute*).

- In favor of **AFlutter** as the etiology of the rhythm in Figure 14-22 — is regular and rapid atrial activity with a peaked upward deflection in *right-sided* lead MCL-1. That said — the atrial rate of 230/minute is a bit *below* the usual *atrial* rate range for *untreated* AFlutter (*of 250-350/minute*) — and the expected "sawtooth" pattern of AFlutter is *missing* in this lead.
- We are *not* told IF this patient is taking an antiarrhythmic agent (*such as flecainide, amiodarone, sotalol, etc.*) that might slow the atrial rate of flutter. We are also *not* told if the patient is taking Digoxin (*less likely in 2013 than in the past — though still a possibility to ask about*).
- In favor of **ATach** (*Atrial Tachycardia*) **with 2:1 AV Block** — is the matrial rate of 230/minute (*which is below the usual range for untreated AFlutter — but within the upper range for atrial tachycardia*) — and the *isoelectric* baseline (*rather than sawtooth*) in this lead.

▶ **BOTTOM Line:** It is *impossible* to be certain of the rhythm diagnosis solely from the rhythm strip seen in Figure 14-22 *without* the benefit of additional information.

- The clinical reality — is simply that *neither* rate *nor* baseline appearance (*sawtooth* vs *isoelectric baseline*) have been shown to reliably distinguish between ATach vs AFlutter.

- Obtaining a **12-lead ECG** may help (*it might reveal a typical sawtooth pattern in other leads*).
- Knowing IF this patient was on some *rate-slowing* antiarrhythmic agent (*which would favor AFlutter*) and/or was taking Digoxin (*which would increase concern about digoxin toxicity*) is critically important.

▶ *Clinical* **NOTE** *and* **Perspective:** Assuming this patient is not on Digoxin — the terminology used to describe the arrhythmia seen in Figure 14-22 is far *less* important than the overall clinical concepts involved. This is because what used to be classified as *"atrial tachycardia"* in non-digoxin toxic patients is now often referred to as an *"atypical"* **form** of **AFlutter**.

- Included within the broad category of *"atypical"* **AFlutter rhythms** are various types of atrial tachycardias that may arise from *anywhere* within the atria or neighboring pulmonary veins.
- Some atrial tachycardias may be "focal" or automatic (*often recognizable by non-sinus P wave appearance — "warm up" phenomenon until the ectopic tachycardia is established — relatively slower rate — and on occasion slightly variable P-P intervals*).
- *Other* atrial tachycardias may be much faster, perfectly regular, lack an isoelectric baseline — and be clinically *indistinguishable* from AFlutter based on ECG appearance.

- **Clinical *"Take-Home"* Point:** While we admittedly cannot be certain whether the arrhythmia in <u>Figure 14-22</u> (*on page 152*) represents ATach <u>or</u> AFlutter — *initial* treatment considerations will be the *same* once Dig toxicity has been ruled out (*pp 156-157*). From a non-specialist perspective — longterm management will also be similar (ie, *EP referral if the arrhythmia is persistent or recurs*).

☞ **AFlutter:** *Is it AFib? – AFlutter – or "Fib-Flutter"* ?

The rhythm shown in <u>Figure 14-23</u> often defies classification. The initial portion of this tracing resembles the sawtooth pattern of AFlutter. On the other hand, erratic undulations in the baseline during the latter portion of this rhythm strip are clearly more suggestive of the coarse *fib waves* of atrial fibrillation. As a "compromise" — the term ***"AFib-Flutter"*** has been proposed.

- Despite anatomic imperfection (*a rhythm is <u>either</u> AFib or AFlutter*) — descriptive use of the term "AFib-Flutter" accurately conveys the ECG picture of atrial activity *intermediate* between AFib <u>and</u> AFlutter.
- Strictly speaking — the initial portion of the rhythm in <u>Figure 14-23</u> does <u>not</u> qualify as "atrial flutter" because atrial activity is *too* fast (*over 350/minute in parts*); irregular; and <u>not</u> consistent in atrial morphology. That said — We would accept as "correct" an interpretation of the rhythm in Figure 14-23 as <u>either</u> AFib (*here with a very slow ventricular response*) – <u>or</u> – "AFib-Flutter". The point to emphasize is that in the *absence* of consistent regular flutter activity *throughout* the rhythm strip — a rhythm such as that seen in <u>Figure 14-23</u> *behaves clinically* as if it was AFib.

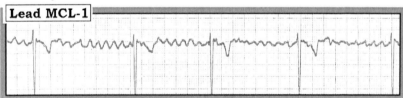

Figure 14-23: AFib with very *slow* ventricular response. Alternatively — one might classify this rhythm as "AFib-Flutter". <u>Clinically</u> — this rhythm *behaves* as AFib (*See text*).

☞ **AFlutter:** *Real or Artifact* ?

The rhythm in <u>Figure 14-24</u> was interpreted as atrial flutter.

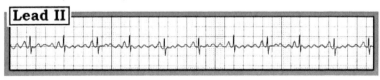

Figure 14-24: This rhythm was interpreted as AFlutter. *Do you agree?*

☞ **Answer to Figure 14-24:** We conclude this group of illustrative tracings with an example of what atrial flutter is not. The rhythm in Figure 14-24 is *not* AFlutter. Instead — an underlying **sinus rhythm** is present. The numerous small undulations that populate the baseline represent **artifact**. Reasons why we *know* this rhythm is *not* AFlutter include the following:

• Distinct sinus P waves are seen preceding each QRS complex with fixed and normal PR interval (***arrows* in Figure 14-25**).

• These normal sinus P waves are *unaffected* by the continuous, *smaller-amplitude* and *irregular* baseline undulations. In fact — sinus P waves are *superimposed* on this baseline artifact.

• *We looked at the patient.* He had an obvious **resting tremor.**

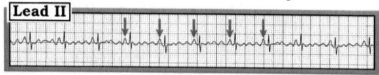

Figure 14-25: Arrows have been added to Figure 14-24, illustrating that sinus P waves are *superimposed* on the smaller amplitude baseline artifact undulations (*See text*).

▶ **BOTTOM Line:** It is *easy* to be fooled by artifact. The *best way* to prevent this from happening is to develop healthy respect for the gamut of *"real appearing"* arrhythmias that artifact distortion may produce.

• ***Looking at the patient*** may provide invaluable insight. Tapping, scratching, coughing, shaking, shivering, seizing and tremor are but a few of the common causes of *artifactual* arrhythmias.

• The frequency of a **resting *Parkinsonian* tremor** is often quite close to the frequency of flutter waves. In addition to observation of the patient — clues that Parkinsonian tremor is the cause of an arrhythmia mimic (*such as that seen in* Figure 14-24) are irregularity of rate <u>and</u> deflection morphology (*whereas both are consistent with atrial flutter*).

Beyond-the-Core: **Typical and *Atypical* AFlutter**

  ⇨ ***Beyond-the-Core ...***

● There is more than a single type of "atrial flutter". With ***typical* AFlutter** (*which makes up over 80% of cases*) — the *sawtooth* pattern of flutter is extremely well visualized in the *inferior* leads and in lead V1. The flutter wavefront almost always manifests CCW (*counterclockwise*) rotation around the tricuspid ring (*ergo alternate designation as* **CTI-dependent** = <u>C</u>avo-<u>T</u>ricuspid-<u>I</u>sthmus-dependent *flutter*). In about 10% of cases — *typical* AFlutter will follow the same path through the atria, but for unexplained reasons with CW (*clockwise*) instead of CCW rotation around the tricuspid ring (ie, *"reverse" typical flutter*). In these patients with "reverse" typical flutter — the *same* leads reveal the diagnosis, but instead of upright flutter waves in V1 there may be a double negative (*W-shaped*) flutter wave in V1.

• The appearance of flutter waves on the surface ECG depends on many factors including pathway through the atria, rotation direction of the impulse (*CCW or CW*), presence of scarring from prior infarction, cardiomyopathy, previous procedure, etc. Realize that even with *"typical"* (*CTI-dependent*) **AFlutter** — flutter waves may be primarily positive, negative or biphasic in inferior leads and V1 (*which are the leads where flutter waves are usually seen best*).

• While <u>not</u> important for non-electrophysiologists to distinguish between the differing ECG appearence of the various types of AFlutter — it <u>is</u> clinically relevant to be aware that *atypical* **AFlutter forms** may be seen in 10-20% of cases, in which the path through the atria is different <u>and</u> AFlutter may be present despite *absence* of a prominent "sawtooth" pattern. As a result — *atypical* AFlutter may be more difficult to recognize on ECG.

▶ *Clinical* **NOTE:** What used to be classified as *"atrial tachycardia"* in non-digoxin toxic patients — is now often referred to as a form of *"atypical"* **AFlutter**. While some atrial tachycardias may be relatively easy to distinguish from AFlutter (*isoelectric baseline, variation in P-P interval, ectopic "warm-up" or "cool-down" period before or after tachycardia*) — this is <u>not</u> always the case.

• *Rapid* atrial tachycardia in a *scarred* atrium may sometimes closely *mimic* AFlutter — such that <u>neither</u> isoelectric baseline <u>nor</u> rate over or under 240/minute serve as distinguishing features.

• *BOTTOM* **Line:** Long-term management of typical and atypical AFlutter rhythms (*including atrial tachycardias*) belongs in the realm of the EP cardiologist. Fortunately — distinction between the various forms of these arrhythmias is <u>not</u> essential by the nonspecialist — <u>and</u> *initial* treatment considerations are essentially the same.

AFlutter: *Treatment Priorities*

➡ *Treatment* Priorities:

● By way of clinical perspective — AFlutter is far *less* common in its clinical occurrence than AFib. That said — there are many similarities in the approach to these 2 arrhythmias, such that it is useful to compare clinical aspects of each (*realizing that distinction between the two is not always clear — and some patients may go back-and-forth from AFib to AFlutter*). We note the following general concepts:

• The *same* **drugs** are used to *slow* the **ventricular response** to *both* AFib <u>and</u> AFlutter (ie, *Diltiazem/ Verapamil; β-blockers; Digoxin*). That said — it will often be *more* difficult to control the ventricular rate of AFlutter with the use of drugs.

- The ***same*** **drugs** are also used for AFib <u>and</u> AFlutter when attempting ***medical*** **conversion** — and/or for *maintenance* of sinus rhythm (ie, *Amiodarone; Sotalol; Propafenone; Flecainaide*). An AV nodal *rate-controlling* agent (*Diltiazem/Verapamil; β-blocker*) will often be used at the same time with patients in AFlutter in hope of avoiding the phenomenon of 1:1 AV conduction that might otherwise arise from slowing the atrial rate of flutter.
- **Ibutilide** (*1 mg IV over 10 minutes; may repeat once*) — works better for converting AFlutter (*~60-70% success*) <u>vs</u> only ~30-40% success with this drug for converting AFib.
- ***Synchronized*** **Cardioversion** — is more effective for converting AFlutter (*it almost always works!*) — compared to a *lower* success rate for acute cardioversion of AFib. **Lower** **energies** (*~50 joules*) usually work for the more organized atrial rhythm of flutter (*vs higher energies that are often needed to cardiovert AFib*).
- ***Longterm*** **Anticoagulation** — <u>is</u> recommended for AFlutter (*although the risk of thromboembolism appears to be less than it is for AFib*).
- Persistent AFlutter is more easily treated (*and more often cured*) with **catheter** **ablation**. Awareness of this fact should *lower* one's threshold for ***referral*** to an **EP** (*Electro<u>P</u>hysiology*) **cardiologist** in the event AFlutter recurs following successful cardioversion.

☞ Realizing that it will often be much *more* difficult to slow the ventricular rate of a patient in AFlutter — initial rate-slowing is most commonly attempted with **IV Diltiazem** (*bolus and infusion — pg 123*):
- <u>**Diltiazem**</u> — Give **~15-20 mg IV bolus**. IF no response — May follow in 15 minutes with a 2nd bolus (*of **~25mg IV***).
- May then start **IV infusion** at **10 mg/hour** to *maintain* rate control (*usual range ~5-15mg/hour range*).
- Alternatively — an **IV β-blocker** could be used *instead* of IV Diltiazem (*page 124*) — especially if increased *sympathetic* tone is a likely.
- Be sure to **replace Mg++** <u>and</u> **K+** (*depletion of one or both of these electrolytes may exacerbate the arrhythmia*).
- Digoxin — is much *less* commonly used in 2013 for treatment of AFlutter than in the past (*though it may help on occasion as a supplemental agent for AFlutter with acute heart failure*).
- ***Synchronized*** **cardioversion** offers a high rate of success in the acute situation. Whether or not to proceed with this intervention in the *acute* setting either initially <u>or</u> if medical treatment fails to adequately control the ventricular response is a decision to be made by the emergency care provider on the scene.

Summary: *Treatment of New-Onset AFlutter*

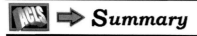 ➡ *Summary*

● Initial priorities and clinical approach to ***new-onset* AFlutter** are in general quite similar to those for AFib:

- Before all else — Ensure the patient with *new* AFlutter is *hemodynamically* stable (*they almost always will be*).
- Look for a **potentially *correctable* underlying cause** of AFlutter (ie, *improving oxygenation in a COPD patient may facilitate spontaneous resolution of AFlutter*).
- Consider early on the need for ***anticoagulation.***
- Optimize fluid balance and electrolyte ($K+$/$Mg++$) status.
- *Slow* the ***ventricular* response** <u>IF</u> it is rapid (*as it most often will be with new-onset AFlutter*). **IV Diltiazem** (*bolus and drip*) — is most commonly used (*although as for AFib — a β-blocker may be used instead*).
- Realize that AV nodal blocking drugs will <u>not</u> always succeed in slowing the ventricular response. <u>IF</u> AFlutter persists despite initial treatment measures (*especially when the ventricular response to AFlutter remains fast*) — referral may be in order. This is because medical conversion (*with drugs such as Amiodarone – Sotalol – Flecainide – Propafenone – Ibutilide*) — and/<u>or</u> nonemergent synchronized cardioversion entail aspects of treatment beyond the scope of the usual noncardiologist emergency care provider.
- If the patient with *new-onset* AFlutter with *rapid* ventricular response shows signs of *hemodynamic* compromise — then *immediately* cardiovert! Acute cardioversion will usually convert the rhythm.
- Realize that precise diagnosis of arrhythmia etiology will <u>not</u> always be possible from assessment of the surface ECG. Some forms of atrial tachycardia with 2:1 AV block may mimic the ECG appearance of AFlutter. Some of these atrial tachycardias develop atrial rates in excess of 240/minute <u>and</u> sawtooth appearance of their baseline that is virtually *indistinguishable* from AFlutter. *NO matter!* Distinction between atrial tachycardia <u>vs</u> AFlutter is *rarely* important in the acute situation. Initial treatment considerations are similar <u>regardless</u> of specific arrhythmia etiology (*pp 156-157*) — <u>and</u> longterm management likewise entails consideration of EP referral *regardless* of whether the arrhythmia persists or recurs.

SVT *Practice* Tracing #5 (*Sinus Tachycardia* — pp 159-162)

 ⇨ **PRACTICE** Tracing:

● The patient is a *hemodynamically* stable adult who presents to the ED with the rhythm shown in Figure 14-26. The **QRS** is *confirmed* to be **narrow** on 12-lead ECG.
• *What* is the Rhythm? — Could this be sinus tachycardia?
• Clinically — *What* should you do next?

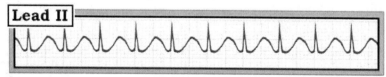

Figure 14-26: The patient is stable. What is the rhythm? *What next?*

What is the Rhythm in Figure 14-26?

 ECG Diagnosis:

● The rhythm in Figure 14-26 is rapid and regular. We are told that a **12-lead ECG** *confirms* **QRS narrowing** in *all* leads. No P waves are seen; the rate is ~150/minute. We have therefore described a *regular* **SVT** *without* clear sign of normal atrial activity. This description should prompt consideration of the **3 entities** to consider in the differential diagnosis of a *regular* **SVT** (Table 14-3 — *previously seen on pages 117, 138 and 147*):

▶ **NOTE:** Because the rate of the *regular* SVT in Figure 14-26 is *close* to 150/minute — the diagnosis could conceivably be *any* of the 3 entities in LIST #2: **i)** Sinus Tachycardia; **ii)** AFlutter; *or* **iii)** PSVT.
• Although we can *not* be certain *which* of the 3 entities in List #2 is the cause of the *regular* SVT in Figure 14-26 — it is *not* essential to know for sure at this point in time, given that the *initial* approach to treatment is fairly similar (*page 160*).

Table 14-3:
Common causes of a *regular* SVT when sinus P waves are *not* clearly evident.

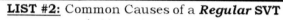

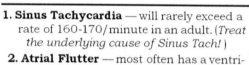

LIST #2: Common Causes of a *Regular* SVT
(*without* sign of *normal* atrial activity)

1. Sinus Tachycardia — will rarely exceed a rate of 160-170/minute in an adult. (*Treat the underlying cause of Sinus Tach!*)
2. Atrial Flutter — most often has a ventricular rate *close* to 150/minute.
3. PSVT (*or AVNRT*).

KEY *Clinical* Points: *Regarding Sinus Tachycardia*

KEY *Clinical* Points:

● Definitive treatment of this patient who is stable **will depend on: i)** the *clinical* setting; and ii) what the *actual* **rhythm diagnosis** of Figure 14-26 happens to be.

- As long as the patient remains alert, stable, and able to tolerate the rhythm *without* undue symptoms — there is clearly **no** **need** for immediate electrical therapy.
- Get a **12-lead ECG** (*may reveal atrial activity elsewhere*).
- IF one *had* to immediately know what the rhythm was — Consider a **vagal maneuver** (*pp 118-120*) — which hopefully will *transiently* slow the rate (*and allow diagnosis*) — and/or which may even convert the rhythm if it is PSVT.
- Consider Adenosine or other AV nodal *rate-slowing* medication (ie, *Diltiazem/Verapamil; β-blocker — pp 121-124*).
- Alternatively — One might **"Do Nothing"** for the immediate moment. This is the course of action we would favor IF we thought the rhythm in Figure 14-26 was most likely to be sinus tachycardia ...

🖙 **Sinus Tachycardia:** *A Tincture of Time ...*

No treatment was given for this patient. A few minutes later — the rhythm in **Figure 14-27** was recorded on the monitor.
- What has *now* happened?

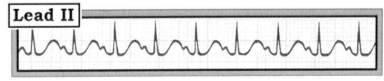

Figure 14-27: Follow-up lead II rhythm strip a few minutes later from the patient initially in the *regular* SVT rhythm seen in Figure 14-26. What has *now* happened? (*See text*).

🖙 **Answer to Figure 14-27:** The **regular** SVT previously seen in Figure 14-26 has slowed. An upright (*sinus*) P wave is now clearly seen to precede *each* QRS complex with fixed PR interval. This defines Figure 14-26 as having been **sinus** tachycardia (*See* **Figure 14-27** *on page 161 for comparison*).

- This case highlights why we *include* sinus tachycardia among the causes of a **regular** SVT in **LIST #2** (Table 14-3). Sometimes (*when the rate is fast*) — Sinus P waves may be hidden within the preceding ST-T wave.

> ▶ **PEARL:** IF you clinically think the *regular* SVT rhythm you are confronted with is *likely* to be sinus tachycardia — then *BE AWARE* that the rate should **slow** in **gradual** fashion as the underlying condition(s) are corrected. Remembering this point will often facilitate making the diagnosis with a tincture of time ...

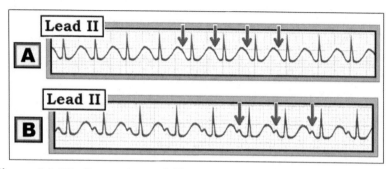

Figure 14-28: Comparison of <u>Figures 14-26</u> *and* <u>Fig. 14-27</u>. Initially (*with Figure 14-26*) — all that could be said was that there was a *regular* SVT at ~150/min *without* clear sign of normal sinus P waves. With a **tincture of time** (*a few minutes later*) — there is slight *slowing* of the rate with resultant separation of sinus P waves from the preceding T wave. This confirms the etiology of this rhythm as sinus tachycardia (*See text*).

Sinus Tachycardia: *Clinical PEARLS*

 ➡ *Clinical Pearls:*

● Sinus Tachycardia is usually an *easy* diagnosis to make: The rhythm is sinus (*defined by an upright P wave in lead II*) – <u>and</u> – the heart rate is *faster* than 100/minute.

• All bets are off in children — for whom sinus rates *over* 100/minute may be *normal* in certain age groups.

• The **formula** for **estimating maximal exercise heart rate** (*and therefore the maximal rate for sinus tachycardia*) = **220 – age**. As a result, a 25-year old male may theoretically attain a sinus tachycardia rate as high as 195/minute during full physical activity (*such as a short-distance sprint*). In contrast — a 40-year old adult might only be able to attain a rate of 180/minute (*220 – 40*). ● <u>BUT</u> — these rates represent maximal **exercise** heart rate (*which is clearly more than the usual upper rate for sinus tachycardia in a patient presenting to the ED or office*). As a **general rule** — sinus tachycardia in a **horizontal adult** (ie, *an adult being seen in the ED, hospital or office*) — will usually **<u>not</u> exceed 150-to-160/minute**.

▶ **NOTE:** This is *not* to say that you will never see sinus tachycardia in an adult patient at a rate faster than 150-160/minute — but rather to suggest that you *strongly consider* **some *other* cause** for a *regular* SVT rhythm than sinus tachycardia <u>IF</u> heart rate in an adult is ≥**170/min**.
• *Remember:* **Children** may have sinus tachycardia at much faster rates (*of 200/minute or more*)!

☞ Sinus Tachycardia: *Clinical Caveats in ECG Diagnosis*

As is the case for ECG assessment of *any* sustained cardiac arrhythmia — Use of a **12-lead ECG** may prove invaluable for confirming the suspected diagnosis. We draw attention to several **caveats** to be aware of in the ECG diagnosis of sinus tachycardia:
• The PR interval generally *shortens* as heart rate increases. As a result — a small upright deflection with a "PR interval" that looks to be fairly *long* in a *regular* SVT rhythm (ie, *placed midway within the R-R interval between QRS complexes*) — is usually <u>not</u> a sinus P wave!
• With rare exceptions — Lack of a clear upright P wave in lead II should suggest that the rhythm is <u>not</u> sinus (*regardless of whether or not upright P waves are seen in other leads*).
• VT may occasionally manifest 1:1 *retrograde* V-A conduction. As a result — Seeing "P waves" in a WCT rhythm does <u>not</u> necessarily mean the rhythm is sinus. This is especially true <u>IF</u> such P waves are *not* upright in lead II preceding each QRS with a fixed and normal PR interval.

Sinus Tachycardia: *Treatment Priorities*

 ⇨ *Treatment* **Priorities:**

● *Sinus* Tachycardia may occur in any age group. In general — Sinus Tachycardia is a **physiologic response** to other factors rather than a primary arrhythmia per se. There are **numerous potential causes** (ie, *acute illness; fever; dehydration; hypoxia; blood loss; shock; drugs; etc.*).
• *Optimal* **management** entails *finding* <u>and</u> **correcting** the *underlying* **cause.** A patient in septic shock develops sinus tachycardia as a **compensatory mechanism** in the body's attempt to increase cardiac output (*IV Fluids plus antibiotics constitute the treatment of choice*).
• Synchronized cardioversion is <u>contraindicated</u> for sinus tachycardia (*this could be a lethal mistake*). Similarly — Use of *rate-slowing* drugs (*Diltiazem-Verapamil; β-blockers*) is generally <u>not</u> indicated in the *acute* situation.
• **Exceptions** (*in which β-blocker therapy may be indicated in the acute setting*) include: **i)** Sinus tachycardia with large acute *anterior* MI; **ii)** Hyperthyroidism (*thyrotoxicosis*); <u>and</u> **iii)** Pheochromocytoma. Other than this — It is best <u>not</u> to use *rate-slowing* drugs for sinus tachycardia in the acute situation.

Section 15 – Bradycardia/Pacing (*pp 163-169*)

 ***B**radycardia/**P**acing*

● The patient may (*or may not*) be responsive — <u>and</u> may (*or may not*) have an acceptable blood pressure:

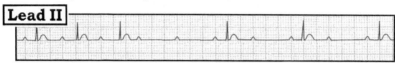

Figure 15-1: Bradycardia — in this case with very slow heart rate. The QRS in this example of bradycardia is *narrow* — <u>and</u> there appears to be regular *atrial* activity. That said — details of QRS width and whether or not P waves are conducting are *secondary* concerns to the most immediate need, which is for assessment of *hemodynamic* status.

- **Rhythm Description** — A "bradycardia" is defined as a cardiac rhythm with an *average* heart rate of *less* than 60/minute.
- **Bedside Pitfalls** — Treat the patient <u>not</u> the monitor! Some patients may be asymptomatic and <u>not</u> in need of acute treatment <u>*despite*</u> surprisingly *slow* heart rates. Unnecessary treatment of bradycardia is <u>not</u> without potential for harm!

☞ ***KEY Clinical* Points** — Regarding the rhythm in <u>Figure 15-1</u> — there appears to be *some* form of AV block. It is difficult to determine the specific *type* of AV block. That said — *It does <u>not</u> matter...*
- The reason it *doesn't* matter what type of AV block is present — is that clinical priorities <u>and</u> **initial** treatment of **bradycardia** are **similar** <u>*regardless*</u> of whether the rhythm in <u>Figure 15-1</u> is 2nd degree AV block (*Mobitz I or II*) <u>or</u> 3rd degree (*complete*) AV block — or for that matter, nothing more than *marked* sinus bradycardia (*AV Blocks are discussed in detail in Section 20 — pp 233-250*).

Bradycardia

  Suggested *Initial* Approach:

● IF the patient with bradycardia is *hemodynamically* stable <u>and</u> *without* symptoms — then *no* immediate treatment is needed (*other than perhaps consideration of "**stand-by**" pacing*).
- Always **Look First** for a **treatable cause** of bradycardia (*especially* **hypoxemia**) in <u>both</u> children <u>and</u> adults!
- Determine <u>IF</u> the patient with **bradycardia** is **symptomatic?** That is — Is there need to treat *now* with drugs/pacing? (*See page 164*).
- Is the patient with bradycardia **hypovolemic?** <u>IF</u> so — cautious fluid challenge may normalize BP.

☞ **IF** *Specific* **Treatment of Bradycardia** is **Indicated**

As already emphasized — No immediate treatment at all may be needed if the patient with bradycardia is *hemodynamically* stable and asymptomatic. *Surprisingly* often — this will be the case. On the other hand — IF the patient with bradycardia IS in need of immediate *specific* treatment, then consider the following:

- **Atropine** — Give **0.5-1.0 mg IV** (*or* IO). May repeat in 3-5 minutes (*up to a total dose of ~3 mg*). We favor trial of Atropine IF the QRS is narrow (*but* not *necessarily if the QRS is wide* and *Pacing is immediately available*).

- **Pacing** — May consider **TCP** (*Trans-Cutaneous Pacing*) even before (*or simultaneously with*) giving Atropine IF bradycardia is severe and TCP is available (*See page 167*).

- Use of a **Pressor** if hypotension is more severe. Give *either* **Dopamine** (*beginning at 2-5 µg/kg/minute*) or **Epinephrine**. IF Epinephrine is used to treat bradycardia with hypotension — Do *not* give Epi as a bolus! Instead — it is best to administer Epinephrine by **IV infusion** to treat bradycardia with hypotension (*beginning Epi at 1-2 µg/minute and titrating the dose upward as needed*). The problem is that one *"cannot take a bolus back"* in the event that *adverse* effects occur from giving IV Epineprhine (*See pp 166-167*).

Bradycardia

 ➡ *Beyond-the-Textbook ...*

● The "good news" for **non-PEA Bradycardia** — is that a **pulse** is **present**! Effective treatment options are available — and overall prognosis is far better than for PEA or Asystole.

- Simple measures (*oxygen, effective airway, fluids*) may be all that is needed to successfully treat many patients with bradycardia.

- *Standard* **ACLS treatments** for **Bradycardia** have *not* changed for many years (*Atropine-Pressor-Pacing*). Only the *specific* indications and *sequence* for use have changed.

- Consider the *same* list of **potentially treatable underlying conditions** as given for PEA (*page 175*). These include — **inadequate ventilation** (*tension pneumothorax, right mainstem intubation*); **inadequate circulation** (*hypovolemia from blood loss, dehydration, shock; aneurysmal rupture; pulmonary embolus; cardiac tamponade*); and **metabolic conditions** (*hyperkalemia, acidosis, hypoglycemia, drug overdose, hypothermia*).

▶ NOTE: **ACLS-PM** (*ACLS Provider Manual*) allows **flexibility** in the **treatment** of Bradycardia. ACLS-PM says, "The treatment sequence (= *Atropine-Pacer-Dopamine/Epinephrine*) is determined by severity; Move quickly through the sequence if symptomatic; *Multiple* interventions may be needed simultaneously; Pacing may be used *before* Atropine when symptoms are more severe".

Bradycardia: *What are the Usual Slow Rhythms?*

The term *"bradycardia"* entails recognition of a rhythm with a rate of <u>less</u> than 60/minute. This encompasses a variety of rhythms:
• Sinus bradycardia (*with or without sinus arrhythmia*).
• The AV blocks (*Section 20 — pp 233-250*).
• Sinus pauses (*and periods of sinus arrest*).
• *Slow* AFib <u>or</u> various **escape rhythms** originating from the AV Node, His, or ventricles *in response* to the slow rate.

▶ **NOTE:** While the above cited entities cover a wide spectrum of arrhythmias — the **common** denominator is a **slow ventricular rate.** Clinical assessment and initial management are similar when *any* of these causes of bradycardia are encountered in an *acute* situation.

Bradycardia: *KEY Clinical Points*

 ➡ *KEY Points*

● We emphasize the following points about the bradycardic rhythms:
• The **rate ranges** cited here relate to **adults.** Norms for rate are generally faster in children (ie, *the normal resting heart rate in a child less than 1 year old is between 80-120/minute*).
• The *clinical* situation is **KEY.** Certain individuals (ie, *physically fit young adults — especially endurance athletes*) may have normal *physiologic* bradycardia (*with sinus rates as slow as 35-45/minute*). No intervention at all is needed in such healthy individuals.
• In contrast (*despite falling within the "normal" range*) — a heart rate of 70-80/minute would be *inappropriately* slow (= **relative** bradycardia) for a patient in shock who should be tachycardic as a normal *compensatory* response.
• Is there **"symptomatic" bradycardia?** That is — Are **signs** <u>or</u> **symptoms** present as a direct <u>result</u> of the *slow* rhythm? One looks for: **i)** chest pain; **ii)** shortness of breath; **iii)** hypotension; **iv)** mental confusion; **v)** weakness/fatigue; **vi)** *new-onset* heart failure; <u>and/or</u> **vi)** syncope or presyncope (*See also pp 51-52*).

▶ **NOTE:** Bradycardia is *less likely* to be the **cause** of **symptoms** — IF the rate is **over 50/minute** in a patient at rest. That said — bradycardia may be the cause of symptoms IF heart rate does not appropriately increase with exercise (*as may often occur in an older patient with sick sinus syndrome or drug-induced bradycardia*).

 Use of Atropine for Bradycardia

Atropine is <u>*not*</u> benign. Especially in the setting of acute ischemia or infarction — resultant acceleration of the sinus rate may prove

deleterious by increasing myocardial oxygen demand (*which may precipitate tachyarrhythmias including VT!*).
- Atropine works best for treating bradycardia due to increased **vagal tone** (ie, *during the early hours of acute inferior infarction*).
- We would generally <u>not</u> use Atropine to treat a patient with acute *inferior* MI — <u>IF</u> he/she was *asymptomatic* with a heart rate of 50/minute <u>and</u> a seemingly stable BP of 80-90mm Hg (*Cautious infusion of IV fluids may help; bradycardia is likely to be transient in this situation*).
- We *would* use Atropine — <u>IF</u> the above patient was symptomatic. Sometimes **"ya just *gotta* be there"** (*at the bedside*) — to determine <u>IF</u> a patient with a rate of 40-50/min <u>or</u> BP of 80-90 is in need of *immediate* treatment <u>vs</u> simple awareness and *treatment "readiness"*.

▶ **NOTE:** Atropine *works best* for **narrow** QRS bradycardia — especially with **Mobitz Type I** (*AV Wenckebach*) **2nd Degree AV block.**

- Atropine works by a *parasympatholytic* effect that increases the rate of SA node firing — as well as improving conduction through the AV node. Since the usual site of AV Wenckebach is *at* the AV node — Atropine is often effective (*especially during the early hours of acute inferior infarction*). In contrast, since the level of block in Mobitz Type II is usually situated *below* the AV node — Atropine is *unlikely* to work with this conduction disorder.
- Atropine may be problematic with *ischemic-induced* AV block because of *increased* myocardial demand that **resultant tachycardia** may produce.

▶ **NOTE:** By increasing *atrial* rate — AV conduction may *paradoxically* worsen *after* giving Atropine. That is, at an atrial rate of 60/min — 1:1 AV conduction (*ventricular rate = 60/min*) may be possible. However, with *atropine-induced* atrial rate increase to 80/min — *no more* than 2:1 AV conduction may now be possible through a diseased or ischemic AV node (*resulting in an overall reduced ventricular rate of only 40/minute*).

- Each patient may respond differently (*Individualize your treatment!*).
- *Don't* use less than 0.5mg Atropine per dose in adults (*may theoretically produce paradoxical slowing*).

☞ Use of a *Pressor* Agent for Bradycardia

Dopamine and Epinephrine are the ACLS "pressor agents" of choice for bradycardia. In our opinion — **_Pressors_** are **2nd-line** to either Atropine or Pacing when a pulse is present. This is because of their potential to *aggravate* the situation (*due to their adrenergic effect*) <u>and</u> the reality that *neither* Dopamine *nor* Epinephrine alone are likely to satisfactorily treat symptomatic bradycardia.
- Give **IV Fluids** *prior* to pressors <u>IF</u> hypovolemia likely.
- In cases when Atropine is either ill-advised *or* fails <u>and</u> pacing is *not yet* available — Our preference for bradycardia *with* pulse is to give

Dopamine (*begin* at **2 µg/kg/minute**; **titrate upward** *as needed based on clinical response*)**.**
- Although prior "doctrine" for giving Dopamine cited *renal-* or *pressor-specific* doses — in reality there is significant variation between patients as to *what* Dopamine dose will produce *which* hemodynamic effect (*ergo start low; titrate up as needed*).
- While **Epinephrine** is our pressor agent of choice for *pulseless* cardiac arrest (*VFib/PEA/Asystole*) — We prefer Dopamine (*as above*) when an increase in BP is the priority.
- IF **Epinephrine** is used to treat *symptomatic* bradycardia <u>with</u> pulse — Be sure to give **Epi** as an **IV infusion** (*and <u>not</u> as an IV bolus!*). You *cannot* take a bolus back ... — whereas more gradual catecholamine infusion is easily titratable (*and easily stopped if excessive tachycardia results*). **Begin Epi** at **1-2 µg/minute**; titrate up as needed.
- Vasopressin is <u>not</u> used to treat bradycardia with pulse.
- IF a pressor <u>is</u> used to treat *symptomatic* bradycardia — Try to **minimize** the time that you use this **treatment**. You may be able to *reduce* the rate of Epinephrine/Dopamine infusion soon after hemodynamics improve (*and correcting other factors may allow you to stop the pressor*).

☞ Use of *Pacing* for Bradycardia

Development of **TCP** (<u>*Trans-Cutaneous*</u> <u>*Pacing*</u>) has dramatically changed the approach to emergency treatment of bradycardia. Favorable points regarding use of this device are:
- Rapidity of application (*and ease of use*) / Lack of invasiveness.
- Effective cardiac pacing in a *majority* of cases (*albeit discomfort when TCP is used in conscious patients*). But — most modern defibrillators have pacing capability <u>and</u> we *no longer* need to depend on arrival of an operator skilled in placing a *transvenous* pacemaker!

▶ NOTE: **TCP** is a **temporizing** measure (*to "bridge" the gap in time until a transvenous pacer can be placed*). The beauty of TCP is ready availability (*TCP may be implemented within seconds!*). This allows **"stand-by"** use (ie, **pacing "readiness"**) at the bedside *if/as* needed.

- There <u>are</u> times when need for transvenous pacing can be *avoided* by TCP *pacing* "readiness" (ie, *IF worrisome bradycardia spontaneously resolves — as might occur with acute inferior MI and transient 3rd-degree AV block*). ● ***Bottom* Line:** Bradycardia <u>with</u> a pulse is often very treatable. Attention to the clinical situation defines *need* for treatment <u>and</u> the preferred *sequence* for interventions.

<u>Pacing CAVEATS: *Is there Capture?*</u>

☞ *Pacing* Caveats:

● Effective TCP capture <u>*can*</u> be obtained in many (*not all*) patients. That said — there are pitfalls inherent in the process of determining IF effective *electrical* <u>and</u> *mechanical* capture are occurring. Consider the 4 rhythm strips shown in **Figure 15-2**:

• Is there *effective* capture for the rhythm strips in <u>Figure 15-2</u> ?
• *How can you tell?* <u>Clinically</u> — What should you do?

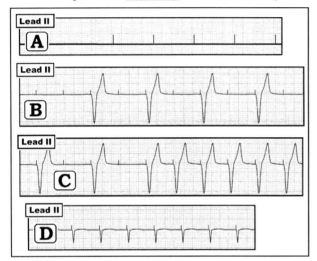

Figure 15-2:
Pacing caveats.
Is there effective
capture for
rhythm strips
A,B,C, and D?
(*See text*).

☞ **Answer to Panel A** (*in Fig. 15-2*): The underlying cardiac rhythm in Panel A is asystole. Pacer spikes are seen at a rate of 75/minute (*occurring every 4th large box*) — but there is *no* sign of capture.

• **Suggested Approach:** Increase current (*gradually from ~50ma up to a max of 200 ma*); correct other factors (ie, *acidosis, hypoxemia*). Treat asystole.

Panel A:

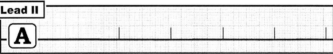

☞ **Answer to Panel B** (*in Fig. 15-2*): The pacer rate is ~100/minute. There is now *electrical* capture of *every-other*-beat in Panel B (*as evidenced by a wide QRS complex with broad T wave occurring after every-other pacing spike*).

• **Suggested Approach:** Since there now <u>is</u> sign of ventricular capture (*at least for every-other pacing spike*) — increasing current further will hopefully result in capture of every spike. Increase current (*up to a max of 200 ma*); correct other factors (ie, *acidosis, hypoxemia*).

Panel B:

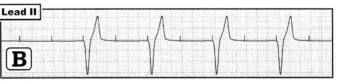

☞ **Answer to Panel C** (*in Fig. 15-2*): Each pacer spike in Panel C now captures the ventricles by the end of this rhythm strip (*evidenced by a wide QRS complex after each spike, followed by a broad, oppositely directed T wave*).

- *Suggested* **Approach:** Look for objective signs to confirm that pacing is working clinically (*Check for pulse and BP; pulse ox pleth wave;* and *ET CO2 readings that should improve if the pacemaker is truly effective*).

Panel C:

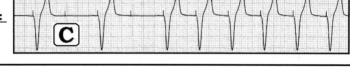

☞ **Answer to Panel D** (*in Fig. 15-2*): The rhythm in Panel D shows a *regularly-occurring* negative deflection after each pacing spike. That said — We suspect this may be **pacer** **artifact** and *not* indicative of true ventricular capture.

- Verifying that *true* ventricular capture has occurred with external pacing is at times easier said than done. Reasons for this include the *indirect* nature of external pacing and a tendency for *electrical* artifact to be produced by the electrical activity generated from the pacemaker.

Panel D:

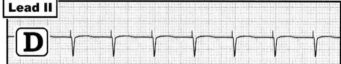

● Electrical artifact is usually *"blocked out"* from the ECG monitor (*by integrated pacemaker software that eliminates a 40-to-80msec period that occurs just after the pacer spike from the ECG recording*). BUT on occasion — a portion of this electrical artifact may persist *beyond* the *blockout* period. When this happens — the electrical artifact that regularly appears on the ECG monitor at fixed interval immediately following each pacer spike may *"masquerade"* as ventricular capture. It is important *not* to be fooled into thinking these *"phantom"* QRS complexes represent true capture. In addition to awareness of this phenomenon — You can **verify** that **ventricular** **capture** has **truly** **occurred** by:

- Being *SURE* the QRS after each pacing spike is *wide* and has a tall *broad* T wave. In contrast — the QRS of *electrical artifact* is narrow and does *not* have any T wave!
- Palpating a pulse with each paced complex (*and being certain not to confuse wishful thinking from pacer-generated muscle twitching as a "pulse"*).
- Checking for other evidence of perfusion (*Can you get a BP? Is there now a pulse ox pleth wave? –* and *– Does ET CO2 increase as it should if the pacer is truly effective?*).

Asystole

● The patient is *unresponsive* in the following rhythm. *No* pulse. *No* spontaneous respiration:

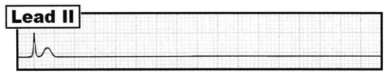

Lead II

Figure 16-1: Asystole (*confirmed by the patient being pulseless and unresponsive*).

• **Rhythm Description** — Flat line rhythm in a patient who is unresponsive *without* a pulse.

• **Bedside Pitfalls** — Keep in mind *other* potential causes of a *flat* line rhythm (ie, very *"fine"* V Fib that may *masquerade* as asystole; *loose* electrode leads/*disconnected* monitor; signal gain *turned way down*).

(☞ **KEY Clinical Points** — Although prognosis is *dismal* when asystole is the cause of *out-of-hospital* arrest — the outcome is <u>not</u> necessarily as uniformly fatal when this rhythm is seen in a hospital setting (*less time until recognition;* **some causes** *of asystole such as excessive vagal tone; hypoglycemia; hypothermia; drug overdose may be* **reversible!**).

Asystole

 ➡ **Suggested *Initial* Approach:**

● Therapeutic interventions for asystole are limited. In addition to **high-quality BLS** — ACLS-PM (*Provider Manual*) recommends **2 drugs** = Epinephrine *and/or* Vasopressin. While fully acknowledging the overall low chance for survival — there *are* some options to consider:

• **Epinephrine** — Our preference as the *initial* pressor agent to use. Begin with **1 mg IV** (or IO). Repeat every 3-5 minutes. Might consider **HDE** in selected patients (*See page 173*).

• *Consider* **Vasopressin** — Give a *one-time* dose of **40U IV**/IO. ACLS-PM allows for use of Vasopressin *instead of* the 1st or 2nd Epinephrine dose (*page 173*).

• *Consider* **Atropine** — Bicarb — Aminophylline (*See pp 173-174*).
  . *Consider* Pacing (*page 173*).

• Consider the *same* list of **potentially treatable underlying conditions** as given for PEA (*See Section 17 — page 175*).

Asystole: *Potentially "Fixable" Causes*

Whatever chance there may be for saving the patient with asystole — will be greatly improved IF one can find and *correct* a treatable cause. The list of *"potentially fixable"* **causes** is similar to that for the patient with PEA (*or VFib for that matter*). Consider the following:

- *Inadequate* **Ventilation** — pneumothorax (*especially tension pneumothorax*); right mainstem intubation.
- *Inadequate* **Circulation** — hypovolemia from blood loss, dehydration, shock; aneurysmal rupture; pulm. embolus; cardiac tamponade.
- *Metabolic* **Conditions** — hyperkalemia, acidosis, hypoglycemia, drug overdose, hypothermia.

▶ NOTE: **ACLS-PM** (*ACLS Provider Manual*) summarizes **treatable causes** of cardiac arrest (*be this from VT/VFib — Asystole/PEA*) by use of **6 H**'s and **5 T**'s:

- **6 H's:** — **H**ypoxia; **H**ypovolemia; **H**ypothermia; **H**+ ion (*acidosis*); **H**ypoglycemia; and **H**yper- *or* **H**ypoKalemia.

- **5 T-s:** — **T**oxins (*including drug overdose*); **T**amponade (*cardiac*); **T**ension Pneumothorax; **T**hrombosis *that is* **Pulmonary** (*embolus*) or **Coronary** (*acute MI*).

Clinical **Perspective:** *Prevalence of Asystole/PEA/VFib*

 ➡ *Clinical* **Perspective:**

⬤ As discussed on page 5 — the *incidence* of **VFib** as the **mechanism** (*initial rhythm*) of **cardiac** arrest has been decreasing in recent years. This holds true for *both* in-hospital and *out-of-hospital* arrests. At the same time — the *incidence* of **Asystole/PEA** as the initial rhythm in cardiac arrest has been increasing. A majority of cardiac arrests now manifest Asystole/PEA as the *initial* mechanism. Clinical implications of these trends are obvious:

- Reasons why the overall incidence of **VFib** is *decreasing* include: **i)** Prompt evaluation with timely reperfusion of patients with acute STEMI (*ST Elevation Myocardial Infarction*); **ii)** Greater public awareness of the need to seek help/call 911 for *new-onset* chest pain; **iii)** More rapid evaluation of chest pain patients who rule out for acute MI — with earlier initiation of treatment for coronary disease; **iv)** More widespread use of ICD (*Implantable Cardioverter-Defibrillator*) devices as treatment for patients with severe heart failure and/or malignant arrhythmias.
- Reasons why *at the same time* the overall incidence of **Asystole/PEA** is *increasing* relate to how common these *"nonshockable"* **rhythms** have become as the **terminal** event in *chronically* ill patients with *multiple* underlying co-morbidities, who have often been kept alive

only by extraordinary treatment measures (*long-term use of venti-lators, pressor drugs, hyperalimentation and extended use of broad spectrum antibiotics*).

- **Prognosis** for cardiac arrest with a **"shockable" rhythm** (*VT/VFib*) as the mechanism is **far better** than when the initial rhythm is a *"nonshockable"* rhythm such as Asystole or PEA. This is especially true if VT/VFib arise as a primary electrical phenomenon in a patient who does not have irreversible underlying heart disease.
- In contrast — When the *precipitating* mechanism of cardiac arrest is **Asystole** or **PEA** in a *chronically* ill patient — the likelihood of *suc-cesssful* resuscitation that is sustained to the point that the patient will *leave* the hospital with intact neurologic status becomes *exceed-ingly* small. That said — on occasion, asystole may be rapidly recognized — <u>and</u>, if *promptly* treated — even reversible! (*See below*).

Asystole: *Beyond-the-Textbook*

  ⇒ ***Beyond-the-Textbook ...***

⬤   As emphasized — overall prognosis for cardiac arrest with asystole as the mechanism is extremely poor. This is the reason ACLS-PM has *removed* pacing <u>and</u> atropine from asystole treatment protocols.

- IF asystole is found as the *initial* rhythm with OOH (*Out-of-Hospital*) cardiac arrest — the *realistic* chance for successful resuscitation is virtually *nil*. This is because *irreversible* cerebral and myocardial injury has almost certainly occurred by this point ...
- *Special* circumstances (ie, *cold-water drowning in a young child*) may provide *rare* exception to the above statement — but in general, OOH asystole is lethal.
- The above said — on occasion **asystole** *may* be a *reversible* rhythm IF it occurs <u>in</u> the hospital, and IF it is promptly recognized and treated.
- **Profound *vagal* stimuli** (*as may occur during prolonged emesis* or *during a procedure such as endoscopy; pulling a chest tube; pulling a central IV line; cardiac cath when injecting the coronary arteries*) <u>have</u> been shown to precipitate marked bradycardia <u>and</u> *even* asystole. In such circumstances — prompt cessation of the stimulus <u>and</u> treat-ment with **Atropine**, Epinephrine *and/or* pacing offer a surprisingly good chance for successful resuscitation.

☞ **Asystole: *A Practical Clinical Approach***

ACLS-<u>PM</u> does *not* alter recommendations for asystole based on presumed cause, whether the event was witnessed <u>or</u> duration of asystole.

- Atropine and pacing are *no longer* recommended by ACLS-PM because they are "unlikely to have benefit" (<u>not</u> *because they are harmful*).
- Most studies on pacing *delayed* intervention until after other treatments failed (*at which time nothing is likely to work*).

⬤ As a result of the unfortunate clinical reality of likely *lethal* outcome if nothing is done – <u>and</u> – awareness that there <u>are</u> occasional instances when prompt recognition and treatment of asystole may be lifesaving (ie, *profound vagal stimuli in a monitored patient*) — We suggest consideration of the interventions below.

> ▶ **NOTE:** We do <u>not</u> routinely advocate these interventions — but rather present them to enhance the clinical armamentarium of the *thinking* clinician for those instances in which there is *some* likelihood that they may be effective.

• **Atropine** — <u>is</u> reasonable to try in *selected* patients <u>IF</u> presumed duration of asystole is *not* prolonged <u>and</u> increased vagotonia seems likely to have a role. Give **1 mg IV** (*or* IO). May repeat in 1-3 minutes (*up to a total dose of 3 mg*).

• **Pacing** — is reasonable (*if not preferable*) to try <u>IF</u> it can be promptly started for witnessed (*monitored*) asystole.

• *Neither* pacing nor atropine is likely to work for prolonged *out-of-hospital* asystole (*especially if arrest is unwitnessed*). They are not recommended in this setting.

• **Epinephrine** <u>*plus*</u> **Vasopressin** — Data are lacking regarding *potential* for **synergistic effect** using <u>*both*</u> Epinephrine <u>*plus*</u> Vasopressin in cardiac arrest. Use of both drugs <u>is</u> reasonable (*slightly differing mechanisms of action*) in *selected* patients for whom the treating clinician feels potential for successful resuscitation exists. Little is lost by this approach given the otherwise dismal prognosis.

• Data are also lacking regarding the *"maximum dose"* of **Epinephrine** for asystole. As a result — a rationale can be made for empiric trial of increasing Epinephrine doses (*2,3,5mg*) in *selected* patients = **HDE** (**H**igher-**D**ose **E**pinephrine).

> ▶ **NOTE:** We do <u>not</u> favor routine use of HDE. Similarly — We do <u>not</u> favor routine use of *both* Epinephrine *plus* Vasopressin for all cases <u>IF</u> arrest is prolonged, prognosis appears dismal, <u>and</u> irreversible brain damage appears likely. We merely present these as options that *may* be considered.

• **Bicarb** — may at times be considered (*page 174*).
• **Aminophylline** — *might* be considered (*page 174*).

• Insight to the likelihood that a patient may respond to treatment may be provided by **capnography** (*pp 18-20*). Prognosis is exceedingly poor — IF **ET CO2** (*End-Tidal CO2*) values **persist <10mm Hg** after more than 20 min of CPR. In contrast — progressively *rising* ET CO2 values with ongoing CPR may be an indication to *continue* intensive therapy.

> ▶ **NOTE:** The finding of asystole as the initial rhythm of cardiac arrest is *no longer* viewed as a relative contraindication to **therapeutic** hypothermia — IF ROSC (*Return Of Spontaneous Circulation*) occurs but the patient fails to wake up (*pp 12-13*).

 Asystole: *Use of BICARB*

ACLS-PM *no longer* routinely recommends Sodium Bicarbonate in the cardiac arrest algorithm. The initial acidosis in cardiac arrest is primarily respiratory (*especially during the first 5-10 minutes*). Giving Bicarb during these initial minutes may paradoxically *worsen* intracellular acidosis (*despite improving ABG pH values*). That said — there <u>are</u> select circumstances when *empiric* **BICARB** (~1 mEq/kg = ~1-1.5 amps) may be reasonable and should *at least* be considered:
- **Hyperkalemia** (*Bicarb is a treatment of choice*)!
- **Tricyclic Overdose** — to alkalinize to a pH value of ~7.45-7.55 in select severe cases of tricyclic overdose.
- ***Preexisting* Metabolic Acidosis**.
- Perhaps (?) for *refractory* cardiac arrest *after* ~5-10 min of resuscitation — <u>IF</u> pH is *still* low (<7.25) and *nothing* else is working ...

 Asystole: *Use of Aminophylline*

ACLS-PM has *never* mentioned use of Aminophylline in its algorithms. Theoretically — there is a rationale for considering Aminophylline in treatment of bradyarrhythmias (*and in years past there were positive reports with use in some ischemic-related forms of AV block*).
- Aminophylline is a **competitive antagonist** of **Adenosine**. Endogenous adenosine (*ADP/ATP*) is produced and released by myocardial cells as a mediator of *ischemic/hypoxemic-related* asystole or bradycardia (*Aminophylline may reverse the rate-slowing effect of endogenous ATP*). That said — studies of bradyasystolic arrest have *not* shown improved survival with use of Aminophylline.

▶ **NOTE:** We do <u>not</u> favor routine use of **Aminophylline** in bradyasystolic arrest. That said — it *might* be tried in *selected* cases (**250 mg IV** *— over 1-2 min; may repeat*). There would seem to be little to lose ...

PEARL: One instance in which Aminophylline <u>is</u> an agent of choice is for ***adenosine-induced* persistent *extreme* bradycardia**. This might occur if a heart transplant patient is inadvertently given Adenosine to treat SVT (*since adenosine half-life is prolonged and resultant bradycardia may therefore persist in such patients*).
- Most of the time — the *ultra-short* half-life of IV Adenosine (*less than 10 seconds!*) — results in very short duration of bradycardia (*almost always resolving in less than 30-60 seconds*).
- Aminophylline may also be life-saving <u>IF</u> *extreme* bradycardia/asystole develops during an adenosine or Lexiscan stress test (*as a competitive antagonist — aminophylline may reverse adenosine-induced extreme bradycardia*).

▶ **Asystole *Bottom* Line:** *Overall* prognosis for asystole is unfortunately poor. That said — *early* intervention may help on occasion in selected cases (*especially if asystole is witnessed, promptly treated,* <u>and</u> *a reversible cause is identified*)

PEA

● The patient is *unresponsive* in the rhythm below. There is *no* palpable pulse.

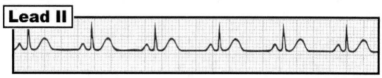

Figure 17-1: PEA (*confirmed by the absence of a palpable pulse*).

• **Rhythm Description** — PEA (*Pulseless Electrical Activity*) is an *organized* rhythm on the monitor of a patient with *no* palpable pulse.
• **Bedside Pitfalls** — *Whenever* the rhythm changes on the monitor — Be *SURE* to check for a pulse. IF no pulse is palpated — then the rhythm is PEA!

▶ **NOTE:** A *wide* tachycardia rhythm *without* a pulse is *not* PEA (*even though "no pulse" is felt*). Instead — Presume *pulseless* VT and shock!

KEY Points: *Potentially "Fixable" Causes of PEA*

 KEY *Clinical* Points:

● Clinically — Whatever chance there might be for saving a patient with PEA will be greatly enhanced IF one can find and correct a treatable cause. The list of ***"potentially fixable"* causes** is similar to that for the patient with asystole (*or VFib for that matter*). Consider the following:
• ***Inadequate* Ventilation** — pneumothorax (*especially tension pneumothorax*); right mainstem intubation.
• ***Inadequate* Circulation** — hypovolemia from blood loss, dehydration, shock; aneurysmal rupture; pulm. embolus; cardiac tamponade.
• ***Metabolic* Conditions** — hyperkalemia, acidosis, hypoglycemia, drug overdose, hypothermia.

▶ NOTE: **ACLS-PM** (*ACLS Provider Manual*) summarizes **treatable causes** of cardiac arrest (*be this from VT/VFib — Asystole/PEA*) by use of **6 H**'s and **5 T**'s:

• **6 H's:** — **H**ypoxia; **H**ypovolemia; **H**ypothermia; **H**+ ion (*acidosis*); **H**ypoglycemia; and **H**yper- or **H**ypoKalemia.

• **5 T-s:** — **T**oxins (*including drug overdose*); **T**amponade (*cardiac*); **T**ension Pneumothorax; **T**hrombosis *that is* **Pulmonary** (*embolus*) or **Coronary** (*acute MI*).

PEA: *Suggested Initial Approach*

 ➡ Suggested *Initial* Approach:

● The key premise for the approach to PEA is to identify a *precipitating* cause that can hopefully be corrected. Recommended interventions include the following:

- **High-quality** BLS (*since PEA by definition is a nonperfusing rhythm*).
- **Epinephrine** — The *only* drugs recommended for PEA by ACLS-PM are pressor agents (*Epinephrine or Vasopressin*). We favor starting with Epinephrine. Begin with **1 mg IV** (*or* IO). Repeat every 3-5 minutes. Consider **HDE** (*page 177*).
- *Consider* **Vasopressin** — Give a *one-time* dose of **40 U IV**/IO (*ACLS-PM allows for use of Vasopressin instead of the 1st or 2nd dose of Epinephrine*).
- Look for a potentially *treatable* **Cause** (*pg 174*). Realistically — finding and "fixing" the cause(s) of PEA holds the key for successful resuscitation and survival.
- *Volume* infusion — as *empiric* trial (*since hypovolemia is perhaps the most common potentially correctable cause of PEA*).
- Pacing — is *not* routinely indicated for PEA (*page 178*).
- Atropine — is *not* routinely indicated for PEA (*page 178*).
- *Consider* Bicarb — IF PEA is thought to result from acidosis — hyperkalemia — *and/or* tricyclic overdose (*page 178*).

PEA: *Beyond-the-Textbook*

 ➡ *Beyond-the-Textbook ...*

● The incidence of **PEA** as the mechanism (*initial rhythm*) of cardiac arrest has increased dramatically in recent years. Together with asystole — PEA/Asystole is now the most common mechanism of cardiac arrest. **Overall prognosis** for PEA is **extremely poor** — especially when PEA develops as the *terminal* event in a chronically ill patient with multiple co-morbidities who has *only* been kept alive by ongoing extraordinary measures (*longterm use of ventilators, pressor drugs, hyperalimentation, extended use of broad spectrum antibiotics*).

- In contrast — the *chance* for **survival** (*with intact neurologic status*) is **not negligible** IF: **i)** PEA occurs in-the-hospital and is *promptly* recognized; **ii)** High-quality CPR is *immediately* started; and **iii)** a potentially *treatable* cause of PEA is recognized and corrected.

▶ **NOTE:** The disorder known as **"PEA"** — is part of a **spectrum**. By definition — PEA rhythms entail **electrical** activity (*ECG rhythm on monitor*) but **NO palpable pulse**.

- That said — at least some *meaningful* cardiac contraction is surprisingly often present (*as detectable by Echo or by pulse with Doppler obtained during resuscitation).* The definition of "PEA" is still satisfied in such cases — because mechanical activity is <u>not</u> sufficient to produce a *palpable* pulse (*nor to generate effective cardiac output*).

☞ PEA: *Use of Epinephrine* and/or *Vasopressin*

The only 2 drugs that ACLS-PM (*Provider <u>M</u>anual*) recommends for treatment of PEA are Epinephrine and Vasopressin. We draw attention to the following:

• There is no evidence for superiority of one drug over the other. We favor starting with Epinephrine — but ACLS-PM allows for *either* drug to be tried first.

• Data are lacking regarding *potential* for **synergistic effect** using <u>both</u> Epinephrine <u>plus</u> Vasopressin in cardiac arrest. Use of both drugs <u>is</u> reasonable (*slightly differing mechanisms of action*) in *selected* patients for whom the treating clinician feels potential for successful resuscitation exists. Little is lost by this approach given the otherwise dismal prognosis of PEA.

• Data are also lacking regarding the **"maximum dose"** of **Epinephrine** for PEA. As a result — a rationale can be made for empiric trial of *increasing* Epinephrine doses (*2,3,5mg*) in *selected* patients = **HDE** (**H**igher-**D**ose **E**pinephrine).

▶ **NOTE:** We do <u>not</u> favor routine use of HDE. Similarly — We do <u>not</u> favor routine use of *both* Epinephrine *plus* Vasopressin for all cases <u>IF</u> arrest is prolonged, prognosis appears dismal, <u>and</u> irreversible brain damage appears likely. We merely present these as options that *may* be considered for the patient with PEA who is not responding.

☞ PEA: *Predicting the Chance for Recovery*

A number of clinical parameters may be used to provide insight as to which patients with PEA have greater likelihood of responding to treatment. *Realistic* chance for *recovery* from PEA is enhanced when one or more of the following are seen. Recognition of these signs encourages continued intense resuscitation:

• Evidence of *meaningful* mechanical activity (*cardiac contraction seen on Echo; detection of pulse by Doppler; well-formed pulse oximetry pleth waveform*).
• Presence of an *organized* ECG rhythm (*especially if the QRS is narrow* <u>and</u> *conducting P waves are seen*).
• *Improving* ET CO2 values *during* resuscitation.
• **Identification of** a readily **treatable cause** of **PEA** (*especially if recognized relatively early in the process*).

☞ PEA: *Benefit of Doing a STAT Echocardiogram*

When available — *Consider* use of **stat Echo** <u>*during*</u> resuscitation. Potential benefits derived from doing an Echo on the patient with PEA include (*See also page 17*):

- Determination <u>IF</u> there is meaningful cardiac contraction (*albeit inadequate to produce a palpable pulse*).
- Ready detection of pericardial (*or pulmonary*) effusion.
- Detection of acute pulmonary embolism (*that may be amenable in certain select centers to emergency thrombectomy or lytic therapy*).
- Detection of regional wall motion abnormalities (*might suggest acute MI that could benefit from immediate cath and reperfusion*).
- Diagnosis of acute dissecting aneurysm (*that might be amenable in select centers to emergency surgery*).
- Then again — *stat* Echo may simply demonstrate that PEA is <u>*not*</u> due to a correctable cause given the location, personnel, and circumstances of the case at hand. This in itself may be comforting to know (*and provides insight for the difficult decision-making process regarding how long to continue resuscitation efforts*).

☞ PEA: *Use (or Not) of Pacing – Atropine – Bicarb –*

ACLS-PM does <u>*not*</u> routinely recommend Pacing, Atropine or Bicarb for PEA. This is because *none* of these interventions have been shown to appreciably increase survival. That said — We feel there <u>*are*</u> certain PEA situations in which these interventions might be life-saving:

- **Pacing** — may be life-saving for **drug overdose** (*in which myocardium is healthy but conduction temporarily impaired by myocardial depressant drug effect*).
- **Atropine** — may help <u>IF</u> the rate of the PEA rhythm is *very* slow (*especially if increased vagal tone is causative*). Give **1 mg IV** (*or* IO). May repeat in 1-3 min (*up to a total dose of 3 mg*). That said — Atropine *rarely* reverses PEA (*and is <u>not</u> routinely recommended for PEA unless there is marked bradycardia thought to be due to vagal tone*).
- **Bicarb** — *may* be indicated for PEA <u>IF</u> there is: **i)** severe acidosis that caused the PEA; **ii)** *marked* hyperkalemia; <u>or</u> **iii)** severe tricyclic drug overdose.

PEA: *Bottom Line*

 ➡ *Bottom Line*

🔵 *Overall* prognosis for PEA is in general quite poor <u>*unless*</u> you are able to find and fix the *underlying* cause. In the meantime — **Continue high-quality CPR** with *ongoing* pressors (*Epinephrine/Vasopressin*).

- *Continue* to **look** for a **precipitating** cause that you may be able to correct.

Section 18 – Escape *and* Premature Beats (*pp 179-195*)

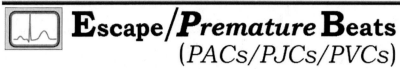

Escape/*Premature* Beats
(PACs/PJCs/PVCs)

● The *underlying* rhythm in <u>Figure 18-1</u> is sinus — as determined by the first 3 beats in this lead II rhythm strip. **Beats #4**, **6** and **8** all occur *earlier* **than expected** (ie, *they are premature beats*).

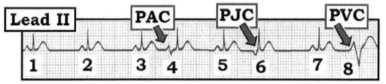

Figure 18-1: Sinus rhythm with *premature* beats (*See text*).

☞ *Premature* Beats: *Description*

Premature beats are QRS complexes that interrupt the underlying rhythm by occurring *earlier* than expected. They are of **3 basic types:**

- **PACs** (**P**remature **A**trial **C**ontractions) — when the underlying rhythm is interrupted by an early beat arising from somewhere in the atria *other* <u>than</u> the SA node. As a result — P wave morphology of a PAC will usually differ in some way from P wave appearance of normal sinus beats (*as seen for* **beat #4** in <u>Figure 18-1</u>). Most often the impulse from a PAC will be conducted with a *narrow* **QRS complex** that is *identical* in appearance to that of normal sinus-conducted beats.

- **PJCs** (**P**remature **J**unctional **C**ontractions) — when the underlying rhythm is interrupted by an early beat arising from the *AV Node*. Most often the impulse is conducted with a *narrow* **QRS** that is at least similar (*if not identical*) in appearance to that of normal sinus-conducted beats. The **P wave** in **lead II** is *negative* or **absent** (*Note the negative P wave with short PR interval preceding* **beat #6** *for the PJC in* <u>Figure 18-1</u>). PJCs are much *less* common than PACs.

- **PVCs** (**P**remature **V**entricular **C**ontractions) — when the underlying rhythm is interrupted by an early beat arising from the *ventricles*. PVCs are *wide* and have an **appearance** that is *very* **different** from that of normal sinus-conducted beats. PVCs are **not** **preceded** by a *premature* **P** wave (*as seen for* **beat #8** in <u>Figure 18-1</u>).

KEY Points: *Premature Beats*

☞ **KEY** *Clinical* **Points:**

● The significance of premature beats depends on a number of factors including the *type* of beat — whether it occurs in *isolation* or in runs — and most importantly, on the *clinical* **setting** in which such beats occur. For example, some patients manifest hundreds (_even thousands!_) of PVCs each hour that are of no prognostic significance (_and need <u>not</u> be treated_). In contrast — development of **frequent new-onset PVCs** with **runs** in a patient with acute _ischemic_ chest pain _is_ cause for concern <u>and</u> _may_ need treatment (ie, _with Amiodarone or other antiarrhythmic_).

- Assess the patient with premature beats for **_extracardiac_ factors** (_caffeine, alcohol, cocaine, amphetamines,_ <u>and</u> _OTC sympathomimetics such as cough/cold preparations_). Try to _eliminate_ these if possible.

- Also assess for potential **_exacerbating_ factors** (ie, _heart failure, hypoxemia, acidosis, hypokalemia/hypomagnesemia, ischemia_). Premature beats often resolve <u>IF</u> these factors can be corrected or eliminated.

- **PACs**/PJCs per se are usually benign (_although if frequent, they may precipitate various types of SVT rhythms_). Specific drug treatment of PACs/PJCs is usually <u>not</u> needed. Instead — emphasis should be placed on **correcting _other_** exatracardiac _and/or_ potentially exacerbating **factors** that may be predisposing the patient to having PACs/PJCs.

- **PACs** are far _more_ common than **PJCs**. That said — the clinical significance of these two forms of premature _supraventricular_ beats is virtually _identical_ — so it is rarely important clinically to distinguish between the two.

- **PVCs** are potentially of greater clinical consequence than PACs or PJCs. This is because under certain circumstances — the occurrence of PVCs at an _inopportune_ moment in the cardiac cycle may _precipitate_ a run of VT. The risk of this occurring depends on multiple factors, including presence of **underlying _heart_ disease** _plus_ potential contribution from the extracardiac _and/or_ exacerbating factors described above.

- **_Isolated_ PVCs** are most often benign. Even if frequent _and/or_ in short runs (ie, _non-sustained_ VT) — they are almost always benign <u>IF</u> the patient does <u>not</u> have underlying heart disease. Treatment is _only_ indicated if PVCs produce symptoms (_a **β-Blocker** is typically the drug of choice_).

- In contrast — **_Repetitive_ PVCs** (_couplets/runs of VT_) become cause for concern when they occur in patients who <u>do</u> have _underlying_ heart disease — especially <u>IF</u> the VT produces symptoms such as syncope <u>or</u> there is evidence of _acute_ ischemia.

- There now <u>is</u> an effective treatment for patients with chronic **malignant _ventricular_ arrhythmias** (ie, _symptomatic VT with associated hypotension, syncope/presyncope, or sudden death_). **_Such patients should be referred_** for consideration of an **ICD** (_<u>I</u>mplantable <u>C</u>ardioverter-<u>D</u>efibrillator_). Although longterm antiarrhythmic therapy (ie, _with amiodarone, procainamide or other agent_) may be used as an adjunct — drug treatment alone (_without an ICD_) is _ineffective_ for reducing the risk of sudden death from malignant ventricular arrhythmias. On the contrary — longterm antiarrhythmic therapy _without_ ICD backup may paradoxically _increase_ the risk of sudden death in a small but important subset of patients (***proarrhthmia***). This is why patients with chronic malignant ventricular arrhythmias should in most instances be referred.

▶ **NOTE:** Most patients with single or repetitive premature beats do *not* have malignant ventricular arrhythmias. Cardiology (*including EP*) referral is <u>not</u> needed for appropriate ambulatory management of most of these patients. The problematic cases can be referred.

☞ Concise *Clinical* Summary: *Treatment Considerations*

As should be apparent from the clinical points emphasized thus far — correlation of the arrhythmia with symptoms (*or lack thereof*) – <u>and</u> – the patient's history (*underlying heart disease or not*) — are *KEY* to formulating an optimally appropriate therapeutic plan.

- **Isolated *premature* beats** (*be they PACs, PJCs, or PVCs*) — are most often benign. Identification and correction of precipitating or exacerbating factors may be all that is needed. With rare exceptions — use of drugs is <u>not</u> advised for treatment of isolated or infrequent premature beats (*PACs,PJCs,PVCs*).
- Cardiac arrhythmias are *generally* of much *less* concern in the absence of underlying heart disease.
- In contrast — timely assessment and management of patients with **malignant *ventricular* arrhythmias** (*runs of VT associated with symptoms*) is essential for optimal outcome. Section 07 (*pp 63-69*) details specific treatment considerations in the acute setting for the patient with *known* VT. Outside of the acute setting — most patients identified as having malignant ventricular arrhythmias should be referred (*Further details extend beyond the scope of this book*).

Premature Beats: *Beyond-the-Textbook*

 ➡ *Beyond-the-Textbook ...*

● Armed with the above basic premises for management of premature beats — We devote the remainder of this Section and the next (*Section 19 on pp 196-202*) to increasing awareness about a number of *additional* concepts regarding **ECG *recognition*** of premature beats, late beats — and associated arrhythmias. We aim to address the following:

- Why P wave morphology of PACs is usually (*but not always*) different from P wave morphology of normal sinus beats.
- Why this matters clinically?
- What determines what the P wave of a PAC will look like?
- How to distinguish between PACs <u>vs</u> PJCs <u>vs</u> PVCs?
- How to distinguish between premature <u>vs</u> *escape* beats?

☞ PACs: *A Closer Look*

As shown for beat #4 in <u>Figure 18-1</u> (*page 179*) — a **PAC** occurs when the underlying rhythm is interrupted by an early beat arising from somewhere in the atria *other than* the SA node (**Figure 18-2**).

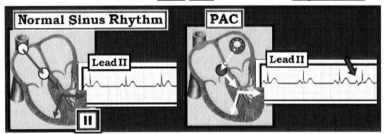

Figure 18-2: Normal sinus rhythm (*left*) <u>vs</u> what happens with a PAC. Ventricular activation occurs early (*prematurely*) with a PAC due to an *early-occurring* impulse arising from another site in the atria. Note the *different* P wave morphology for the PAC compared to sinus P waves (*arrow over the 4th P wave on the right*). The P wave of a PAC looks *different* because it arises from a *different* site in the atria.

☞ The **appearance** (*P wave shape* <u>and</u> *PR interval*) of **PACs** may **vary**. What the P wave will look like — will depend on *from* **where** in the atria the **impulse** is **arising** (<u>Figure 18-3</u>).
- Most often the impulse will be conducted with a **narrow QRS** that is **identical** in **morphology** to normal *sinus-conducted* beats.
- Occasionally — especially *early-occurring* PACs may arrive at the ventricles at a time when a portion of the ventricular conduction system has *not yet* recovered. In such cases — the QRS complex may be *widened* due to **aberrant conduction** (*See Section 19 — pp 196-202*).

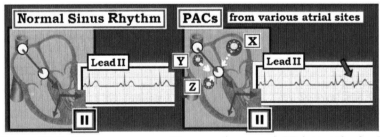

Figure 18-3: The appearance (*P wave shape* <u>and</u> *PR interval*) of a PAC will depend on the location from where in the atria the impulse arises. Consider what PACs arising from sites X, Y or Z might look like?

☞ **Figure 18-3** schematically illustrates how a *different* **atrial site** of origin might affect **P wave appearance** of a PAC.
- The reason the **normal *sinus* P wave** is **upright** (*positive*) in **lead II** — is that the overall direction of atrial activation (*as the impulse*

travels from SA node — through both atria — to AV node) moves *toward* lead II (*which anatomically lies at +60 degrees*).

- **PAC-X** — should show *some* **positivity** (*perhaps like the biphasic PAC under the arrow in* Figure 18-3) — since the *overall* direction of its path en route to the AV node moves *toward* lead II. That said — P wave morphology of **PAC-X** will clearly differ from P wave morphology of normal sinus beats because PAC-X arises from a *different* site (*in the left atrium vs the upper right atrial location of the SA node*) — and its path toward the AV node will follow a different trajectory.

- **PAC-Y** — will be *all* **upright**. It should look *very much* **like** a **normal sinus P wave** — because it arises from a site that anatomically is *very close* to the SA node.

- **PAC-Z** — may be **negative**. IF a PAC arises from *low* **down** in the **atria** (*Z in* Figure 18-3) — its path (*as atrial depolarization spreads up to the left and right atria*) may be directed *away* from lead II. As a result — a **low atrial PAC** may look *indistinguishable* from a **PJC!**

☞ *Advanced* Concept: *Why P Wave Morphology Matters*

When a PAC arises from a site *close* to the SA node (*like* **PAC-Y** *in* Figure 18-3) — any ECG change that occurs in P wave morphology may be subtle. In this case — *more* than a *single* monitoring lead may be needed to detect such subtle change. Awareness of this clinical reality provides but one more example of how obtaining a **12-lead ECG** may assist in arrhythmia diagnosis. Distinction between sinus arrhythmia — vs sinus rhythm or sinus arrhythmia with PACs — vs wandering atrial pacemaker may sometimes *not* be possible *unless* one has access to a *simultaneously* recorded 12-lead tracing (**Figure 18-4** — *on pg 184*):

- *Sinus* **Arrhythmia** – will manifest *identical* P wave morphology for all P waves (*since by definition — all impulses arise from the same place, which is the SA node*). Sinus P waves are *upright* in lead II (*page 22*). The R-R interval will vary with sinus arrhythmia — sometimes markedly (*pp 24-25*).

- *Sinus* **Rhythm** or *Sinus* **Arrhythmia** *with* **PACs** — will manifest *identical* sinus P waves except for *early-occurring* beats, which can be identified as PACs by their *differing* P wave morphology. That said — it may at times be exceedingly challenging to try to distinguish between baseline variation in R-R interval from sinus arrhythmia — vs sinus arrhythmia with PACs that only manifest *minimal* variation in P wave morphology compared to normal sinus beats (Figure 18-4).

☞ Clinical *Bottom* Line: *Variation in P Wave Morphology*

Most of the time — subtle variations in P wave morphology as seen in **Figure 18-4** will *not* matter clinically. We present these variations primarily to illustrate the reason why P wave morphology may change (Figure 18-3) — as well as to emphasize the potential benefit of obtaining a **12-lead ECG** as possible *whenever* the etiology of an arrhythmia is in question.

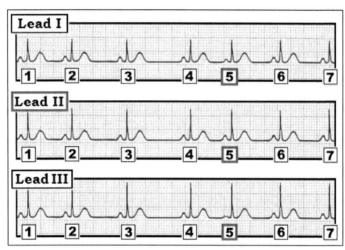

Figure 18-4: Use of *additional* leads to distinguish between sinus arrhythmia <u>vs</u> PACs. Rhythm strips are *simultaneously* recorded in leads I, II and III. Although **beat #5** clearly occurs *earlier* than other beats in this tracing — the *similar* morphology of *all* P waves in **lead II** makes it difficult to determine <u>IF</u> slightly *early* occurrence of beat #5 reflects the *underlying* sinus arrhythmia <u>or</u> is due to a PAC. It is *only* when we look at **simultaneously recorded leads I** and **III** — that a definite difference in P wave morphology for beat #5 is seen. One could <u>not</u> have known that beat #5 is a **PAC** if *only* lead II had been used ...

▶ **NOTE:** Use of multiple leads for assessing P wave morphology is an *advanced* concept. *Do <u>not</u> be concerned* if the above goes beyond the level of arrhythmia interpretation you wish to attain.

- Realize that yet a *final* layer of complexity may be introduced beyond that illustrated by **Figure 18-4** — <u>IF</u> ***baseline* artifact** is present (*as it so often is when ECGs are obtained on acutely ill patients*). In such cases — the clinician needs to further distinguish between variations in P wave morphology that may be due to artifact <u>vs</u> changes that are *real* due to shift in the atrial site of origin for the beat(s) in question.
- Distinction between sinus arrhythmia <u>vs</u> sinus arrhythmia with PACs <u>vs</u> wandering atrial pacemaker is in many cases merely of academic interest. This is because immediate specific treatment is rarely indicated for any of these rhythm disturbances. That said — an example of when distinction between sinus <u>vs</u> ectopic P waves *does* make an important clinical difference is in differentiation between sinus tachycardia <u>vs</u> **ectopic *atrial* tachycardia**. Recognition of a *change* in P wave morphology is usually essential for the diagnosis of atrial tachycardia. Whereas treatment of the much more common sinus tachycardia focuses on identification and correction of the underlying precipitating cause — specific treatment <u>will</u> *often* be needed for *symptomatic* atrial tachycardia. <u>IF</u> seen in a patient taking digitalis —

atrial tachycardia almost always indicates digoxin toxicity. When seen in a patient not on digitalis — specific antiarrhythmic treatment (ie, *with amiodarone or other drug*) is indicated.

☞ *Distinction Between* PACs <u>*vs*</u> *"Escape"* Beats

The *KEY* to recognizing *premature* beats (*PACs,PJCs,PVCs*) — is their **timing** (*early occurrence*) with respect to the *underlying* rhythm. Contrast the timing of *premature* beats with what is seen below in **Figure 18-5**. — Is the *different-looking* P wave for **beat #5** a PAC?

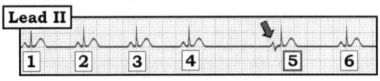

Figure 18-5: Distinction between PACs <u>vs</u> escape beats. Does beat #5 occur *earlier* or *later* than expected? (*See text*).

☞ **Answer to Figure 18-5:** The *underlying* rhythm in Figure 18-5 is sinus — as determined by the presence of regular upright P waves preceding beats #1-*thru*-#4 with a constant (*and normal*) PR interval.
- It should be obvious that **beat #5** is **late**. As a result (*by definition*) — beat #5 can *not* be a "PAC", since it is *not* "premature".
- Instead — beat #5 is an ***"escape"* beat**. Beat #5 in Figure 18-5 is a good thing! Sinus conduction fails after beat #4. If not for the atrial escape beat (*beat #5*) — the pause may have been *much* longer...

● We *know* the **site** of **escape beat #5** in Figure 18-5 is **atrial** — because: **i)** The QRS is narrow (*and identical in morphology to the QRS of normal sinus beats*); *and* **ii)** Beat #5 is preceded by a P wave that looks *different* than the sinus P wave (*arrow in Figure 18-5*).
- Note that **sinus rhythm** resumes after *slight* delay with **beat #6**.
- The duration of the **brief pause** (*between beats #4-to-5*) is **1.4 seconds** (*7 large boxes*). Clinically — pauses *less* than 2.0 seconds are common and usually *not* of concern.

☞ PJCs: *A Closer Look*

As was shown at the beginning of this Section (*in* Figure 18-1 *on page 179 for beat #6*) — a **PJC** occurs when the *underlying* rhythm is interrupted by an early beat arising from the AV node. We schematically illustrate the sequence of activation with a PJC in **Figure 18-6** (*page 186*). The left panel in this Figure distinguishes PJC activation from what occurs with a PAC (*in which the early-occurring impulse arises from a site in the atria and travels toward rather than away from the AV node*).

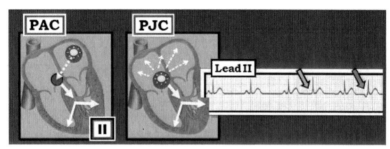

Figure 18-6: Comparison of what happens with a **PAC** (*left*) <u>vs</u> what happens with a PJC (*right panel*). Ventricular activation occurs early (*prematurely*) with a PAC due to an *early-occurring* impulse arising from a site in the atria *other than* the SA node. In contrast, with a **PJC** (*right panel*) — the early impulse arises from the AV node. As a result — there is *retrograde* activation of the atria at the same time there is *forward* propagation of the impulse to the ventricles (*See text*).

☞ With a **PJC** — the early beat arises from *within* the AV node. From there it travels down the Bundle of His and over the normal conduction pathway as it activates ventricular myocardium. As a result — the premature impulse with a PJC is usually conducted with a **narrow QRS** complex that is **similar** (*or identical*) in appearance to *sinus-conducted* beats.

- The **P wave** in **lead II** with a **PJC** will either be **negative** <u>or</u> **absent** (*arrows in* <u>Figure 18-6</u>). Rarely a *negative* P wave may be seen immediately *after* the QRS with a PJC. But by far — the **most common** situation is for there to be **no P wave** preceding the *early-occurring* narrow QRS that is a PJC.
- There are exceptions to the statement that with PJCs the QRS complex will be narrow. That is — there may be *baseline* QRS widening (*from preexisting bundle branch block*) – <u>or</u> – the PJC may occur so early in the cycle that it conducts with aberration. That said — the vast majority of the time, the **QRS complex** with a **PJC** will be **narrow** and *at the least* look very similar to the QRS complex of normal *sinus-conducted* beats.

▶ <u>PEARL</u> (*Advanced Concept*): On occasion — the **QRS** of a **PJC** may be **similar** but **<u>not</u>** identical to the QRS of normal sinus beats. This is because the AV node is *not* a homogenous structure. Instead — a PJC may arise from *different* parts of the AV node (ie, *from the top, sides, or bottom of the AV node*). This may result in a **minimal** (*yet often noticeable*) **variation** in QRS morphology of the PJC. Once *out* of the AV node — normal conduction resumes through the Bundle of His, bundle branches, and Purkinje fibers.

- The above *advanced* concept is illustrated in **Figure 18-6** — in which the **1st PJC** (*1st arrow*) manifests a narrow QRS that is *slightly taller* than the QRS of all other beats in this tracing. Note that the 2nd PJC in this tracing (*2nd arrow*) manifests a QRS that is *identical* to the QRS of normal sinus beats.

- Recognizing subtle differences in QRS morphology between sinus and AV nodal beats <u>is</u> challenging. For the ***more advanced* interpreter** — this concept may be of *invaluable* assistance when interpreting complex arrhythmias in which subtle differences in QRS morphology reveal which beats are nodal escape <u>vs</u> sinus-conducted.

▶ **SUMMARY re ECG *Recognition* of PJCs:** PJCs are *supraventricular* beats that occur *earlier-than-expected* and arise from the AV node. The QRS complex of a PJC will usually be narrow (*unless the patient has underlying bundle branch block* <u>or</u> *manifests aberrant conduction*). QRS morphology will <u>either</u> be *identical* to that of normal *sinus-conducted* beats <u>or</u> very similar to sinus beats. PJCs may be preceded by a *negative* P wave in lead II <u>or</u> manifest *no* P wave at all (*Rarely a negative P wave may follow the QRS in lead II*).

☞ ***Distinguishing Between* PJCs *vs* Low Atrial PACs**

The etiology of *early-occurring* beats that are preceded by a *negative* P wave in lead II is often open to question. Can YOU tell <u>IF</u> the 2nd early beat in **Figure 18-7** (*2nd arrow in Figure*) is a **PAC** <u>or</u> **PJC?**
- Clinically — *Does it matter* if the beat under the question mark in Figure 18-7 is a PAC or PJC? If not — *WHY* not?

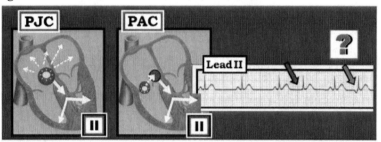

Figure 18-7: Differentiating between a PJC (*left panel*) <u>vs</u> a *low atrial* PAC (*right panel*). In either case — a *negative* P wave may be seen to precede the *early-occurring* QRS complex in lead II (*See text*).

☞ **Answer to Figure 18-7:** There is a tendency for providers to call any *early-occurring* supraventricular (*narrow-complex*) beat a "PJC" if it is preceded by a *negative* P wave in lead II.
- Much of the time — this well-intentioned tendency is inaccurate.
- Clinically — *it doesn't matter*.

● There are **3 types** of ***premature* beats**: **i) PACs** (*arising from a site in the atria*); **ii) PJCs** (*arising from the AV node*); <u>and</u> **iii) PVCs** (*arising from a site in the ventricles*). <u>IF</u> the *early-occurring* beat has a ***narrow***

QRS complex — then it is *either* a PAC or a PJC (*since the QRS will be wide with a PVC*).

• Clinically — **PACs** are *far more common* than PJCs. As a result, on a *statistical* basis — the chances are far greater that a *narrow* premature beat will be a PAC rather than a PJC.

• IF the site of the premature beat arises from *low down* in the atria (*right panel in* Figure 18-7) — then the path of atrial depolarization may be perceived as moving *away* from the direction of lead II (*thereby writing a negative P wave in lead II*).

• That said — **It doesn't really matter** IF the *narrow* premature beat is a PAC or PJC — because clinical consequences of these two types of premature beats are the same (*pp 179-181*).

▶ **Beyond-the-Core:** One may suspect that IF the *narrow* premature beat has a *negative* P wave preceding it with a very *short* PR interval — that it is more likely to be a PJC. Conversely — one might anticipate a PAC to be more likely IF the negative P wave in lead II has a longer PR interval. While these suppositions are probably true — the clinical reality is that relative length of the PR interval from the negative P to the premature QRS complex is *not* reliably predictive of site of origin. That said — discussion is academic *because it doesn't matter* clinically.

🖙 **Escape** Beats: *Identifying Narrow-Complex Escape*

As previously emphasized — **timing** is the key parameter for distinguishing between *premature* vs *escape* beats. Consider the events in the 2 tracings shown below in **Figure 18-8**:

• What is **beat #5** in *both* Tracing A and Tracing B ?

• Is the P wave that precedes beat #5 in Tracing B conducting?

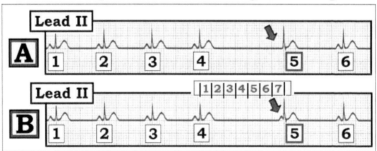

Figure 18-8: *Narrow-complex* escape beats. Why is QRS morphology of beat #5 in each tracing *slightly different* than QRS morphology of normal sinus beats? Is the P wave that just precedes beat #5 in Tracing B conducting? (*See text*).

🖙 **Answer to Figure 18-8:** The *underlying* rhythm in Figure 18-8 is sinus — as determined by the presence of regular upright P waves preceding each of the first 4 beats with a constant (*and normal*) PR interval.

- **Beat #5** in *both* Tracings A and B of Figure 18-8 is **late**. As a result (*by definition*) — beat #5 can *not* be either a "PAC" or "PJC", since it is *not* "premature".
- Instead — beat #5 is an **"escape" beat**. Beat #5 in Figure 18-8 is a *good* thing! Sinus conduction *fails* after beat #4. If not for this escape beat (*beat #5*) — the pause may have been *much* longer...

☞ Focusing first on **Tracing A** in **Figure 18-8**: The QRS complex of beat #5 is narrow. It is *not* preceded by any P wave. As a result — we *know* this escape beat *must be* arising from **within** the **conduction system**. Possibilities include the AV node, bundle of His, or from one of the major fascicles of the bundle branch system. Practically speaking — precise location of the escape site does *not* really matter since initial clinical management will be the same *regardless* of the site.

- Sinus rhythm resumes in Tracing A after *slight* delay with **beat #6**.
- *Beyond-the-Core:* QRS morphology of escape beat #5 is similar but *not quite* identical to QRS morphology of normal sinus beats (*beat #5 is slightly taller than sinus beats — and it has a small narrow s wave that sinus beats don't*). It is not at all uncommon for QRS morphology of escape beats from the AV node or His/fascicles to differ slightly from QRS appearance of normal sinus beats.

☞ Looking next at **Tracing B** in **Figure 18-8**: The QRS complex of beat #5 is again narrow. This time beat #5 is preceded by a P wave — albeit the PR interval *preceding* the QRS of beat #5 in Tracing B is far **too short to conduct**.

- The P wave preceding beat #5 in Tracing B is *not* a "PAC" — because this P wave is not premature.
- We surmise instead that a brief **sinus pause** (*of 7 large boxes =1.4 seconds*) ensues after beat #4. The sinus node finally recovers — but *before* the P wave preceding beat #5 in Tracing B is able to conduct to the ventricles, an **escape** beat occurs.
- That the **QRS** complex of escape beat #5 in Tracing B is **narrow** tells us the escape focus must be arising from a site **within the ventricular conduction system**. Possibilities include the AV node, bundle of His, or one of the major fascicles of the bundle branch system.
- *Beyond-the-Core:* The R-R interval preceding escape beat #5 in Tracing B is 7 large boxes. This corresponds to an **escape rate** of ~**43/minute** (300/7). Given that the *normal* AV nodal *escape* rate range in adults is *between* 40-to-60/minute — this presumed escape rate could be consistent with *either* an AV nodal escape site – or – a site from *lower down* in the ventricular conduction system.
- Normal sinus rhythm resumes in Tracing B after *slight* delay with **beat #6**.

☞ *Identifying WIDE Complex Escape Beats*

Up until now — the QRS complex of the escape beats we have illustrated (*in Figures 18-5 and 18-8*) were *narrow* beats.
• What is beat #5 in **Figure 18-9**? — What happens *after* beat #5?

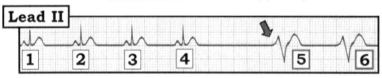

Figure 18-9: *Wide-complex* escape beats. From where does the escape focus arise? (*See text*).

☞ **Answer to Figure 18-9:** The *underlying* rhythm in Figure 18-9 is sinus — as determined by the presence of regular upright P waves preceding beats #1-*thru*-#4 with a constant (*and normal*) PR interval.
• **Beat #5** in <u>Figure 18-9</u> is **late**. Beat #5 is therefore an *"escape"* **beat**.
• The QRS complex of beat #5 is wide. It is *not* preceded by any P wave. Beat #5 in Figure 18-9 is therefore a ***ventricular* escape beat**.
• Once again, beat #5 in <u>Figure 18-9</u> is a *good* thing! Sinus conduction *fails* after beat #4. If not for this escape beat (*beat #5*) — the pause may have been *much* longer ... ●**NOTE:** Unlike the case for Figures 18-5 and 18-8 — *no* P waves are seen after this ventricular escape beat. Instead, another ventricular complex ensues (*beat #6*) — suggesting *protective* emergence of a **ventricular *escape* rhythm**. Additional rhythm strips would be needed to know for sure — but an R-R interval of 5 large boxes (*as seen between beats #5-to-6 in Fig. 18-9*) would correspond to **AIVR (**<u>*A*</u>*ccelerated* <u>*Idio*</u><u>*V*</u>*entricular* <u>*R*</u>*hythm*) at a rate of 60/minute (*300/5=60*). *— See page 195 —*

☞ *Escape* Beats: *KEY Points*

We have already emphasized the *beneficial* aspects of "escape" — namely, that <u>IF</u> the impulse from above *fails* to occur (*for whatever reason*) — that an *"escape"* **beat** (*or an* **escape** *rhythm*) may arise as a **protective mechanism** to prevent a *prolonged* pause or asystole. As is the case for escape beats — there are **4 possible sites** for *escape* **rhythms**. These include:
• from a site in the **Atria**.
• from a site in the **AV Node**.
• from a site <u>*below*</u> the AV node, yet still <u>*within*</u> the conduction system (ie, *from the His or from a major bundle branch fascicle*).
• from the **Ventricles**.

● Practically speaking — we can determine the **probable *escape* site** based on consideration of **3 factors: i)** QRS width and morphology of the escape beat complex; **ii)** rate of the escape rhythm; <u>and</u> **iii)** whether

the escape rhythm is associated with P waves that are conducting. Consider the **4 *escape* rhythms** in **Figure 18-10**.
• What is the *probable* site of escape in *each* case?

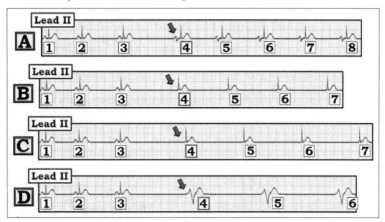

Figure 18-10: The 4 basic types of escape rhythms. (*See text*).

📚 **Answer to Figure 18-10:** Each of the 4 tracings in Figure 18-10 begins with 3 *sinus-conducted* beats. There follows a *brief* pause — with onset of an *escape* **rhythm** beginning with beat #4:

• **Tracing A** — The escape rhythm is regular with a *narrow* QRS complex. The QRS complex during the escape rhythm looks *identical* to the QRS during sinus rhythm. Each QRS complex during the escape rhythm is preceded by a P wave of *different* morphology compared to the first 3 sinus beats. The R-R interval for beats #4-thru-8 is 5 large boxes. This suggests an **atrial escape rhythm** at 60/minute.

• **Tracing B** — The escape rhythm is regular with a *narrow* QRS complex. The QRS during the escape rhythm looks *identical* to the QRS during normal sinus rhythm. *None* of the escape beats are preceded by P waves. The R-R interval for beats #4-*thru*-7 is 6 large boxes. This corresponds to an escape rate of 50/minute (*300/6=50*) — and suggests that beats #4-*thru*-7 represent a **junctional escape rhythm** at a rate *within* the usual 40-60/minute range for AV nodal escape.

• **Tracing C** — The escape rhythm is regular with a *narrow* QRS complex. Close attention to QRS morphology during the escape rhythm suggests a slight difference in morphology compared to the QRS of normal sinus beats (*slightly taller R wave plus addition of a narrow s wave for escape beats*). There are *no* P waves during the escape rhythm. The R-R interval for beats #4-*thru*-7 is 7 large boxes, corresponding to an escape rate of ~43/minute. We can <u>not</u> be sure IF the site of escape is *at* the level of the AV node <u>or</u> *below* the AV node (*but still within the conduction system*). Fortunately — this distinction is <u>not</u> important clinically for initial management.

- **<u>Tracing D</u>** — The escape rhythm is regular with a **wide** QRS that looks very *different* from the QRS of normal sinus beats. There are *no* P waves during the escape rhythm. The R-R interval for beats #4-*thru*-6 is 9 large boxes, corresponding to a rate just over 30/min. This suggests a ***slow idioventricular* escape rhythm** at a rate *within* the usual 20-40/minute range for ventricular escape.

☞ PVCs: *A Closer Look*

We conclude this Section 18 on *Escape/Premature* Beats with a closer look at PVCs (<u>P</u>remature <u>V</u>entricular <u>C</u>ontractions). A **PVC** occurs when the *underlying* rhythm is interrupted by an early beat arising from a site in the left or right ventricle. We schematically illustrate this in **Figure 18-11**.

- PVCs are recognized by **QRS widening** (*morphology very different from that of normal sinus beats*) — <u>and</u> by **lack** of a **preceding** P wave.

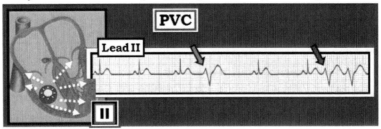

Figure 18-11: A PVC is an *early* beat arising from the left or right ventricle. The QRS of a PVC is wide and *not* preceded by a premature P wave. The 4th beat shown here is a single PVC (*1st arrow*). A ventricular couplet (*2nd arrow*) is seen after the 6th beat (*See text*).

☞ Under normal conditions — conduction through the ventricles is fast over the *normal* pathway (*from AV node — to His — thru bundle branches*). **Conduction *slows* dramatically** (*and the QRS widens*) with a **PVC** (*1st arrow in* <u>Figure 18-11</u>) — because the impulse arises from *outside* the normal pathway.

- One or more PVCs may occur in a row (*2nd arrow highlighting the ventricular couplet in* <u>Figure 18-11</u>).
- Note the ***slight* pause** *following* the 1st PVC in <u>Figure 18-11</u>. This "compensatory pause" is often seen because the next sinus P wave is *unable* to be conducted to the ventricles (*this next sinus P wave falls somewhere within the T wave of this 1st PVC — which is within the absolute refractory period*). Most PVCs will manifest *at least* a slight pause before the sinus beat that follows.
- Note also that the ***coupling* interval** (*distance between the preceding sinus beat and the PVC*) changes for the PVCs highlighted by the arrows in <u>Figure 18-11</u>. Most of the time the coupling interval for

PVCs originating from the same ventricular focus will be the same (*Exceptions exist beyond the scope of this book*).

▶ **Beyond-the-Core:** As implied in Figure 18-11 — the depolarization wavefront originates from the site in the ventricles of the PVC. From there it *spreads* throughout both ventricles. On occasion, after arriving at the AV node — the impulse will be conducted back (*retrograde*) to the atria. When this happens, a *negative* P wave may be seen *after* the PVC in lead II. As may be anticipated — retrograde conduction back to the atria will *reset* the timing of the next sinus P wave.

• Retrograde conduction to the atria does *not* always occur. For simplicity — **Figure 18-11** does not show retrograde atrial conduction.

▶ **PEARL Beyond-the-Core:** Awareness that retrograde atrial conduction *may* occur with ventricular rhythms helps to explain why *non-sinus* atrial activity can sometimes be seen with WCT (*Wide-Complex Tachycardia*) rhythms. Unless there is clear evidence of a *definite* sinus P wave (*upright in lead II with fixed and normal PR interval*) — Always assume a WCT rhythm is VT <u>until</u> proven otherwise (*regardless of whether or not there is suggestion of atrial activity before or after the QRS in other leads during the tachycardia*).

☞ **PVC Definitions: *Repetitive Forms and Runs of VT***

Clinically — the occurrence of **repetitive PVCs (*2 or more in a row*)** — is of much more concern than **isolated PVCs** (*pp 179-181*). In addition to clinical assessment of the patient (ie, *for underlying heart disease; associated medical conditions; electrolyte imbalance; hypoxemia; etc.*) — one aims to assess the *relative* frequency of PVCs — QRS morphology (*uniform or multiform*) — coupling interval — <u>plus</u> the rate and duration of any runs. We define these parameters by means of the 2 rhythms strips shown in **Figure 18-12**:

• Describe the ventricular ectopy seen in Figure 18-12?

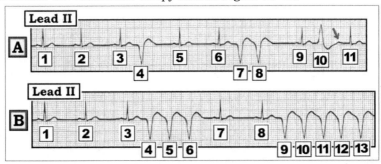

Figure 18-12: Underlying sinus rhythm with various forms of ventricular ectopy. (*See text for description of all PVC forms*).

☞ The **underlying** rhythm for both A and B in Figure 18-12 is **sinus** — as determined by the first 3 beats in each rhythm strip. Numerous forms of ventricular ectopy follow. In **Tracing A**:

- **Beat #4** in Tracing A — is an **isolated** PVC. It is followed by a *brief* pause before resumption of sinus rhythm with beat #5.
- **Beats #7** and **#8** — represent a **ventricular** couplet. Note that the coupling interval (*distance between beat #6 and beat #7 in Tracing A*) and QRS morphology of this ventricular couplet are the *same* as was seen for the initial PVC in the tracing (*beat #4*). Once again, a brief pause follows the 2nd PVC in the couplet (*beat #8*) until resumption of sinus rhythm with beat #9.
- **Beat #10** in Tracing A — is another **isolated** PVC. Note that QRS morphology of beat #10 is very *different* from QRS morphology of all other ventricular beats on these 2 tracings. Because there is more than a single QRS shape for the PVCs seen in Figure 18-12 — we say there are **"multiform" PVCs**. It is common for patients with underlying heart disease to manifest *multiform* PVCs. Their presence does *not* necessarily forebode a worse prognosis than for uniform PVCs. Sinus rhythm resumes at the end of Tracing A with beat #11. Note that there is virtually no pause following this last PVC (*beat #10*).
- *Beyond-the-Core:* The reason there is barely any pause following this last PVC (*beat #10*) — is that the next sinus impulse (*arrow in Tracing A*) falls *beyond* the refractory period and is able to conduct to the ventricles. In fact — it conducts to the ventricles with a *prolonged* PR interval due to an *advanced* concept known as **"concealed" conduction** (*presumed retrograde conduction from the PVC that we do not see on the surface ECG delays forward conduction of the next sinus beat*).

▶ **BOTTOM Line:** Do not be concerned about the concept of "concealed conduction" if it is beyond what you have encountered. What is important — is to recognize that there are **multiform PVCs** in Tracing A — and that a brief pause usually (*but not always*) follows isolated PVCs or the last PVC in a run.

☞ The first 3 beats in **Tracing B** again manifest *underlying* sinus rhythm.

- **Beat #4** in Tracing B begins a **ventricular salvo** or **triplet** (*3 PVCs in a row*). Note *uniform* ventricular morphology for this salvo. The **definition** of **"VT"** (*Ventricular Tachycardia*) is **3** (*or more*) **PVCs in a row** — so technically there is a 3-beat run of VT beginning with beat #4 in Tracing B. The coupling interval at the onset of the run (*distance between beat #3 and beat #4*) and QRS morphology during the run is similar to that for all PVCs in Figure 18-12 *except for* beat #10. Note that the R-R interval during this 3-beat run is approximately 2 large boxes in duration. This corresponds to a ventricular rate for this salvo of ~150/minute.
- **Beat #9** in Tracing B begins a **longer** run of **VT**. In fact — we have *no idea* of how long this run will last since Tracing B was cut off after

beat #13! We would describe beats #9-*thru*-13 as a **5-beat run** of *uniform* VT at a *rate* of ~**150/minute**.

☞ The last 2 terms to introduce are **NSVT** (*Non-Sustained Ventricular Tachycardia*) *vs* **sustained VT**. The difference between the two is that NSVT *spontaneously* terminates after a period of time — whereas *sustained* VT does not.

• There is no universal agreement regarding the *amount of time* that determines that a run of VT is "sustained". Among the definitions that have been used are VT lasting for 15 seconds — for 30 seconds — or for long enough to produce symptoms.

• Optimal description of ventricular ectopy will therefore entail defining the *number* of beats in the run of VT — *regularity* of the run — QRS *morphology* — the ventricular *rate* — <u>and</u> if clinically the run was (*or was not*) accompanied by symptoms.

• Without seeing what follows after beat #13 in Tracing B — it is impossible to know if this 5-beat run of *uniform* VT constitutes NSVT or "sustained" VT.

☞ A final *"escape"* rhythm: — *AIVR* —

We close Section 18 with a reminder about a special *"escape"* rhythm = **AIVR** (*Accelerated IdioVentricular Rhythm* = **Figure 18-13**).

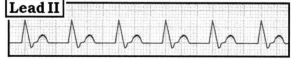

Lead II

Figure 18-13: AIVR (*previously discussed on pg 52*).

● As noted for Tracing D in <u>Figure 18-10</u> (*pg 191*) — the usual rate of an **idioventricular *ventricular* escape rhythm** is **20-40/minute**. In contrast — ***ventricular* "tachycardia"** is usually much faster (*at least 130/minute*). Ventricular rhythms *in between* this range (ie, *between ~60-120/minute*) are generally referred to as **"AIVR"** — since they are *"accelerated"* compared to the usual ventricular escape rate (*of 20-40/min*) — but *not quite as fast* as a VT rhythm likely to produce *hemodynamic* consequence.

• **AIVR** generally occurs in one of the following settings: **i)** as a rhythm during cardiac arrest; **ii)** in the monitoring phase of acute MI (*esp. with inferior MI*); <u>or</u> **iii)** as a *reperfusion* arrhythmia (*following thrombolytics, angioplasty, or spontaneous reperfusion*). The rhythm is often *transient* <u>and</u> treatment is usually *not* needed <u>IF</u> the patient is stable.

• **AIVR** is often an ***"escape rhythm"*** — that arises because *both* the SA and AV nodes are *not* functioning. <u>IF</u> treatment is needed (*because loss of atrial "kick" results in hypotension*) — Atropine is the drug of choice (*in hope of speeding up the SA node to resume its pacemaking function*). AIVR should *not* be shocked *nor* treated with Amiodarone/Procainamide — since doing so might result in asystole ...

Section 19 – Blocked PACs *and* Aberrancy (*pp 196-202*)

 # Blocked PACs /Aberrancy

● Most premature *supraventricular* beats (*PACs or PJCs*) will be conducted normally to the ventricles (ie, *through the normal AV nodal pathway with a narrow QRS complex that looks similar or identical to sinus beats*). That said — PACs (*and PJCs*) are <u>not</u> always normally conducted. Instead — these *premature* beats may sometimes occur *so early* in the cycle as to be **"blocked"** (*non-conducted*) — <u>or</u> **conducted with aberration** because the conduction system is *either* in a total *or* partial refractory state. <u>**Figure 19-1**</u> illustrates these **3 possible ways** in which a **PAC** (*or PJC*) may manifest:

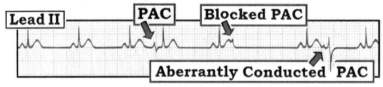

Lead II — PAC — Blocked PAC — Aberrantly Conducted PAC

Figure 19-1: A premature beat (*PAC or PJC*) may manifest in one of 3 ways. It may: **i)** be conducted normally (*with a narrow QRS complex that looks similar or identical to sinus conducted beats*); **ii)** be "blocked" (*non-conducted*); or **iii)** be conducted with a wider and *different-looking* QRS complex (*aberrant conduction*).

The goal of this Section 19 is to discuss why premature supraventricular beats may conduct aberrantly (*or not conduct at all*) — <u>and</u> to highlight awareness of these events on ECG. Recognition of blocked or aberrant PACs/PJCs may be important clinically because:

• *Blocked* PACs may be followed by a pause that *simulates* AV block.
• *Aberrantly* conducted PACs may result in QRS widening that simulates ventricular ectopy. An *aberrantly* conducted run of SVT may *simulate* VT.

▶ **NOTE:** For simplicity (*as well as because PACs are so much more common than PJCs*) — we will refer primarily to PACs for the rest of this Section discussing aberration and non-conduction.
• Realize the PJCs may also be blocked or conducted with aberration.

☞ *Refractory* Periods: *Why a PAC is Blocked or Aberrant*

After the ventricles have been electrically depolarized — there is a period of time known as the ***"refractory period"*** during which the ventricles cannot be activated again until recovery (*repolarization*) has occurred. Different portions of the ventricular conduction system have slightly differing durations of refractoriness.

- The **ARP** (*Absolute Refractory Period*) — encompasses that period within which *no part* of the conduction system has yet recovered. We schematically illustrate the ARP by the solid *box* extending through the large initial portion of the ST-T wave in **Figure 19-2**.
- The ARP is followed by a shorter **RRP** (*Relative Refractory Period*) — during which a portion (*but not all*) of the ventricular conduction system has recovered (*schematically illustrated by the diagonal lined box in* Figure 19-2).

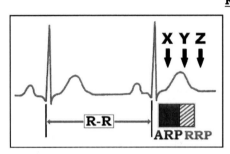

Figure 19-2: Absolute and relative refractory periods (*ARP and RRP*). A PAC occurring during the ARP (ie, *at point X*) cannot be conducted. A PAC occurring during the RRP (*point Y*) may be conducted with aberration. Only a PAC occurring after the refractory period is over (*at point Z*) will be conducted normally (*See text*).

☞ How a PAC will (*or will not*) be conducted is a function of *where* the PAC occurs in relation to the **absolute** and **relative Refractory Periods** (*ARP and RRP*).

- A **PAC** occurring at **Point Z** in Figure 19-2 — will be **conducted normally** (*because it occurs after the refractory period is over*).
- A **PAC** occurring at **Point X** — will be **blocked** (*non-conducted*) because it occurs so early that it falls *within* the ARP (*during which time no impulse can be conducted*).
- A **PAC** occurring at **Point Y** — will be **conducted** with **aberrancy** because it occurs during the RRP (*when part of the ventricular conduction system has recovered — but part has not*).

☞ Coupling Interval: *Role in Determining PAC Conduction*

We have already defined the "coupling interval" with respect to PVCs (*page 192*). We use a similar concept when assessing PACs — in which the **coupling interval** is measured from the onset of the preceding QRS until the onset of the premature P wave. ● **Figure 19-3** (*on page 198*) numbers the beats that were seen in Figure 19-1. The lower portion of this Figure measures the coupling interval for each of the 3 PACs that are seen.

- The **PAC** that occurs **earliest** in Figure 19-3 is seen to notch the T wave of beat #5. This PAC has a coupling interval of **0.19 second**. It is **blocked** (*non-conducted*) — because it presumably occurs during the ARP (*point X in* Figure 19-2).

- The **PAC** that has the *longest* **coupling interval** in Figure 19-3 is beat #4. This PAC has a coupling interval of **0.36 second**. It is **conducted** normally (*with a QRS complex identical to that of other normal sinus beats*) — because it presumably occurs after the refractory period is completely over (*as does point Z in* Figure 19-2).
- The **last PAC** on this tracing (*beat #7*) — has an **intermediate coupling interval** of **0.28 second**. Note that although this QRS complex initially looks the same as normal sinus beats (*it begins with a slender upright R wave*) — that it ends with a deep and widened S wave. This last PAC is **conducted** aberrantly (*with a QRS complex in the pattern of a left anterior hemiblock*). It presumably occurs during the RRP (*as does point Y in* Figure 19-2).

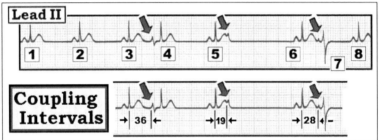

Figure 19-3: Measurement of coupling intervals for the 3 PACs that are seen on this tracing. The shorter the coupling interval — the earlier in the refractory period that the premature P wave occurs (*See text*).

☞ QRS Morphology of *Aberrant* Beats

Practically speaking – *aberrant* conduction is most likely to take the form of *some* type of bundle branch block *and/or* hemiblock pattern. The most common pattern seen is **RBBB** (*Right Bundle Branch Block*) **aberration** — which may occur with or without hemiblock.

- The reason aberrant beats most often conduct with a RBBB pattern is illustrated in **Figure 19-4** (*on page 199*). As shown in this Figure — the refractory period of the right bundle branch tends to be *longer* than the refractory period for either hemifascicle of the left bundle branch. As a result, a premature supraventricular impulse (*PAC or PJC*) arriving at the ventricles is much more likely to find the right bundle branch still in a refractory state — than it is to find part or all of the left bundle branch refractory.

▶ **NOTE:** The above generality that the refractory period of the RBB (*right bundle branch*) tends to be longest is _not_ necessarily true for all patients under all circumstances. For example — ischemia, hypoxemia, electrolyte imbalance or other associated medical conditions may all influence relative conduction properties of one or the other conduction fascicles. We can therefore state the following (*page 199*):

- **RBBB aberration** — is the **most common pattern** of aberrant conduction seen. Awareness of this fact is extremely helpful diagnostically because of the very characteristic (*and easily recognizable*) QRS morphology of typical RBBB (*See 'Rabbit Ears' below*).
- That said — virtually **any combination** of bundle branch block or hemiblock aberration is possible. This includes RBBB with or without LAHB or LPHB (*Left Anterior or Left Posterior HemiBlock*); isolated LAHB or LPHB; or pure LBBB (*Left Bundle Branch Block*) aberration.

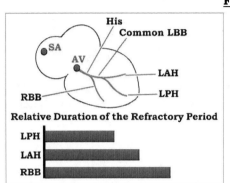

Figure 19-4: Explanation for the frequency of RBBB aberration. Of the 3 conduction fascicles — refractory period of the RBB (*right bundle branch*) tends to be longest in most individuals. As a result – a PAC (*or PJC*) arriving at the ventricles is most likely to find the RBB still in a refractory state, and conduct with RBBB aberration. LAHB and LPHB aberration are both *less* common — because refractory period of the LAH (*left anterior hemifascicle*) and LPH (*left posterior hemifascicle*) are both usually *shorter* than that of the RBB (*See text*).

☞ **RBBB Aberration: *Looking for 'Rabbit Ears'***

As emphasized in Section 08 (*pp 81-82*) when discussing ECG diagnosis of WCT (*Wide-Complex Tachycardia*) rhythms — the *only* QRS morphology with **high specificity** for **aberrant conduction** is the presence of a **typical RBBB pattern** in a **right-sided lead** (*lead V1 or MCL-1*). Recall of this pattern may be facilitated by the concept of a **taller *right* "rabbit ear"** (Figure 19-5):

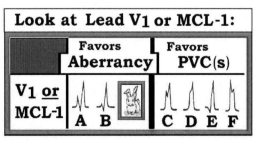

Figure 19-5: Use of QRS morphology in a right-sided lead (*V1 or MCL-1*) to distinguish between PVCs vs aberrant conduction. Only a *typical* RBBB pattern (*rsR' with taller right rabbit ear*) is predictive of aberration (*A or B*). Any other pattern (*C, D, E, F*) predicts ventricular ectopy.

● The **best** way to **prove aberrant conduction** is by demonstration of a **premature P wave** *preceding* the widened complex. The challenge arises if no PAC is seen — or if uncertainty exists about the presence of a premature P wave.

- Additional support that a widened beat is *aberrantly* conducted may be forthcoming <u>IF</u> *typical* **RBBB morphology** is seen in a right-sided lead (*lead V1 or MCL-1*). Thus, the presence of **an rsR' complex** (*with taller right 'rabbit ear'* <u>and</u> *S wave that descends* <u>below</u> *the baseline*) — **strongly** suggests a **supraventricular etiology** due to RBBB-type *aberrant* conduction (*A or B in* <u>Figure 19-5</u>).
- In contrast — **_any other_ QRS morphology** in lead V1 or MCL-1 **_favors_ ventricular ectopy** (*C,D,E or F in* <u>Figure 19-5</u>).

▶ **CAVEAT:** This criterion is strict. Only a *typical* **RBBB pattern** in lead V1 or MCL-1 (**A or B** *in* <u>Figure 19-5</u>) suggests aberrant conduction. *Any other* QRS pattern in V1 or MCL-1 suggests ventricular ectopy (*PVCs, VT*) as the reason for QRS widening.

☞ Aberrant Conduction: *Applying the Criteria*

The QRS complex of beat #4 in **Figure 19-6** is wide and occurs early. We can say with **100% confidence** that beat #4 in this short *right-sided* (*MCL-1*) lead rhythm strip is a **PAC** with QRS widening due to **aberrant conduction**. — *How can we be so sure?*

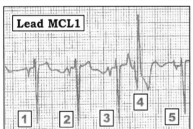

Figure 19-6: Beat #4 in this short MCL-1 lead rhythm strip is an aberrantly conducted PAC. What findings seen here allow us to say this with certainty? (*See text*).

☞ **Answer to Figure 19-6:** As already emphasized — the *BEST* way to prove *aberrant* conduction is by demonstration of a *premature* P wave *preceding* the widened complex. A **PAC** is clearly seen to **notch** the **T wave** of **beat #3** in <u>Figure 19-6</u>.

- Although the rhythm strip in Figure 19-6 is admittedly short – <u>and</u> – there IS some variation in ST-T wave morphology for normal sinus beats #1 and #2 — the presence of a premature P wave in the T wave of beat #3 is *unmistakable* by its tall peaked appearance that clearly differs from P wave morphology of other sinus beats on this tracing.
- Additional support that **beat #4** is an **aberrantly conducted PAC** is forthcoming from assessment of its morphology. Note the typical **rsR' pattern** that is *highly* suggestive of RBBB conduction in this *right-sided* lead MCL-1 (*similar to A in* <u>Figure 19-5</u>). It is extremely rare for ventricular ectopy to produce this typical RBBB pattern with similar *initial* deflection to normal sinus beats (*in the form of a slender upright small r wave*) — clean descent of the S wave to *below* the baseline — and terminal R' with taller *right* rabbit ear.

▶ **_Beyond-the-Core:_** One exception in which typical RBBB-type morphology may be seen with VT is when there is a **_fascicular_ VT**. In such cases of this relatively uncommon form of VT — the impulse arises from a site in the ventricles in close proximity to either the left anterior or posterior hemifascicles. The result is a _regular_ WCT rhythm _without_ P waves that _resembles_ RBBB with either LAHB or LPHB. The QRS complex is usually not greatly prolonged with fascicular VT (_most often between 0.11-to-0.14 second_). Many of these patients are younger and less likely to have underlying heart disease than the usual patient with ischemic VT. Clinically — it may _not_ be possible to distinguish between _fascicular_ VT vs SVT with _aberrant_ conduction from a _single_ 12-lead tracing.

• Awareness of _fascicular_ VT as a distinct type of VT may be important for the advanced provider. Despite its _ventricular_ origin — **_fascicular_ VT may respond** to **Adenosine**. This is one of the key reasons why Adenosine is now recommended as the _initial_ drug for treatment of a hemodynamically _stable_ WCT of _uncertain_ etiology (_See pp 58-62_).

SUMMARY: _Blocked PACs/Aberrant Conduction_

 ➡ **_Summary_**

⬤ Although most _premature_ supraventricular beats (_PACs or PJCs_) will be conducted _normally_ to the ventricles — awareness that _very_ early occurrence of PACs (_or PJCs_) may result in either _non-conduction_ of the impulse — or aberrant conduction with QRS widening may be invaluable for understanding a number of complexities in arrhythmia interprettation. Many of these concepts that are covered in this Section 19 are _advanced_ — but we also include basic principles applicable for _any_ level provider. **In Summary:**

• There are 3 types of _early-occurring_ beats: **PACs – PJCs – and PVCs** (_Section 18 — pp 179-195_). While not dangerous per se as an isolated occurrence — _premature_ beats may present difficulties in arrhythmia diagnosis.

• _Very early_ PACs/PJCs may be "blocked". This may result in a brief pause that simulates bradycardia or AV block. **The commonest cause of a pause is a blocked PAC.** This is far more common than any form of AV block. _Blocked_ PACs are often overlooked. They are usually _easy_ to recognize if looked for ...

• _Early-occurring_ PACs/PJCs may also result in QRS widening due to **_aberrant_ conduction** IF the premature impulse occurs during the _relative_ refractory period. On occasion — a run of _aberrantly_ conducted wide beats may occur that _simulates_ VT. Recognition that the 1st beat in the run — or that _other_ beats on rhythm monitoring are clearly _aberrant_ may be invaluable for distinguishing between VT vs SVT with aberrant conduction.

- The **best way to prove *aberrant* conduction** is by demonstration of a ***premature* P wave** *preceding* the widened complex. This will *not* always be possible — but when you <u>*can*</u> confidently identify that the *widened* beat(s) is preceded by a *premature* P wave — you have virtually *excluded* ventricular ectopy including VT as the cause.
- Support that a *widened* beat (*or widened run*) reflects aberrant conduction may be forthcoming from ***assessment*** of **QRS morphology**. The easiest (*and most helpful*) pattern to recognize is that of *typical* RBBB aberration in a *right-sided* lead (*V1 or MCL-1*). One looks for an rsR' with similar *initial* deflection to normal beats — S wave that descends to *below* the baseline — and terminal R' with taller *right* rabbit ear (<u>Figure 19-5</u> *and* <u>Figure 19-6</u>). Assume ventricular etiology (*PVCs,VT*) until proven otherwise for <u>*any*</u> deviation from this typical RBBB pattern.
- **Always assume that a beat** (*or a run of beats*) **is "guilty"** (ie, *a PVC, VT*) **<u>until</u> proven otherwise**. The onus is on proving aberrant conduction (*and <u>not</u> the other way around*).

➡ **PRACTICE Examples:**

● What follows is a series of **Practice Rhythm Strips** with goal of reinforcing the essential arrhythmia concepts covered in this section on *Blocked/Aberrant PACs.* Although clearly *not* an exhaustive compendium of clinical examples on this topic — our hope is that review of these examples will increase your appreciation <u>and</u> comfort level in recognizing and applying the principles summarized on pages 196-202.

 • For each of these 14 *Practice* Tracings (*pp 203-232*) — Assess the rhythm using the **Ps,Qs,3R Approach**.
• **HINT:** Each tracing illustrates an important principle related to the concept of *blocked* PACs/*aberrant* conduction.
• Our *explained* interpretations follow.

● ***Practice* Tracing #1:** Interpret the rhythm in Figure 19A-1 using the *Ps,Qs,3R* Approach. The patient is *hemodynamically* stable.
• What are beats #3,7,11 and 12? — *How certain* are you of your diagnosis? (**HINT:** *See pp 196-202 as needed for assistance*).

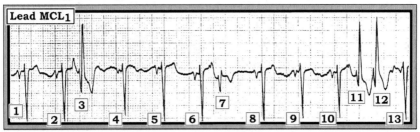

Figure 19A-1: *Practice* Tracing #1.

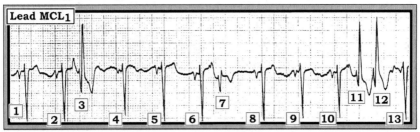 **Answer to Tracing #1:** Although there is some baseline artifact — the underlying rhythm in this *right-sided* MCL-1 lead is sinus, as suggested by the presence of sinus P waves with *fixed* PR interval preceding beats #1,2,4,5,6,8,9,10.
• It is easiest to start with the 1st *widened* complex (**beat #3**) — that we can definitively comment on. This beat occurs early. It is clearly preceded by a *premature* P wave that spikes the T wave of beat #2 (**Figure 19A-2**). Beat #3 manifests an rSR' with taller *right* rabbit ear in this MCL-1 lead. These features are **diagnostic** of **aberrant conduction**.
• Knowing of definite presence of an *aberrantly* conducted PAC facilitates interpretation of the other widened beats on this tracing. Despite some variation in ST segment morphology among sinus beats in this tracing (*due to baseline artifact*) — there is no mistaking that *each* of the early beats is preceded by a *notch* in the preceding T wave (*arrows preceding beats #3,7,11 in* **Figure 19A-2**). Thus, we can

confidently say that beats #11,12 are also conducted with RBBB aberration — and beat #7 is a PAC conducted with *incomplete* RBBB aberration.

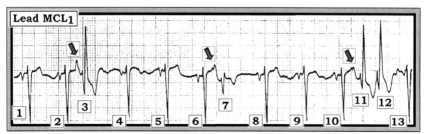

Figure 19A-2: Arrows have been added to Figure 19A-1 to highlight the PACs that notch the preceding T waves. Beats #3,11,12 all manifest RBBB aberration. Beat #7 manifests *incomplete* RBBB aberration.

➡ *Clinical* **PEARL:** As emphasized on page 198 — *aberrant* conduction is most likely to take the form of *some* type of bundle branch block *and/or* hemiblock pattern.

- Although RBBB aberration is by far the most common form of aberrant conduction (*since the refractory period of the right bundle branch tends to be longer than other conduction fascicles in most patients*) — *any* combination of bundle branch block or hemiblock aberration is possible (Figure 19-4 *on page 199*).
- *Beyond-the-Core:* Note the *smaller* rSr' complex for beat #7. This morphology in a *right-sided* lead (ie, *with a relatively small r' right rabbit ear*) is typical for incomplete RBBB. The negative T wave of beat #7 is also consistent with what one expects with *incomplete* RBBB.

▶ **NOTE:** There is considerable **baseline** artifact on this tracing. Despite this — there is *little* doubt from the *unmistakable* peaking of T waves prior to *widened* beats plus characteristic RBBB-morphology that this tracing represents frequent PACs with *aberrant* conduction.

Practice Tracing #2:

 ➡ **PRACTICE Tracing:**

● Interpret the rhythm in <u>Figure 19A-3</u> by the **Ps,Qs,3R Approach**. The patient is *hemodynamically* stable.
- Note that beat #4 manifests an rsR' pattern with taller right rabbit ear. Is this an *aberrantly* conducted beat?

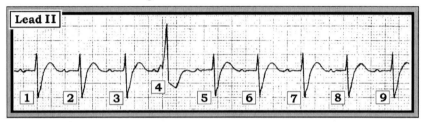

Figure 19A-3: *Practice* Tracing #2.

☞ **Answer to Tracing #2:** This rhythm strip emphasizes several *KEY* principles discussed in this Section 19 (*pp 196-202*):
- Although beat #4 manifests an rsR' pattern with taller *right* rabbit ear — the lead being monitored is **not** a **right-sided lead**. Assessment of QRS morphology for a RBBB pattern *only* counts when the rsR' is seen in a *right-sided* lead (*MCL-1 or V1*). Lead II is of *no help* in assessment for RBBB aberration (*pp 198-200*).
- Although a P wave *does* precede beat #4 in <u>Figure 19A-3</u> — this P wave is *not* premature! Instead — it occurs right on time (*arrows in* **Figure 19A-4**). The fact that the P wave preceding beat #4 occurs precisely on time actually **proves** that **beat #4** is a **PVC**! It normally takes 0.22 second for sinus P waves to conduct on this tracing. The P wave preceding beat #4 simply did *not* have enough time to conduct — because something (*a PVC*) arose *before* this atrial impulse impulse could make it through the normal conduction system.
- There is no "reason" for aberrant conduction in <u>Figure 19A-4</u>. Beat #4 occurs relatively *late* in the cycle (*at a time when one would expect the conduction system to no longer be in a refractory state*).

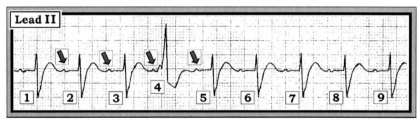

Figure 19A-4: Arrows have been added to <u>Figure 19A-3</u> to highlight that the P wave preceding widened beat #4 is not premature. Realization that the P-P interval remains constant and that the PR interval preceding beat #4 is too short to conduct *proves* that beat #4 is a PVC.

☞ **Our Interpretation of Figure 19A-3:** Completing our assessment — We'd interpret Practice Tracing #2 on page 205 as follows:

• Sinus rhythm with baseline QRS widening and 1st degree AV block (*PR interval = 0.22 second*). Beat #4 is a PVC.

➡ ***Clinical* PEARL:** Use of *calipers* greatly expedites and facilitates the analysis of tracings such as this one!

• An *additional* benefit of using calipers is that you *instantly* look like you *really* know what you are doing!

▶ **NOTE:** The cardiologist who fails to use calipers will overlook (*and misinterpret*) certain complex arrhythmia tracings — *regardless* of whether he/she admits this ...

End-Diastolic PVCs

  ***Beyond*-the-Core ...**

⬤ Beat #4 is sometimes referred to as an ***"end-diastolic"* PVC**. It *does* occur early — but *barely* so. Physiologically — its timing (*occurring relatively late in the cardiac cycle*) corresponds to the period of end-diastole (*during the late ventricular filling phase just prior to the next contraction*).

• Clinically — it is fine if you simply call beat #4 a "PVC". That said — qualifying your description by saying, *"end-diastolic PVC"* conveys to the informed clinician a later occurrence in the cycle for the ventricular ectopic beat.

• ***End-diastolic* PVCs** are often seen in association with AIVR (*Accelerated IdioVentricular Rhythm*) in patients who have recently reperfused an acutely occluded coronary artery (*either spontaneously or following thrombolytics or angioplasty*). Treatment is rarely needed (*these PVCs are usually self-limited — and they may be indicators of the "good news" that reperfusion has occurred!*).

• As might be expected — *end-diastolic* PVCs will often manifest some degree of *fusion* due to their late occurrence in the cycle. As a result — QRS morphology may be *intermittent* between these ventricular beats <u>and</u> the QRS from subsequent sinus P waves that partially conduct.

Practice **Tracing #3:** *Commonest Cause of a Pause*

 ➡ **PRACTICE Tracing:**

● Interpret the rhythm in Figure 19A-5 by the ***Ps,Qs,3R* Approach**. The patient is *hemodynamically* stable.

• Is the cause of the 2 pauses in Figure 19A-5 (*between beats #2-3 and #6-7*) an AV block? In view of the "group beating" that is seen — is this Mobitz I (*AV Wenckebach*) 2nd degree AV block?

• ***Extra* Credit:** What is beat #7?

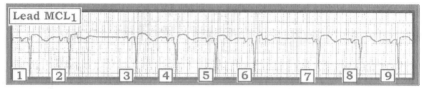

Figure 19A-5: *Practice* Tracing #3.

☞ **Answer to Tracing #3:** The underlying rhythm is sinus. As noted — 2 pauses are seen (*between beats #2-3 and #6-7*). The "mindset" with which we approach interpretation of this tracing is as follows:

• **The commonest cause of a pause is a blocked PAC.** Blocked PACs are far more common than *any* form of AV block. They *will* be found if looked for. Therefore — *whenever* we see a pause on a tracing — we *begin* by looking first for a *blocked* PAC.

• The best way to look for blocked PACs is to closely survey the ST-T wave at the onset of the pause (ie, *the ST-T wave of beats #2 and #6 in* Figure 19A-5). Compare this ST-T wave with the ST-T wave of all normal beats on the tracing (ie, *the ST-T wave of beats #1,3,4,5,7,8,9*). The **arrow** in **Figure 19A-6** highlights a *notch* in the T wave of beat #6 that represents the **hidden blocked PAC**. Note that a similar notch is seen at the onset of the 1st pause in Figure 19A-5 (*in the ST-T wave of beat #2*). Therefore — the cause of the pause in this tracing is that *very early* PACs are occurring during the absolute refracttory period — and are therefore *not* conducted. There is no evidence of any AV block.

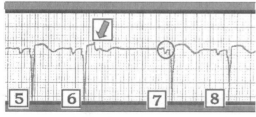

Figure 19A-6: The arrow highlights the *blocked* PAC in the T wave of beat #6. Beat #7 is a junctional escape beat (*See text*).

➡ ***Extra* Credit:** The QRS complex of beat #7 looks identical to the QRS of other normal sinus beats. However, the PR interval preceding beat #7 is *too short* to conduct. Therefore — there is **transient AV**

dissociation. Something else (ie, *an escape beat*) must be occurring *before* the P wave preceding beat #7 has time to conduct to the ventricles. Given *identical* QRS morphology of beat #7 to normal sinus beats in Figure 19A-5 — this escape beat must be arising from the AV node.

• **Junctional *escape* beats** (*like beat #7 in* Figure 19A-5**)** — are commonly seen following brief pauses. Rather than being problematic — their occurrence should be viewed as a "good thing" (*since without the escape beat the pause may have been much longer*).

• *Beyond-the-Core:* Use of calipers reveals that the R-R interval of the 1st pause (*between beats #2-3*) is slightly *longer* than the R-R interval of the 2nd pause (*between beats #6-7*). This explains why beat #3 (*which has slightly more time to recover*) conducts normally (*with normal PR interval*) — whereas beat #7 is a junctional escape beat. (*The sites for the various types of escape beats were reviewed on pages 190-192*).

Practice Tracing #4:

 ⮕ **PRACTICE Tracing:**

● Interpret the rhythm in <u>Figure 19A-7</u> by the ***Ps,Qs,3R* Approach.** The patient is *hemodynamically* stable.

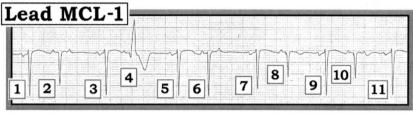

Figure 19A-7: *Practice* Tracing #4.

☞ **Answer to Tracing #4:** There is a LOT going on in <u>Figure 19A-7</u>. Keeping the *Ps,Qs,3R* Approach in mind — we look first to see if *despite* the obvious *irregularity* of QRS complexes there is an **underlying rhythm**. The sequence of analysis we use to interpret this rhythm is as follows:

• There *are* **P waves!** We look next to see if the underlying mechanism of this rhythm is sinus by trying to identify <u>IF</u> there is a *similar* P wave shape with *similar* PR interval preceding a majority of QRS complexes in Figure 19A-7.

• *Open* **arrows** in **Figure 19A-8** identify what looks to be **sinus P waves** preceding beats #1,3,5,7,9 and 11.

• We save analysis of beat #4 for last. We note next that beats #2,6,8 and 10 all occur early. Each of these beats is preceded by a *slightly-different* looking P wave (*lacks the shallow negative component of sinus P waves*). The QRS complex for each of these beats is narrow, albeit slightly different than the QRS of normal sinus beats (*less deep S wave*). Each of these beats is a PAC being conducted with varying degrees of aberrancy.

• A *very early* PAC is seen to notch the T waves of beats #2, 6 and 10. These are **blocked PACs.**

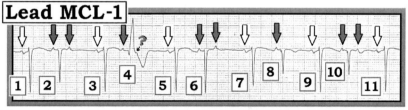

Figure 19A-8: Arrows have been added to <u>Figure 19A-7</u> to facilitate identifying atrial activity. ***Open* arrows** indicate sinus P waves. ***Solid* arrows** indicate PACs. The PACs that notch the T waves of beats #2, 6 and 10 are blocked. Varying degrees of *aberrant* conduction are seen for other PACs (*See text re beat #4 and the question mark that follows it*).

What is Beat #4 in **Figure 19A-8?**
- What about the *Question* Mark that follows this beat?

☞ Since the *"theme"* of <u>Figure 19A-8</u> is **underlying *sinus* rhythm** with very *frequent* **PACs** (*that are <u>either</u> conducted with aberration <u>or</u> non-conducted*) — it becomes likely that widened beat #4 is also *aberrantly* conducted.

- **Beat #4** is also preceded by a *premature* P wave. Despite *not* manifesting a completely typical rsR' pattern of aberration — the qR' tall right rabbit ear *in context* of everything else overwhelmingly favors *aberrant* conduction as the reason for QRS widening of beat #4.
- Given the *repetitive* pattern in <u>Figure 19A-8</u> (*of 2 successive PACs — one aberrant, the other blocked — following most sinus beats*) — We suspect a *blocked* PAC accounts for the little 'hump' in the beginning of the descending ST segment of *aberrantly* conducted beat #4.

➡ *Bottom* **Line:**   Details of whether beat #4 is a PVC or aberrant — <u>and</u> — whether the question mark in <u>Figure 19A-8</u> represents another blocked PAC or not are academically interesting but far *less* important clinically than **"the theme"** — which is that there is **underlying *sinus* rhythm** with extremely *frequent* **PACs** (*2 PACs in a row follow beats #1,6 and 9*).

- Some PACs are blocked — <u>and</u> others are conducted with aberration.
- <u>Clinically</u> — Attention should be placed on considering potential extracardiac *and/or* exacerbating factors that may be causing the frequent PACs (*pp 179-181*).

Practice Tracing #5: *Pseudo-AV Block*

 ⇨ **PRACTICE Tracing:**

⬤ Interpret the rhythm in Figure 19A-9 by the ***Ps,Qs,3R* Approach.** The patient is *hemodynamically* stable.

* Is there 2:1 AV block in Figure 19A-9? If so — Does this represent Mobitz Type I or Mobitz Type II 2nd degree AV block?

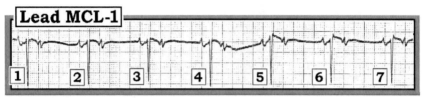

Figure 19A-9: *Practice* Tracing #5.

☞ **Answer to Tracing #5:** At first glance at Figure 19A-9 — there appears to be 2:1 AV block. That said — this is *not* the correct interpretation of this rhythm strip. The "mindset" with which we approach interpretation of this tracing is as follows:

* ***The commonest cause of a pause is a blocked PAC.*** Blocked PACs are far more common than *any* form of AV block. They *will* be found if looked for (*just like we found them in* Figure 19A-5 *on page 207*). Therefore — *whenever* we see one or more pauses on a tracing — we always *begin* by looking first for a *blocked* PAC.
* As will be discussed in Section 20 (*page 237*) — a fundamental criterion for **AV block** is the presence of a **regular** (*or almost regular*) **atrial rhythm.** It is common with AV block to see *minor* irregularity in the P-P interval (*due to underlying sinus arrhythmia or ventriculophasic sinus arrhythmia associated with AV block*). However — such P-P variability should *not* be nearly as much as seen in Figure 19A-9.
* Note below in **Figure 19A-10** — *subtle-but-real* difference in P wave morphology between **sinus P waves** highlighted by **open arrows** (*initial positive then wide negative component*) – vs – **PACs** highlighted by **solid arrows** (*negative-positive-negative triphasic P waves*).

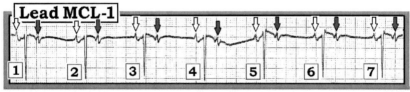

Figure 19A-10: Arrows have been added to Figure 19A-9 to facilitate recognition of sinus P waves (*open arrows*) and PACs (*solid arrows*).

⇨ ***Clinical* PEARL:** This interesting tracing emphasizes how sinus rhythm with atrial bigeminy (*every-other-beat a PAC*) can *mimic* AV block IF PACs occur *so early* as to be non-conducted.

- <u>KEY</u> Point: Remembering that **"the most common cause of a pause is a blocked PAC"** is *invaluable* for preventing you from accepting our initial erroneous impression that <u>Figure 19A-9</u> represents 2:1 AV block.
- AV block is ruled out by the clearly *varying* P-P interval. *Blocked* PACs are confirmed by recognition of different P wave morphologies for sinus beats and the P wave notching each T wave (*open and solid arrows in* <u>Figure 19A-10</u>).
- This patient does *not* need a pacemaker. Instead — attention should be given to potential factors that may be causing frequent PACs (*pp 179-181*).

Practice Tracing #6:

 ➡ **PRACTICE Tracing:**

● Interpret the rhythm in Figure 19A-11 by the **Ps,Qs,3R Approach**. The patient is *hemodynamically* stable.

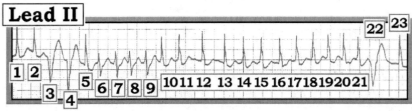

Figure 19A-11: *Practice* Tracing #6.

☞ **Answer to Tracing #6:** A lot is going on in Figure 19A-11. We look first for the presence of an *underlying* rhythm — as this may provide the best clue to the primary problem. We defer assessment of the *different-looking* beats (ie, *beats #3,4 — #6,7,8,9 and #22*) until after we determine the rhythm.

• The **underlying rhythm** in Figure 19A-11 (*as determined by assessment of beats #1,2,5; 10-thru-21 and 23*) is **atrial fibrillation** with a **rapid ventricular response** (*irregularly irregular rapid rhythm — no P waves — normal duration QRS*).

• We strongly suspect that **beats #3, 4** and **22** in Figure 19A-11 are **PVCs**. The QRS complex of each of these beats is wide — very different in morphology from the QRS complex during AFib — and not preceded by premature P waves. Note that a relative pause follows beat #22 — with resumption of rapid AFib occurring with beat #23.

• We strongly suspect **beats #6-thru-9** represent a run of **aberrant conduction**. These beats are *not* overly wide. The initial QRS deflecttion of these beats is *similar* in direction and slope to that of the QRS complex for AFib beats. In addition — the R-R interval between these beats maintains the same *irregularity* as the underlying AFib. Finally — there is no relative pause at the end of the run as AFib resumes with beat #10. That said — We can *not* be 100% certain these beats are aberrant since with AFib we *won't* see any premature P wave ...

• Use of additional monitoring leads (*or obtaining a 12-lead ECG during tachycardia*) — might assist further in assessment of this rhythm.

➡ **Bottom Line:** Clinically — it *doesn't matter* if beats #6-thru-9 represent a run of NSVT (*Non-Sustained Ventricular Tachycardia*) or AFib with *aberrant* conduction. Regardless, the *"theme"* of the rhythm in Figure 19A-11 is **rapid AFib** with at least *some* ventricular ectopy.

• As long as the patient remains stable — management with goal of controlling the rapid rate of this AFib plus *correcting* potential precipitating factors may be all that is needed to improve the clinical situation (*pp 127-132*).

Practice **Tracing #7:** *End-Diastolic PVCs*

 ➡ **PRACTICE Tracing:**

● Interpret the rhythm in <u>Figure 19A-12</u> by the **Ps,Qs,3R Approach**. The patient is *hemodynamically* stable.

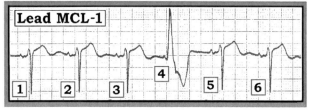

Figure 19A-12:
Practice
    Tracing #7.

☞ **Answer to Tracing #7:** The underlying rhythm in <u>Figure 19A-12</u> is sinus — as determined by presence of P waves with fixed PR interval preceding beats #1,2,3 and #5,6. The question arises as to the etiology of **widened** beat **#4**?

• Initially it appears that beat #4 manifests rsR' morphology. However, closer inspection of this rhythm reveals that this is <u>not</u> the case. Use of **calipers** instantly reveals that the P-P interval remains *constant* throughout the rhythm strip (**Figure 19A-13**).

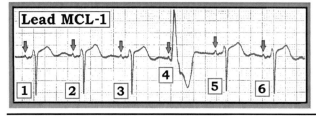

Figure 19A-13:
Arrows added
to Figure 19A-12
show *regular* si-
nus P waves per-
sist throughout.

☞ *Widened* beat #4 is <u>not</u> preceded by a premature P wave. Instead — the P wave preceding this beat occurs right on time (*arrows in* <u>Figure 19A-13</u>). This results in a PR interval preceding beat #4 that is clearly *too short* to conduct — which **proves** that **beat #4** is a **PVC** (*something from below must have occurred <u>before</u> this P wave had a chance to conduct to the ventricles*).

• Rather than rsR' morphology for *widened* beat #4 — this beat manifests a monophasic upright R wave (*a shape consistent with its ventricular origin*). The small positive deflection initially thought to be an r wave (*arrow preceding beat #4 in* <u>Figure 19A-13</u>) is actually the next sinus P wave occurring precisely on time.

➡ <u>*Beyond-the-Core:*</u> Beat #4 may be called as an **"end-diastolic PVC"**. It *does* occur early — but *barely* so (*See page 206*). It is well to be aware of the existence of this type of PVC — so that it is not mistaken for "junctional escape with aberrant conduction". There is no reason for this beat to conduct aberrantly (*it occurs so late in the cycle, long after the refractory period should be over*)

Practice Tracing #8: *The ASHMAN Phenomenon*

⇒ PRACTICE Tracing:

⬤ Interpret the rhythm in Figure 19A-14 by the **Ps,Qs,3R Approach**. The patient is *hemodynamically* stable.
• What is the *underlying* rhythm?
• Is *widened* beat #12 a PVC *or* aberrantly conducted PAC? How *certain* are you of your answer?
• What is the **Ashman** phenomenon?

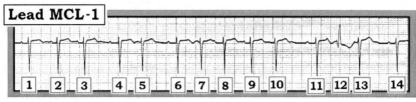

Figure 19A-14: *Practice* Tracing #8.

☞ **Answer to Tracing #8:** The *underlying* rhythm is appears to be sinus — although it is admittedly difficult to determine the underlying sinus rate due to continual irregularity of this tracing.
• The reason we interpret the **underlying rhythm** as **sinus** is the similar P wave morphology and PR interval for beats #4,6,11 and 14.
• There are **multiple** PACs on this tracing. Although P wave morphology seems to change slightly for many of these PACs — it is admittedly difficult to be certain if some of the *earlier-than-anticipated* beats are PACs vs rhythm regularity from sinus arrhythmia. Clinically — it doesn't matter, since **"the theme"** of this rhythm is **sinus** with **multiple** PACs.
• *Beyond-the-Core:* Technically — we can't rule out the possibility of MAT for this rhythm. Our tendency is to favor sinus rhythm with *multiple* PACs as the diagnosis because of similar P wave shape and PR interval for beats #4,6,11 and 14 (*vs continually varying P wave morphology from beat-to-beat that is typical for MAT*). That said — **sinus rhythm with *multiple* PACs** and **MAT** are essentially two points on different ends of the same spectrum. Practically speaking, distinction between these 2 entities does *not* matter — since clinical implications of these two rhythms are virtually the same (*See also* 133-137).
• **Beat #12** — is an **aberrantly conducted** PAC. We are able to confidently make this diagnosis because: **i)** Beat #12 is preceded by a *premature* P wave (*arrow in* Figure 19A-15); **ii)** The *"theme"* of this rhythm is sinus with *multiple* PACs — so it is *more likely than not* that the cause of the single *widened* beat in Figure 19A-14 will also be a PAC; **iii)** Beat #12 manifests typical RBBB morphology (*rsR' with taller right rabbit ear in right-sided MCL-1*); *and* **iv)** Beat #12 manifests the **Ashman phenomenon**.

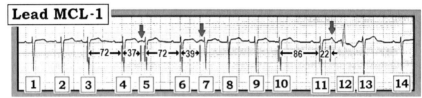

Figure 19A-15: Arrows have been added to Figure 19A-14 to highlight the relative relationship between the coupling interval of the *premature* P waves preceding beats #5, 7 and 12 — <u>and</u> the *preceding* R-R interval. Beat #12 is an *aberrantly* conducted PAC that manifests the **Ashman phenomenon** (*See text*).

☞ The *Ashman* Phenomenon

We have emphasized the role of **PAC *coupling* interval** (*pp 196-198*) in determining whether a PAC will be blocked — conducted normally — <u>or</u> conducted with QRS widening from aberrancy. We expand on *previously discussed* <u>Figure 19-2</u> (*page 197*) with **Figure 19A-16** below — in which consideration is now also given to the *relative* length of the *preceding* R-R interval.

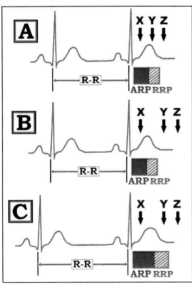

Figure 19A-16: Illustration of the effect that the *preceding* R-R interval exerts on duration of the *subsequent* refractory period. This explains the **Ashman phenomenon**.

- **Panel A** — reproduces <u>Figure 19-2</u> (*pg 197*). It schematically illustrates that a premature impulse (*PAC or PJC*) occurring during the **ARP** (*Absolute Refractory Period* — corresponding to *Point X*) will be **blocked**. In contrast — a PAC (*or PJC*) occurring *after* repolarization is complete (*corresponding to Z in Panel A*) will be conducted normally. **Aberrant conduction** will *only* occur IF a *premature* impulse occurs during the **RRP** (*Relative Refractory Period* — corresponding to Point Y in Panel A).

- Events in **Panel B** — suggest a different clinical situation. Once again — points X, Y and Z represent theoretical timing for 3 PACs. *Premature* impulse X will again be blocked (*since it occurs within the ARP*). This time— <u>both</u> Y and Z fall *beyond* the RRP, so *both* of these premature impulses will be conducted normally to the ventricles.

⬤ **KEY Point:** Whether a *premature* impulse will fall ***within* the RRP** (*and conduct with **aberration***) — will also be determined by length of the R-R interval immediately *preceding* the anomalous (*widened*) beat. This is because **duration of the refractory period is directly proportional to the length of the preceding R-R interval.** When heart rate slows (*as it does in* **Panel C** *of* Figure 19A-16) — the *subsequent* ARP and RRP will *both* be prolonged.

• **Panel C** — shows the effect of rate slowing on conduction of the 3 PACs from Panel B. *Premature* impulse X will again be blocked (*it occurs within the ARP*). Premature impulse Z will again be conducted normally (*it occurs after the refractory period is over*). However, **premature impulse Y** (*which in Panel B had occurred after repolarization was complete*) — will now be conducted with aberrancy (*since the preceding longer R-R interval has now prolonged the RRP*).

➡ *Clinical* **PEARL:** The cycle-sequence manipulation illustrated by events in **Panel C** is referred to as the **Ashman Phenomenon.** We synthesize this phenomenon into a concise *easy-to-remember* format:

• **"The funniest-looking (**ie, *most aberrant*) **beat** is **most** likely to **follow** the **longest pause"** (*Grauer – 1992*).

☞ We magnify events from Figure 19A-15 below in **Figure 19A-17.** Note that the "funniest beat" (*beat #12*) follows the *longest* pause (*the R-R interval between beats #10-11*). Therefore — in addition to the **very short coupling interval** of **0.22 second** for the PAC *preceding* beat #12 (*solid arrow*) — the relatively *longer* preceding R-R interval favors conditions that predispose to *aberrant* conduction (*via the* **Ashman phenomenon**). Cycle-sequence comparison for *other* PACs in Figure 19A-17 (*open arrows*) is not nearly as favorable for aberrant conduction.

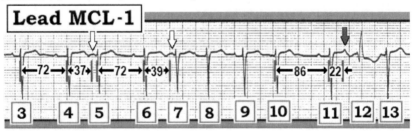

Figure 19A-17: Magnification of part of Figure 19A-15 (*See text*).

▶ *Beyond-the-Core:* Utilization of the **Ashman phenomenon** may be extremely helpful diagnostically when applied to assessing wide beats in arrhythmias obtained from patients who are in **sinus rhythm**.

• Be aware that the Ashman phenomenon is of **uncertain value** with **AFib** (*Atrial Fibrillation*). This is because the length of the R-R interval in AFib is continually influenced by another phenomenon known as **concealed conduction**, in which *variable* penetration of the 400-to-600 atrial impulses that arrive each minute at the AV node with AFib affects conduction in a way that the preceding R-R interval *no longer* accurately reflects the duration of the subsequent refractory period.

Practice Tracing #9: *Ashman in AFib*

 ➡ PRACTICE Tracing:

● Interpret the rhythm in Figure 19A-18 by the **Ps,Qs,3R Approach**. The patient is *hemodynamically* stable.

• What is **beat #13**? — Is the **Ashman phenomenon** present**?**

• Can you also explain the slightly different appearance of beats #4 and #7 compared to most other beats on the tracing?

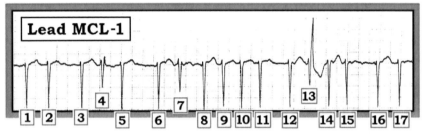

Figure 19A-18: *Practice* Tracing #9.

Answer to Tracing #9: The *underlying* rhythm in Figure 19A-18 is *irregularly* irregular. The QRS complex for most beats on the tracing is narrow. No P waves are seen. Therefore — the *underlying* rhythm is **AFib** with a **relatively *rapid* ventricular response**.

• Beat #13 occurs relatively early. QRS morphology manifests a **typical RBBB pattern** with rSR' complex showing similar initial deflection (*upright*) as for normal beats <u>and</u> taller *right* rabbit ear (Figure 19-5 — *pg 199*). This characteristic appearance of **beat #13** strongly suggests this beat is *not* a PVC, but is instead an **aberrantly conducted** supraventricular impulse.

• **Beats #4** and **#7** in this tracing also look different than normally conducted beats. They both manifest an rSr' pattern, albeit not quite as pronounced as for beat #13. We strongly suspect the appearance of beats #4 and 7 reflects *aberrant* conduction with a pattern of *incomplete* RBBB.

• <u>Clinically</u> — it probably matters *little* whether beats #4, 7 and 13 represent isolated PVCs <u>vs</u> aberrant conduction of several AFib impulses. In either case — the **primary problem** is **rapid AFib** in a hemodynamically stable patient. As a result — management priorities rest with trying to find and "fix" the *precipitating* cause of AFib <u>and</u> with *controlling* the ventricular response. Regardless of the etiology of beats #4, 7 and 13 — it is likely that widened complexes will decrease in frequency (*or resolve completely*) once the ventricular rate of AFib is controlled.

➡ **Beyond-the-Core:** At first glance, beats #4, 7 and 13 all appear to manifest the **Ashman phenomenon** — in that these slightly *widened* and *different-looking* beats all follow a relatively *longer* preceding R-R interval (*pp 215-217*). That said — we cautioned against reliance on the Ashman phenomenon in the setting of AFib because of the possibility of *concealed* conduction (*See our Beyond-the-Core Comment on page 217*).

- Definitive diagnosis of *aberrant* conduction is also more difficult in the setting of AFib — because one loses the diagnostic utility of identifying a premature P wave (*since there are no P waves with AFib*).

- Despite these caveats — we estimate a **greater than** 90% **likelihood** that beats #4, 7 and 13 all represent **aberrantly** conducted AFib impulses because of their highly characteristic appearance. Specifically — **beat #13** in Figure 19A-18 looks *identical* to B in **Figure 19-5** (*that we reproduce below from page 199*) in that **beat #13** manifests an rsR' with S wave that descends *below* the baseline and taller *right* rabbit ear (*R'*) in a *right-sided* lead (*such as MCL-1*).

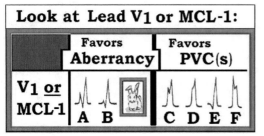

Figure 19-5: Use of QRS morphology in a right-sided lead (*V1 or MCL-1*) to distinguish between PVCs vs *aberrant* conduction. Only a *typical* RBBB pattern (*rsR' with taller right rabbit ear*) is predictive of aberration (*A or B*). Any other pattern (*C, D, E, F*) predicts ventricular ectopy (*reproduced from pg 199*).

Practice Tracing #10: *Compensatory Pauses*

 ⇒ <u>PRACTICE</u> Tracing:

● Interpret the rhythm in <u>Figure 19A-19</u> by the **Ps,Qs,3R Approach**. The patient is *hemodynamically* stable.
• Beats #3 and #12 occur early and look somewhat different. Are these beats PVCs or *aberrantly* conducted PACs?

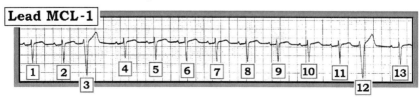

Figure 19A-19: *Practice* Tracing #10.

☞ **Answer to Tracing #10:** The *underlying* rhythm is **sinus** — as determined by the presence of regular *narrow-QRS* complexes at a rate of ~80/minute. Each sinus beat is preceded by a P wave with fixed PR interval in this *right-sided* MCL-1 lead.
• There are **2 *different-looking* beats** (*#3 and #12*). Although at first glance, QRS morphology of these beats superficially resembles that of normal sinus beats (*both manifest an rS complex*) — the QRS complex of beats #3 and #12 is definitely *widened* <u>and</u> the *slope* of the initial r wave upslope is different (*slower rising*). Beats #3 and #12 are <u>not</u> preceded by premature P waves. These beats are **PVCs** (*Premature Ventricular Contractions*) — despite the fact that they superficially resemble normal sinus beats in morphology.

⇒ <u>KEY</u> **Point:** A *premature* beat is presumed **"guilty"** (ie, *ventricular in origin*) <u>until</u> proven otherwise. Beats #3 and #12 in <u>Figure 19A-19</u> are wide — premature — <u>and</u> *not* preceded by P waves. Even *before* assessing QRS morphology — this combination of findings makes it **almost certain** that these beats are **PVCs**.

☞ ***Compensatory* Pauses**

A *brief* pause will often be seen following premature beats. This is *not* unexpected. Premature *supraventricular* complexes (*PACs,PJCs*) typically conduct through much or all of the atria — resulting in a "reset" of sinus node activity. As a result — the next sinus impulse will be delayed.
• The amount that the next sinus P wave will be delayed after a PAC or PJC is variable — depending on speed and degree of conduction through the atria <u>and</u> conduction properties of the sinus node. For example — sinus node recovery time may be especially delayed in

patients with sick sinus syndrome (*which is why prolonged sinus pauses so commonly follow a run of tachycardia in such patients*).
- PVCs may or may not conduct retrograde (*backward*) to the atria. When PVCs do not conduct retrograde — then the sinus node will not be "reset". As a result — the sinus node will continue to "fire" at its regular intrinsic sinus rate. Regular sinus P waves continue on time. The sinus P wave that occurs at about the time of the PVC will *not* be conducted (*since the PVC renders the ventricle refractory to impulses from above*). However, the *next* sinus P wave will occur and conduct *precisely* on time. As a result — there may be a **full compensatory pause** with this PVC (**Figure 19A-20**).

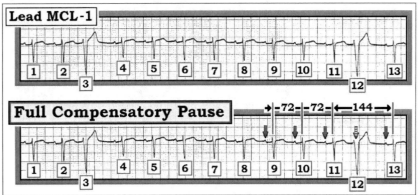

Figure 19A-20: Addition of arrows with measurement of intervals from the rhythm previously shown in Figure 19A-19. The 2 **PVCs** in this tracing (*beats #3 and #12*) manifest a **full compensatory pause.**

▶ **NOTE:** Our reason for the following *detailed* explanation of compensatory pauses is that this concept is still often cited as a criterion for distinguishing between PACs <u>vs</u> PVCs. Unfortunately, this concept is so problematic as to virtually **invalidate** its clinical utility. Nevertheless, because of *continued* common usage — it remains important to be aware of this phenomenon.

- **Figure 19A-20** illustrates that the 2 PVCs in Figure 19A-19 (*beats #3 and 12*) — manifest a **full compensatory pause**. That is — sinus P waves are regular throughout with a consistent R-R interval of **0.72 second** (*solid arrows*). The pause that contains each PVC in Figure 19A-20 is *precisely* **twice** the normal R-R interval = **1.44 second.**
- The reason the pause in Figure 19A-20 is *fully* compensatory — is that the sinus P wave that occurs at about the time of the PVC (*striped arrow*) is <u>not</u> conducted (*since the PVC will have rendered the ventricles momentarily refractory to conduction from above*). However, the *next* sinus P wave (*the P wave preceding beat #13*) occurs on time — <u>and</u> can now be conducted. The result is that the pause that *contains* the PVC is *exactly* twice the normal R-R interval.

⬤ The reason the **concept** of *compensatory* **pauses** is *problematic* is:

- **i)** A significant percentage of PVCs <u>do</u> conduct retrograde to the atria. When this happens — the SA node *will* be "reset" — <u>and</u> the pause containing the PVC will *no longer* be exactly twice the sinus R-R interval;

- **ii)** PACs that "reset" the SA node may *by chance* result in a pause that lasts as long as the time for two R-R intervals; <u>and</u>

- **iii)** *Beyond-the-Core:* Even when PVCs do *not* conduct retrograde far enough to reset the SA node — they may *partially* conduct far enough retrograde to prolong the *subsequent* PR interval (*via concealed conduction*). This will affect duration of the R-R interval containing the PVC.

▶ **Bottom Line:** Be aware that there <u>is</u> a *full* compensatory pause for the 2 PVCs in <u>Figure 19A-20</u>. This does provide some additional support that beats #3 and 12 are PVCs. That said — Realize that looking to see IF the pause following a premature beat is fully compensatory or not will *at most* be of *very limited* diagnostic utility.

Practice **Tracing #11: "Birds" of a Feather**

 ⇒ **PRACTICE Tracing:**

● Interpret the rhythm in Figure 19A-21 by the *Ps,Qs,3R* **Approach.** The patient is *hemodynamically* stable.
• What are beats #6,7,13 and 14? *How certain* are you of your answer?

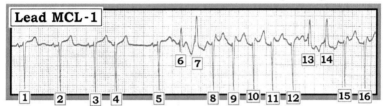

Figure 19A-21: *Practice* Tracing #11.

Answer to Tracing #11: We approach interpretation of this complex rhythm strip by once again looking first for an *underlying* rhythm:
• The **underlying rhythm** is **sinus** — as determined by **beats #1,2,3.** The QRS complex for these first 3 beats is *narrow* — and each of these beats is preceded by a P wave with a *fixed* and normal PR interval. Therefore — *it all begins* with **normal sinus rhythm** at a rate of ~80/minute.
• **Beat #4** — occurs early and appears to be a **PAC.** The QRS complex of beat #4 is narrow and looks *identical* to the QRS of normal sinus beats. We suspect the subtle notch in the *preceding* T wave of beat #3 represents a *premature* P wave (*1st slanted arrow with question mark in* **Figure 19A-22**).
• There is slight *reset* of the sinus node — with resumption of sinus rhythm (*after a brief non-compensatory pause*) by **beat #5.**
• **Beat #6** — is the *KEY* to interpreting this rhythm! Beat #6 occurs early. It is clearly *preceded* by a **premature P wave** that notches the T wave of preceding beat #5 (*solid vertical arrow in* Figure 19A-22). The QRS complex of beat #6 is wider and looks different than the QRS of normal sinus beats. However, it is *not* overly wide (*0.11 second at most*) — it has an *identical* initial deflection as normal sinus beats (*small thin upright r wave*) — and it manifests *typical* RBBB morphology (*rSR' with taller right rabbit ear*). These features are overwhelmingly in favor of beat #6 being an **aberrantly conducted PAC.**

Figure 19A-22: We have magnified the initial part of Figure 19A-21. Arrows have been added to indicate *premature* P waves. Beat #4 and beat #6 are PACs. Beat #6 is *aberrantly* conducted.

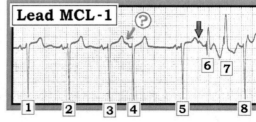

☞ The *"Birds of a Feather"* Concept

We _know_ beat #4 in Figure 19A-22 is a premature supraventricular impulse. Subtle notching (*slanted arrow*) in its preceding T wave that is *not* seen in the smooth T waves of sinus beats #1 or 2 strongly suggests that beat #4 is a PAC.

- The *"Birds of a Feather"* **concept** simply states that IF a certain rhythm phenomenon occurs in one part of a tracing — that it is likely to occur again in other parts of the tracing (*or in subsequent tracings*). This provides additional support that the apparent notch in the T wave of beat #5 is real (*not artifact*) — and that beat #6 is also a PAC.

● Did You Recognize the *Ashman* Phenomenon?

Final confirmation that beat #6 is an *aberrantly* conducted PAC is forthcoming from recognition of the **Ashman phenomenon** (*page 216*).

- The "essence" of the Ashman phenomenon — is that *"the funniest beat is most likely to follow the longest pause"*. In Figure 19A-21 — the *longest* pause on the tracing (*the pause between beats #4-5*) sets up conditions for aberrant conduction by *prolonging* the relative refractory period of the *subsequent* beat. This makes it that much *more* likely that the premature P wave preceding beat #6 will conduct with aberrancy, whereas the premature P wave preceding beat #4 (*which has a shorter preceding R-R interval*) conducts normally.

● Interpretation of the Rest of the Tracing:

Once established that we are 100% confident beat #6 is an *aberrantly* conducted PAC — we can use this information to complete our interpretation.

- By the *"birds of a feather"* concept — it is extremely likely that the *other* widened beats in Figure 19A-21 that manifest *similar* rSR' QRS complexes are *also* aberrantly conducted supraventricular impulses. Therefore — _all_ QRS complexes in Figure 19A-21 appear to be *supraventricular* — and **beats #6,7,13,14** are **aberrantly conducted**.
- Knowing that _all_ QRS complexes in Figure 19A-21 are supraventricular tells us that following resumption of sinus rhythm with beat #5 — a run of a rapid *ever-so-slightly* **irregular SVT** occurs (*beats #6-thru-16*). As often happens with *new-onset* SVT — this run of tachycardia is initiated by a premature atrial impulse (*solid vertical arrow*) — that presumably occurs during the atrial "vulnerable" period. There are no definite P waves during the run after beat #6 — although deflections in the ST-T waves in many of the beats suggests there may be atrial activity. We suspect beats #7-*thru*-16 represents a **run** of **rapid AFib** precipitated by a PAC (*beat #6*) — or possibly a run of AFlutter in process of deteriorating to AFib.

➡ _Bottom_ Line: This is a *challenging* rhythm strip. While complete interpretation of all aspects of this tracing extends beyond the level of the less experienced provider — **the way to *approach* interpretation** is relevant to all:

- When confronted with a complex rhythm strip — Start by attending to those parts of the rhythm that you *can* comfortably identify. We always look first to see IF there is an *underlying* rhythm. We *know* Figure 19A-22 begins with sinus rhythm (*beats #1,2,3*).

- We *know* beat #4 is a premature *supraventricular* impulse (*PAC or PJC*).

- Awareness of the basic principles of *aberrant* conduction should alert to the likelihood that the notch preceding the first *widened* beat (*solid vertical arrow*) is likely to represent a PAC buried within the preceding T wave. Recognition of *typical* RBBB morphology for beat #6 (*with taller right rabbit ear*) — supports the premise that beat #6 is an *aberrantly* conducted PAC.

- Use of the *"birds of a feather"* concept should then suggest that *other* wide beats in the tracing are likely to *also* be aberrantly conducted.

- We are left to explain the slightly *irregular* SVT in the latter half of the rhythm strip. P waves are lacking. One has to presume this is *rapid* AFib ...

Practice Tracing #12:

 ➡ **PRACTICE Tracing:**

● Interpret the rhythm in Figure 19A-23 by the ***Ps,Qs,3R* Approach**. The patient is *hemodynamically* stable.

- **HINT:** Figure 19A-23 was obtained from the *same* patient whose rhythm we discussed on pages 223-225. *Does knowing this help* in determining what beats #10,11 are likely to be?
- What is your ***differential diagnosis*** for the 4-beat **run** of **widened beats** that begins with beat #13?

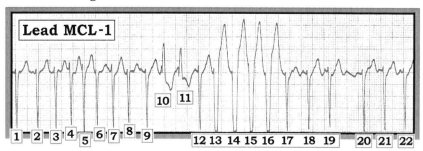

Figure 19A-23: *Practice* Tracing #12.

☞ **Answer to Tracing #12:** Attaining a level of comfort in assessing rhythm strips such as that shown in Figure 19A-23 is our principal reason for writing Section 19. This rhythm is rapid — it contains wide beats of differing QRS morphology — and it is clearly of concern as a potentially *life-threatening* arrhythmia. That said — We approach assessment of this rhythm <u>and</u> clinical management of this patient in the *same* manner we approach *all* arrhythmias:

- ***Is the patient hemodynamically stable?*** We are told that he/she is. This means (*by definition*) — that we *at least* have a moment of time to further assess the rhythm. Be ready to cardiovert at *any* time <u>IF</u> the patient decompensates — but as long as the patient remains stable <u>and</u> is tolerating the tachycardia, it is worth spending a moment in further assessment of the rhythm. Treatment is far *more* likely succeed (*and avoid adverse effects*) — <u>IF</u> we can figure out what the tachyarrhythmia is.
- ***Assess*** the rhythm **by** the ***Ps,Qs,3R* Approach**. Since more than one element is present (ie, *there are at least 3 different QRS morphologies*) — Start by assessing what you <u>*know*</u>, and leave more difficult parts of the arrhythmia for later. Is there an ***underlying* rhythm**?

▶ **NOTE:** There will often be rhythm strips that *even the experts* are uncertain about. Figure 19A-23 is one such example — in which we admittedly did not know for sure what this rhythm was until *after* the patient was successfully treated.

☞ Begin assessment of Figure 19A-23 with the ***Ps,Qs,3R* Approach**:

- We note that the ***predominant* QRS morphology** is a ***narrow* rS complex** (*small slender initial r wave; deep S wave*). This rS pattern is seen for all beats on the tracing *except for* beats #10,11 and #13-*thru*-16. We ***defer*** assessment of these *different-looking* widened beats (*#10,11; #13-16*) until later. Instead — Focus first *solely* on beats with the *predominant* QRS morphology to determine the underlying rhythm.
- The ***underlying* rhythm** in Figure 19A-23 appears to be ***rapid* AFib**. We arrive at this conclusion from assessing **beats #1-*thru*-9** at the *beginning* of the rhythm strip. The QRS complex of these beats is *narrow* — the rhythm is fast and *irregularly* irregular and *no P waves* are seen. *Rapid* AFib (*albeit at a slightly slower rate*) is also seen for **beats #17-*thru*-22** at the *end* of the rhythm strip.
- We now ***return*** to assess the ***different-looking* widened beats** (*#10,11; #13-16*) that we previously deferred. QRS morphology of **beats #10,11 in Figure 19A-23** looks familiar! These beats are virtually *identical* in morphology to beats #6,7 in Figure 19A-21 (*on page 223*) that we previously identified as being *aberrantly* conducted. By the ***"birds of a feather"*** concept (*pg 224*) — it is virtually certain that **beats #10,11** in Figure 19A-23 are also ***aberrantly* conducted**.

▶ **NOTE:** Even if we did *not* have access to the prior rhythm strip from page 223 on this patient — we would still guess that **beats #10,11** in **Figure 19A-23** are **likely** to be ***aberrantly*** conducted because: **i)** these beats are *not* overly widened and they manifest *typical* RBBB morphology (*rSR' with taller right rabbit ear*) that is characteristic of aberrant conduction; and **ii)** there is a "reason" for aberrancy — in that beat #10 in Figure 19A-23 occurs relatively *early* in the cardiac cycle (*with a relatively short coupling interval at a time when the ventricles are likely to still be partially refractory*).

☞ We are left with the task of assessing **beats #13-*thru*-16** in **Figure 19A-23**. Each of these beats is widened with a QS morphology. The differential diagnosis for these 4 beats is that of a **WCT** (*Wide-Complex Tachycardia*) without sign of atrial activity = **VT** *vs* **SVT with aberrant** conduction. As always — assume VT *until* proven otherwise. In the meantime — *Treat* the patient accordingly.

➡ **KEY *Clinical* Point:** Even IF beats #13-*thru*-16 in Figure 19A-23 do represent VT — these beats are *not* the primary arrhythmia problem of this patient who remains *hemodynamically* stable. Instead — the primary arrhythmia problem is *rapid* AFib.
- It is likely that *regardless* of the etiology of these beats — they will go away (*or at least occur less often*) once the rate of AFib is controlled. Initial management should therefore focus on rate control of underlying *rapid* AFib.

Beyond-the-Core: *Rapid AFib with RBBB* <u>and</u> *LBBB Aberration*

  Beyond-the-Core ...

⬤ IF your assessment of the rhythm in **Figure 19A-23** was *rapid* AFib with some *aberrant* conduction and a 4-beat run of *presumed* VT — You are doing *very* well and should be commended! That said — our *Beyond-the-Core Answer* is that we **suspect** beats **#13-*thru*-16** in this tracing are also **aberrantly conducted** because:

- **Reason #1:** Beats #13-*thru*-16 maintain the *same* pattern of *irregular* irregularity seen *throughout* the entire tracing <u>without</u> even *brief* pause at the *onset* of the 4-beat run (*beat #13*) <u>and</u> *without* any pause at the end of the run after beat #16 (*See blow-up* **Figure 19A-24** *below*).
- **Reason #2:** = *"Birds of a Feather"* — since we see other clear evidence of *aberrant* conduction on this tracing (*beats #10,11*).
- **Reason #3:** *Rapid* AFib is an extremely common "setting" for aberrant conduction to occur. ⬤***Advanced* PEARL:** If ever you see clear RBBB aberrancy in a *right-sided* lead for a patient with *rapid* AFib in which a *single* normally conducted beat (*beat #12*) is *sandwiched* between abrupt transition from ***RBBB* aberration** to a QS pattern of WCT — the run of beats with QS morphology (*beats #13-thru-16 in Panel B*) is almost certain to represent a run of ***LBBB* aberration** (*Marriott*).

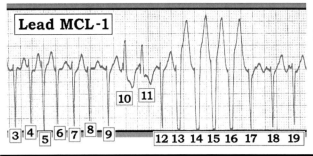

Figure 19A-24: *Blow-up* view of Figure 19A-23 (*See text*).

➡ ***Bottom* Line:** This is one of the most *challenging* rhythm strips in this entire book. The most important message to convey is that accurate interpretation of all aspects of each rhythm strip is <u>not</u> necessary in order to begin effective treatment. For this particular case — it wasn't until *after* this patient was treated that we were able to confirm LBBB aberration for beats #13-*thru*-16 in Figure 19A-24 by finding a prior tracing from this patient showing sinus rhythm with a PAC manifesting *identical* QS morphology in lead MCL-1 for the *aberrant* beats.

- *Regardless* of whether your assessment of <u>Figure 19A-23</u> was rapid AFib with *aberrant* conduction <u>or</u> *rapid* AFib with a 4-beat run of <u>either</u> VT <u>or</u> WCT of *uncertain* etiology — *initial* treatment of this hemodynamically *stable* patient should be the same (ie, *enacting measures to address the cause* <u>and</u> *control the rate of the primary arrhythmia problem, which is the rapid AFib*).

Practice Tracing #13: — *"12 Leads are Better than One"*

 ⇨ **PRACTICE** Tracing:

● Interpret the rhythm in Figure 19A-25 by the ***Ps,Qs,3R* Approach**. The patient is *hemodynamically* stable.
- Does Figure 19A-25 show atrial trigeminy (*every 3rd beat a PAC*)?

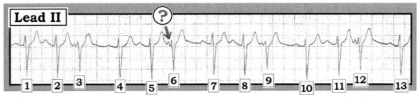

Figure 19A-25: *Practice* Tracing #13.

☞ **Answer to Tracing #13:** The *underlying* rhythm is **sinus** — as determined by the presence of *upright* P waves with *fixed* PR interval preceding beats #1,2; 4,5; 7,8; 10,11; and 13 in this lead II monitoring lead. The QRS complex of sinus beats is narrow.
- *Every-third-beat* occurs *earlier-than-expected* and looks slightly different. That is — the QRS complex of **beats #3, 6, 9** and **12** each have a *smaller* r wave and *less deep* S wave than do sinus beats. The QRS complex for each of these early beats *looks* to be narrow and *preceded* by a *premature* P wave (***arrow*** in Figure 19A-25). IF this were the case — the rhythm would be **atrial trigeminy** (*every third beat a PAC*).

● **QUESTION:** *Do you agree with the above assessment?*
- HINT #1: Do we have *enough* information from Figure 19A-25 to determine IF the QRS complex of each early beat is *truly* narrow?
- HINT #2: Look at **Figure 19A-26** — in which we have added a *simultaneously* recorded lead I rhythm strip. *Does the QRS of each early beat still look narrow?*

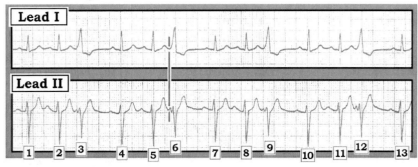

Figure 19A-26: A *simultaneously* recorded lead I rhythm strip has been added to Figure 19A-25. Note from the ***vertical* time line** that the notch which looked to be a premature P wave in Figure 19A-25 is actually the initial part of the QRS complex in *simultaneous* lead I ...

☞ 12 Leads are *Better* than One

We have *intentionally* added this *trick* tracing (Figure 19A-25) to this collection of *Practice* Tracings in order to emphasize a number of important points:

- POINT #1: **12 Leads are *Better* than One.** It is *easy to get fooled* when you are not provided with complete information. Part of the QRS complex may sometimes lie on the baseline. When this happens — the QRS complex may look narrow in one lead — whereas in reality it is actually quite wide. At other times (*as in* Figure 19A-25) — what looks like a preceding "P wave" may actually be the initial part of the QRS complex. Use of a **simultaneously recorded *multilead* rhythm strip** (*or 12-lead ECG*) may be invaluable in such cases for shedding light on the true nature the rhythm being assessed. With the extra information provided by lead I in **Figure 19A-26** — it is now apparent that every *third* beat (ie, *beats #3,6,9,12*) occurs early, is wide, and is *not* preceded by any premature P wave. Every third beat in Figure 19A-26 is therefore a **PVC**. The rhythm is ***ventricular* trigeminy.**

- POINT #2: **Assume that a Premature Beat is "Guilty"** (ie, *a PVC*) **until Proven Otherwise.** Statistically — most early occurring *different-looking* beats that are not clearly preceded by a premature P wave will be ventricular in etiology. We present notable exceptions to this general rule throughout Section 19 with goal of enhancing appreciation and awareness of the many facets of aberrant conduction. However, the *"onus of proof"* always rests with the interpreter to establish that the *abnormal-looking* beat(s) is aberrantly conducted. Until this is convincingly done — **assume** a **ventricular etiology** and treat the patient accordingly. Figure 19A-25 illustrates how you can *not* "prove" aberrant conduction with use of the *incomplete* information provided from a *single* monitoring lead.

Practice Tracing #14: *Rate-Related Aberrant conduction*

 ⇒ *Beyond-the-Core ...*

● Interpret the rhythm in Figure 19A-27 by the **Ps,Qs,3R Approach.** The patient is *hemodynamically* stable.

• Do **beats #4-*thru*-7** in Figure 19A-27 represent a short run of **NSVT** (*Non-Sustained Ventricular Tachycardia*) — *or* are these beats supraventricular with QRS widening due to *aberrant* **conduction?**

• How *certain* are you of your answer? — *What* would be needed to become *more* certain?

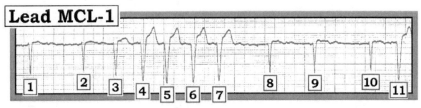

Figure 19A-27: *Practice* Tracing #14.

☞ **Answer to Tracing #14:** We begin assessment of this challenging rhythm strip by looking to see IF there is an **underlying rhythm**. Overall — the rhythm in this *right-sided* MCL-1 monitoring lead appears to be *irregularly* irregular. No P waves are seen. This suggests that the **underlying rhythm** is **AFib**. Fine undulations in the baseline represent "fib waves". The interesting part of the rhythm strip is **intermittent** widening of the **QRS complex**.

• Although at first glance one might be tempted to interpret the run of *widened* beats (*beats #4-thru-7*) as a short run of *ventricular* tachycardia — subsequent rhythm strips proved this *not* to be the case.

☞ *Rate-Related* **Bundle Branch Block**

An alternative explanation for the QRS widening seen in Figure 19A-27 is *rate-related* **BBB** (*Bundle Branch Block*) — in which acceleration of the underlying supraventricular rhythm does not allow adequate time for all fascicles of the conduction system to recover. The result is *intermittent* QRS widening in a pattern of a conduction block (*LAHB; LPHB; RBBB with or without hemiblock; LBBB*). We make the following points regarding *rate-related* **BBB**:

• It is *impossible* to be certain about the diagnosis of *rate-related* BBB from inspection of the single rhythm strip shown in Figure 19A-27. That said — awareness of this entity provides a plausible explanation for why the widened beats in this tracing may be supraventricular.

• Supporting the premise that the *widened* run of **beats #4-*thru*-7** is consistent with *rate-related* **BBB** — QRS morphology of these widened beats manifests the predominantly negative with *rapid* downslope QS complex expected in a *right-sided* lead when LBBB (*Left Bundle Branch Block*) is present.

• Rather than 2 competing rhythms — the **overall *irregular* irregularity** of the rhythm in Figure 19A-27 suggests it is far *more* likely that *all* beats seen represent **AFib**. *Rate-related* BBB characteristically begins when heart rate speeds up a bit — as it does in this tracing.

• Close inspection of **beat #3** reveals that it too is slightly widened. Beat #3 actually represents the onset of LBBB-conduction in this tracing (*albeit with a less complete form of LBBB given its lesser degree of QRS widening*).

• The run of rate-related LBBB conduction continues until **beat #8** — when the rate of AFib slows.

• **Beat #11** at the end of the tracing represents a final widened beat that manifests LBBB-conduction as a result of its *short* coupling interval with beat #10. Realizing that the Ashman phenomenon is *less* reliable in the setting of AFib (*pp 215-219*) — it is of note that a relatively *longer* pause preceded the onset of aberrant conduction for *both* beats #3 and 11 in Figure 19A-27.

▶ **NOTE:** *Subsequent* rhythm strips on this patient proved *beyond doubt* that LBBB conduction *consistently* occurred during periods of more rapid AFib <u>and</u> often began following a relatively *longer* R-R interval. In addition — QRS widening consistently resolved soon after the rate of AFib slowed down.

▬

⇒ *Clinical* **PEARLS:** Of interest (*and further complicating diagnostic recognition of the important but uncommon phenomenon of rate-related BBB*) — are the following clinical points:

• The **rate** of **onset** of **rate-related BBB conduction** is often <u>not</u> the same as the rate where normal conduction resumes. For example — *rate-related* BBB may begin when heart rate exceeds 90 or 100/min — but normal conduction may not resume until heart rate goes back down to 80/minute or less. This explains why serial tracings over time are often needed to make this diagnosis.

• ***Ventricular* rhythms** (*including both slower as well as more rapid versions of VT*) — are **<u>not</u> always *precisely* regular**. This makes it more difficult in cases like this to determine when a run of irregular *widened* beats represents NSVT <u>vs</u> AFib with *rate-related* BBB conduction.

• There will often <u>not</u> be enough information (*prior rhythm strips; 12-lead ECG*) available at the bedside to determine with any certainty that the run of *widened* beats you are looking at represents *rate-related* BBB ...

Section 20 – AV Blocks/AV Dissociation (*pp 233-250*)

 AV **B**locks
/AV *D*issociation

We conclude this *ACLS-2013-Arrhythmia* book with a primer and review on **recognition** of the **AV blocks** (*pp 233-250*). Discussion includes the concept of AV dissociation <u>and</u> its *distinction* from clinically important AV block.
* We highlight what AV block is not (ie, *it is <u>not</u> blocked PACs or marked sinus arrhythmia*). ● Beginning on **page 251** — We illustrate clinical application of these concepts with a series of *Practice* **Rhythms**.

☞ *Clinical* Context: Importance in *Assessing* AV Blocks

Diagnosis of the specific *type* of AV block is *less* important than the **clinical context** in which the AV block occurs. For example — *imme-diate* treatment is *<u>not</u>* always needed in 3rd degree AV block!

* A patient with 3rd degree AV block from acute *inferior* infarction may <u>not</u> necessarily need a pacemaker <u>IF</u> *asymptomatic* <u>with</u> junctional escape at *reasonable* rate and a normal BP. This is because: **i)** such patients may *remain* hemodynamically stable <u>despite</u> complete AV block; <u>and</u> **ii)** AV block in this setting may resolve on its own.
* In contrast — A pacemaker <u>is</u> indicated for *symptomatic* bradycardia that is <u>not</u> readily reversible (*not due to drugs/treatable cause*).
* **Assessment** of **clinical** context is therefore **essential** for determining the *optimal* course of management.

☞ *Blocked* PACs: *Much More Common than AV Block*

It is well to remember the following *KEY* point from Section 19: The **commonest** cause of a **pause** is a **blocked** PAC. <u>IF</u> looked for — blocked PACs <u>will</u> be found *much* more often than *any* type of AV block.
* We illustrate this concept in **Figure 20-1**. Despite two pauses and the presence of group beating — this is <u>not</u> any form of AV block.

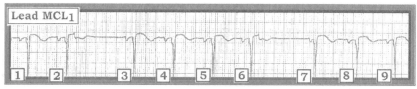

Figure 20-1 (*previously shown as Figure 19A-5 — page 207*): Despite 2 pauses and group beating — this is <u>not</u> any form of AV block. Instead — the *underlying* rhythm is sinus. The notch in the T wave at the beginning of each pause is a **blocked** PAC (*See also pp 196-202; pp 207-208*).

Facilitating Diagnosis

The 3 Degrees of AV Block:

⬤ Diagnosis of the different forms of AV block need *not* be difficult. Simply stated — there are **3 degrees** of AV block:

- **1st degree AV Block** — in which *all* impulses from above (ie, *from the SA node*) are conducted to the ventricles. It is just that they take *longer* than usual to get there (ie, *more than 0.20 second in an adult*).
- **2nd degree AV Block** — in which *some* sinus impulses get through the AV node and are conducted to the ventricles, but others do not.
- **3rd degree** or ***complete* AV Block** — in which *no* sinus impulses get through.

▶ **NOTE:** From a practical, clinical perspective (*as we will see momentarily*) — the diagnosis of <u>*both*</u> 1st degree <u>and</u> 3rd degree AV block is surprisingly easy!

- Awareness of this important concept tremendously facilitates diagnosis of the AV blocks. That is — <u>IF</u> an AV block is present <u>and</u> the block is *neither* 1st degree *nor* 3rd degree — then it <u>must</u> be *some form* of 2nd degree AV block (*See pp 236-240*).

1st Degree AV Block:

⬤ First degree AV block is diagnosed by the finding of a *prolonged* PR interval. This is defined as a **PR interval** that clearly measures **more** than **0.20-0.21 second (**or clearly <u>*more*</u> than 1 LARGE box in duration *on ECG grid paper***)**.

- Practically speaking — **1st degree AV Block** is simply a sinus rhythm with a *long* PR interval (<u>Figure 20-2</u>).
- The ***isolated* finding** of **1st degree AV block** (*even if marked*) is most often *not* clinically significant. This is especially true when a *prolonged* PR interval is seen in an otherwise healthy individual who does not have underlying heart disease. In contrast — *new* 1st degree AV block in a patient with acute evolving infarction (*especially if associated with other new conduction defects*) <u>is</u> clearly cause for concern. *Clinical correlation* is everything!

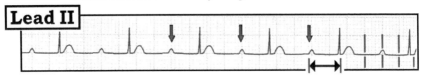

Figure 20-2: Sinus rhythm with **1st degree AV Block**. Each sinus P wave (*arrows*) <u>is</u> conducted to the ventricles; it just that it takes each sinus impulse *longer* to be conducted. Note that the PR interval preceding each QRS is fixed. PR interval prolongation is easily recognized because the PR clearly exceeds 1 *large* box in duration (*vertical lines*).

📖 *Regarding PR Interval Prolongation*

The **PR interval** is defined as the period that extends from the *onset* of atrial depolarization (*beginning of the P wave*) — until the *onset* of ventricular depolarization (*beginning of the QRS complex*).

- The best lead to use for assessing the PR interval is **lead II**. In adults, IF the P wave is *upright* in this lead (ie, *if there is sinus mechanism*) — the PR is considered **normal** IF **between 0.12-*to*-0.20 second**.
- The PR interval is defined as "short" if it measures *less* than 0.12 sec. in lead II (*as may occur with WPW when the AV node is bypassed*). That said — *Some* patients may normally have a PR interval of *less* than 0.12 second *without* necessarily having an accessory pathway.
- Although the *upper* limit of normal for PR interval duration in adults is generally cited as 0.20 second — some individuals normally have PR intervals slightly above this upper range. This is especially true for athletic young adults who often manifest increased vagal tone. As a result — we generally prefer the **PR interval** to be *at least* **0.22 second** before saying that **1st degree AV block** is present.
- Precise determination of a PR interval that falls within the normal range is *not* necessary. Clinically in this situation — it suffices to say that the PR interval is "normal".
- We generally **undercall 1st degree AV block**. This is because the clinical significance of *isolated* 1st degree AV block is usually minimal (*if not negligible*). For the same reason — we have *deleted* the term ***"borderline" 1st degree*** from our ECG vocabulary for PR intervals that measure within the range of 0.19-*to*-0.21 second. Saying that a patient has *"borderline 1st degree AV block"* really says *nothing more* than that the patient almost has a finding that *even if they had*, would usually not mean anything clinically.
- **Norms** for the PR interval (*as well as for QRS interval duration*) are *different* **in children**. Pediatric hearts are smaller. It therefore takes *less* time for the electrical impulse to travel through the conduction system of a child. For example — a PR interval of 0.18 second would be long for an infant. When in doubt about norms for a *younger-aged* patient — upper limits for the PR and QRS intervals should be *looked up* in an age-specific table.

▶ *FINAL* Point: The question is often asked as to ***HOW long*** the **PR interval can be** and ***still* conduct** to the **ventricles?** The answer is *very* long! We have seen PR intervals of *greater* than 1.0 second that still conduct to the ventricles in association with Mobitz I AV block.

- Although it is true that in *most* cases you'll encounter, the PR interval will *rarely* exceed 0.40-*to*-0.50 second — it is possible for the PR interval to be *much* longer than this and still be conducting to the ventricles.

☞ 2nd Degree AV Block (*3 Types*):

● Second degree AV block is traditionally divided into *two* types: Mobitz I and Mobitz II. It is important to emphasize that a **third type** of 2nd degree AV block also exists known as **2:1 AV block**.

- The common denominator for *all* types of 2nd degree AV block is that *some* but <u>not</u> all P waves are conducted to the ventricles.
- We schematically illustrate the 2nd degree AV blocks in **Figure 20-3**:

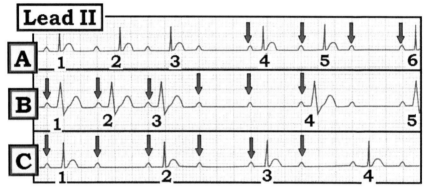

Figure 20-3: The 3 types of 2nd degree AV block. **Panel A** – Mobitz I 2nd degree AV block with *gradual* prolongation of the PR interval until a P wave is dropped (*pg 236*). **Panel B** — Mobitz II with QRS widening and a *fixed* PR interval until sudden loss of conduction with *successive* nonconducted P waves (*pg 238*). **Panel C** — 2nd degree AV block with 2:1 AV conduction. It is impossible to be certain if 2:1 AV block represents Mobitz I or Mobitz II, because we *never* see 2 conducted P waves in a row — <u>and</u> therefore *cannot* tell if the PR interval would progressively lengthen prior to nonconduction <u>IF</u> given a chance (*pp 238-240*).

☞ Mobitz I 2nd Degree AV Block (*AV Wenckebach*)

Mobitz <u>I</u> (*AV Wenckebach*) — is by far the *most* common type of 2nd degree AV block (*accounting for **more than 95%** of cases in our experience*). **Mobitz I** is *recognized* by: **i)** Progressive *lengthening* of the PR interval <u>until</u> a beat is dropped; **ii)** group beating; **iii)** a regular (*or at least fairly regular*) atrial rate; <u>and</u> **iv)** the pause that contains the dropped beat is *less* than twice the shortest R-R interval. These characteristics are known as **"the Footprints of Wenckebach"**. They are all present in **Figure 20-4**:

- There is **"group beating"** in Figure 20-4. This takes the form of 2 groups encompassing beats #1,2,3 and #4,5 (*each group separated by a pause of approximately equal duration between beats #3-4 and between #5-6*).
- The P-P interval is regular (*in this case at a rate of 100/minute*).

- ***Within*** groups — the **PR** interval *progressively* **lengthens** until a beat is dropped. Note the PR interval preceding beat #4 gets longer preceding beat #5 *until* the P wave after beat #5 is nonconducted. The next cycle then begins as the PR interval shortens prior to beat #6.
- The **pause** *containing* the ***dropped*** **beat** in Figure 20-4 is *less* than **twice** the *shortest* **R-R interval**. For example, in the first group of beats in Figure 20-4 — the *shortest* R-R interval is between beats #2-3. The pause that contains the dropped beat (ie, *the pause between beats #3-4*) measures *less* than twice than this R-R interval between beats #2-3.

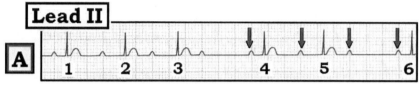

Figure 20-4: Mobitz I 2nd degree AV block. The PR interval progressively lengthens until a beat is dropped (*See text*).

☞ *KEY* **Points:** *The 2nd Degree AV Blocks*

Regarding **Mobitz I** 2nd degree AV block — the level of block usually occurs at the AV node. As a result: **i)** the QRS complex is typically narrow (*unless there is preexisting bundle branch block*); **ii)** the conduction defect may respond to Atropine (*especially if due to acute inferior infarction and treated within the first few hours of onset*); <u>and</u> **iii)** a permanent pacemaker is usually *not* needed.

● In contrast — the less common **Mobitz II** form (*page 238*) is more likely to occur at a *lower* level in the conduction system (*below the AV node*) — often in association with large *anterior* infarction. As a result: **i)** the QRS complex is likely to be wide with Mobitz II; **ii)** Atropine will usually *not* work; <u>and</u> **iii)** permanent pacing is *more* likely to be needed.

- The reason for addition of a **3rd category** (= **2:1 AV conduction**) — is to acknowledge that because you *never* see 2 *consecutively* conducted beats in a row, you *cannot* tell <u>IF</u> the PR interval would progressively lengthen if given a chance to do so. As we will see momentarily — *other* clinical clues may allow us to predict whether 2:1 AV conduction is more likely to be due to Mobitz I *or* Mobitz II. Given that the former condition *rarely* needs pacing whereas the latter *almost always* does — this distinction is very important clinically (*pg 238*).

▶ **PEARL:** The *atrial* **rate** should be **regular** (*or almost regular*) when there is AV block. It is common to see slight variation (*known as* **ventriculophasic sinus arrhythmia**) in the setting of 2nd or 3rd degree AV blocks. However — *marked* P wave irregularity — *change* in P wave morphology — <u>or</u> *prolonged* sinus pauses all suggest some phenomenon *other <u>than</u>* AV block is operative (ie, *blocked PACs; escape rhythms without AV block; sick sinus syndrome; sinus arrest ...*).

☞ Mobitz II 2nd Degree AV Block

The ***Mobitz II*** form of 2nd degree AV block — is recognized by QRS widening <u>with</u> a ***constant* PR interval** for ***consecutively* conducted beats** — <u>until</u> one or more beats are dropped.

- As noted on page 237 — **Mobitz II** occurs *lower* down in the conduction system. As a result — the QRS is usually wide. The problem with Mobitz II is its disturbing tendency to *abruptly* go from regular conduction of P waves to *nonconduction* of multiple P waves in a row, sometimes leading to ventricular standstill. This explains why **pacing** is almost always needed with *true* Mobitz II 2nd degree AV block.
- The features of Mobitz II are illustrated in **Figure 20-5**. Note that the QRS complex is wide. The underlying atrial rate (*P-P interval*) is regular. Following normal conduction of the first 3 beats on the tracing — there is *nonconduction* of multiple subsequent P waves.
- *Unlike* Mobitz I — the **PR interval** remains ***constant*** preceding all QRS complexes that conduct to the ventricles (*beats #1,2,3; #4,5*).

▶ **PEARL:** The *KEY* for diagnosing Mobitz II is that the PR interval remains constant for *consecutively* conducted P waves (*seen for the PR interval preceding beats #1,2,3 in* <u>Figure 20-5</u>).

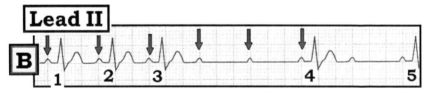

Figure 20-5: Mobitz II 2nd degree AV block. The PR interval is *constant* preceding *all* QRS complexes that *do* conduct to the ventricles.

2nd Degree AV Block with 2-to-1 AV conduction:

☞ 2-to-1 AV Block: *Mobitz I* <u>or</u> *Mobitz II* ?

● The final form of 2nd degree AV block is with 2:1 AV conduction. As with any form of AV block — the atrial rate is regular (*or almost regular*). Every other P wave is conducted (**Figure 20-6**).
- The rhythm in <u>Figure 20-6</u> is <u>*not*</u> complete AV block — because the PR interval preceding each QRS complex is constant. This tells us that *each* P wave on the tracing <u>is</u> being conducted to the ventricles.
- Note that P wave morphology is the *same* for all P waves <u>and</u> the P-P interval remains *regular* throughout <u>Figure 20-6</u> (*arrows*). This *rules out* atrial bigeminy with blocked PACs as the cause for the slow rate and nonconducted P waves (*as was seen for the example of "pseudo-AV-block" presented in* <u>Figure 19A-9</u> *on page 211*). We have therefore established **AV Block** of **2nd Degree** as the cause for the slow rhythm and conduction of only *every-other-P wave* on the tracing.

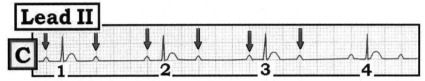

Figure 20-6: Second degree AV block with 2:1 AV conduction. The atrial rate is regular (*arrows*). Every other P wave is conducted to the ventricles. Although *impossible* to be certain IF this example of 2nd degree AV block with 2:1 AV conduction represents Mobitz I or Mobitz II — certain clinical clues may facilitate making this distinction (*See text*).

☞ 2:1 AV Conduction: *Is it Mobitz I or Mobitz II*?

As emphasized throughout Section 15 on Bradycardia — **highest priority** in evaluation and management of a patient with a rhythm such as that seen in <u>Figure 20-6</u> is to **assess *hemodynamic* status:**

- Specific diagnosis of the type of AV block is far *less* important initially than stabilization of the patient — be this with medication (*Atropine, pressor agent*) *and/or* Pacing if/as needed (*pp 163-164*).
- Specific diagnosis of the type of conduction disturbance will <u>not</u> always be possible based on the information (*rhythm strips*) available. Some conduction disturbances simply *defy* classification into "neat degrees" of AV block — especially during the setting of cardiopulmonary resuscitation, in which many of the "rules" for AV block classification are *not* reliably followed (*escape rhythms may be less regular in the "dying" heart*). That said — the general rules discussed in this Section 20 will serve well in most instances.

- We **strongly suspect** the example of **2:1 AV conduction** in **<u>Figure 20-6</u>** represents **Mobitz I** 2nd degree AV block. We say this because: **i)** Mobitz I is so much *more* common than Mobitz II (*accounting for more than 95% of cases in our experience*); **ii)** The QRS complex in <u>Figure 20-6</u> is narrow (*it is usually wide with Mobitz II*); <u>and</u> **iii)** It looks like the PR interval of conducting beats is long. Mobitz I frequently follows *sequential* progression from 1st degree — <u>to</u> Mobitz I 2nd degree — <u>and</u>, then on to 3rd degree AV block (*especially when this conduction defect arises during the early hours of acute inferior infarction*). In contrast — the PR interval for conducted beats with Mobitz II is much more likely to be normal than prolonged.

▶ *Additional* **CLUES:** Serial tracings <u>and</u> the *clinical* setting may provide *additional* clues in support of a diagnosis of Mobitz I. Although possible — it is **rare** for a patient **to go *back-and-forth* between Mobitz I *and* Mobitz II** forms of AV block. Therefore, <u>IF</u> there is clear evidence elsewhere that this patient manifested Mobitz I (*from the patients chart; from ongoing telemetry monitoring*) — then it is highly likely that the 2:1 AV conduction block seen in <u>Figure 20-6</u> also represents Mobitz I.

- Finally — IF 2:1 AV block occurs in association with **acute *inferior* infarction** — then **Mobitz I** is far more likely (*since occlusion of the right coronary artery commonly impedes blood supply to both the inferior wall of the left ventricle* <u>and</u> *the AV nodal artery*). In contrast — acute *anterior* infarction is much more likely to result in Mobitz II.

▶ *Clinical* **NOTE:** Although there is 2:1 AV block in <u>Figure 20-6</u> — the ventricular rate is <u>not</u> overly slow (*the R-R interval is 6 large boxes; the ventricular rate is 50/minute*). As a result — there is an *excellent* chance that this patient may be hemodynamically stable *despite* AV block. Immediate treatment may therefore <u>not</u> be needed.

- IF this patient became hypotensive — initial treatment with Atropine would be reasonable given that the QRS is narrow (*pg 164*).

Complete AV Block

☞ 3rd Degree AV Block

● Complete (*or 3rd degree*) AV block — is said to be present when <u>none</u> of the impulses from above (*P waves*) are able to conduct to the ventricles. In this case — there is **complete AV Dissociation** — because <u>none</u> of the P waves are related to any of the QRS complexes. The result is that **2 *independent* rhythms** are going on. One of these rhythms will be *from* **"above"** (*in the form of regularly occurring sinus P waves*). The *other* ongoing rhythm will be *from* **"below"** (*in the form of an escape rhythm originating <u>either</u> from the AV node, the His, or the ventricles*). Awareness of these features facilitates recognition and understanding of diagnostic criteria for what **3rd degree AV block** <u>is</u> — and *what* it <u>is</u> <u>not</u>:

- With *complete* AV block — <u>none</u> of the impulses from above (*sinus P waves*) are able to penetrate the AV node to arrive at the ventricles. As a result — there is regular (*or almost regular*) atrial activity — <u>and</u> a regular (*or almost regular*) ventricular escape rhythm (**Figure 20-7**).

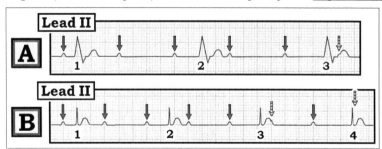

Figure 20-7: Anatomic levels of 3rd degree AV block. **Panel A:** *Complete* AV block at the *ventricular* level. The escape rhythm QRS is wide with an *idioventricular* escape rhythm *between* 20-40/minute. **Panel B:** *Complete* AV block at a *higher* level (*probably in the AV node*) — given the *narrow* QRS escape rhythm at a rate *between* 40-60/minute.

☞ There is **complete AV dissociation** in Figure 20-7 (ie, *none of the regularly occurring P waves are related to any QRS complexes*). As a result — **P waves** are seen to *"march through"* the **QRS**, occurring at all phases of the R-R cycle. This is most easily seen by focusing on each QRS complex for *both* A and B in Figure 20-7 — and seeing that the PR interval *immediately* preceding each QRS *continually* changes.

▶ **NOTE:** The anatomic level of *complete* AV block may vary. Most commonly — the level of block will occur *below* the AV node with a resultant ***ventricular*** escape rhythm (**Panel A** *in* Figure 20-7). When this happens — the **QRS** of the *escape* **rhythm** will be *wide* and the *escape* **rate** will be *between* **20-40/minute.**

☞ The anatomic level of block may occur at a *higher* **level** within the conduction system (*either within the AV node or the Bundle of His*). When this happens — the **QRS** of the *escape* **rhythm** will be *narrow*.
• IF the escape rhythm arises from the **AV node** — the *escape* **rate** will typically be *between* **40-60/min** (*as seen in* **Panel B** *of* Figure 20-7).
• IF the escape rhythm arises from the **Bundle of His** — the QRS complex will again be *narrow*, but the escape rate may be slower. One may therefore surmise the *probable* anatomic level of block based on characteristics of the escape rhythm (*QRS width and escape rate*) — realizing that exceptions may exist in patients with preexisting conduction defects *and/or* influence by medications, hypoxemia, acute ischemia/infarction, etc.

▶ **Clinical NOTE:** More important than the anatomic level of block per se in initial management decision-making is the patient's *hemodynamic* status. For example — a hypotensive patient with altered mental status and *complete* AV block associated with an escape rate of 40/min will still be in dire need of immediate treatment *regardless* of whether the escape rhythm manifests a wide or narrow QRS. That said — knowing the escape rhythm QRS is *narrow* suggests greater potential for reversibility and response to Atropine (*pp 165-166*).

☞ **PEARL: *Recognizing* and *Confirming Complete AV Block***

Most of the time IF the degree of AV block is complete (*3rd degree*) — then **the *ventricular* rhythm should be *at least fairly* regular.** This is because escape rhythms arising from the AV node, the His or ventricles are usually *fairly* regular rhythms. Exceptions may occur during cardiopulmonary resuscitation — but even then, there will usually be a recognizable pattern of ventricular regularity.

▶ **PEARL:** If the ventricular rhythm in a tracing with AV block is *not* regular (*or almost regular*) — then it is likely that at least *some* conduction is occurring (ie, *rather than 3rd degree — there is probably high-grade 2nd degree AV block*). Note that the R-R interval *is* regular for *both* examples of complete AV block in Figure 20-7.

☞ *Confirmation* of *complete* AV block *requires* that **P waves *fail* to conduct *despite*** being given adequate opportunity to do so. Satisfying this requirement provides the evidence needed to distinguish complete AV block from AV dissociation due to other causes. To do this — one must see P waves in *all* phases of the R-R cycle (ie, *having opportunity to conduct* — *but failing to do so*).

- For example, in **Tracing A** of <u>Figure 20-7</u> (*pg 240*) — the P wave hidden within the T wave of beat #3 (*striped arrow*) would *not* be expected to conduct to the ventricles because it occurs during the absolute refractory period. In contrast, virtually *all other* P waves in Tracing A occur at points in the cardiac cycle that should allow opportunity to conduct — yet none of them do. Similarly, in **Tracing B** of <u>Figure 20-7</u> — the P wave that notches the terminal portion of the T wave of beat #3 <u>and</u> the P wave hidden within the QRS complex of beat #4 each occur (*striped arrows*) at a time when conduction is not expected. However, *all other P waves* in Tracing B should have opportunity to conduct — yet fail to do so.

▶ **PEARL:** In order to *guarantee* that P waves will have adequate opportunity to conduct — the rate of the escape rhythm should ideally <u>not</u> exceed 50/minute. Escape rates faster than this often result in inopportune timing of P waves that mitigates against having an adequate opportunity to conduct. In such instances (*when the escape rate is well over 50/min*) — a much *longer* period of monitoring will be needed to ensure that the degree of AV block is complete. Note that the escape rate is <u>below</u> 50/minute for *both* examples of AV block in <u>Figure 20-7</u> — further confirming that the degree of AV block is complete.

AV *Dissociation* vs 3rd Degree AV Block

 # AV Dissociation

● The term, **"*AV dissociation*"** — simply means that for a certain period of time sinus P waves are *not* related to neighboring QRS complexes. That is, the P waves preceding the QRS are <u>not</u> being conducted to the ventricles.

- AV dissociation may be intermittent, recurrent and short-lived – <u>or</u> – it may be persistent/permanent, as occurs with complete AV block.
- **AV dissociation is *never* a "diagnosis"**. Instead — it is a condition caused by "something else". The task for the clinician is to figure out what the cause of AV dissociation is for any given rhythm. This assignment is far more than academic — since *appropriate* management depends on figuring out the cause of AV dissociation. Active treatment may or may not be indicated. For example — optimal treatment of *complete* AV dissociation with an accelerated junctional rhythm due to digitalis toxicity is simple: <u>IF</u> the patient is *hemodynamically* stable — simply *stop* digoxin! No pacemaker is needed

despite that fact that none of the P waves on the tracing may be conducting.

- *Complete* **AV dissociation is _not_ the same as** *complete* **AV block!** This is one of the most commonly *misunderstood* concepts in all of arrhythmia interpretation. Complete AV block is just *one* of 3 possible causes of AV dissociation. Patients with "complete AV dissociation" may actually have *no* degree of AV block at all ...
- Always try to determine *which* of the **3 Causes** of **AV Dissociation** is operative. The 3 possible causes are: **i) AV block** itself (*either from 2nd or 3rd degree AV block*); **ii) Usurpation** — in which P waves *transiently* do not conduct because an *accelerated* junctional or ventricular rhythm takes over the pacemaking function (ie, *"usurps" the rhythm*); _and/or_ **3) Default** — in which a junctional or ventricular *escape* rhythm takes over by *"default"* because the rate of the sinus pacemaker has *slowed down* for whatever reason.

⬤ Consider the rhythm strip shown in **Figure 20-8**. Are the P waves (*slanted arrows in* Figure 20-8) being conducted to the ventricles?
- IF so — Which one or two P waves are likely to be conducting?
- Which P waves are clearly *not* conducting?
- Is there AV block present? If so — what *degree* of AV block?
- **HINT:** Do *any* of the P waves that are not conducting have a "chance" to conduct — yet still *fail* to do so?
- *Extra* **Credit:** What is the *correct* interpretation of this rhythm?

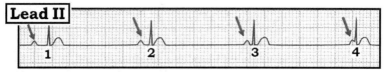

Figure 20-8: Is there AV block? If so — what *degree* of AV block is present? Explain your answer (*See text*).

☞ **Answer to Figure 20-8:** Full interpretation of the rhythm strip shown in Figure 20-8 is problematic because: i) We are *not* provided with information about the clinical setting; _and_ ii) The rhythm strip is short (*just over 4 seconds in duration*) _and_ we do *not* get to see the immediately preceding rhythm strips that are likely to be revealing about what is truly going on. That said — what *can* be stated about the rhythm strip in Figure 20-8 is the following:
- The *underlying* **rhythm** appears to be **sinus** — as suggested by **beat #1** which is preceded by an *upright* P wave with *reasonable* PR interval (*of 0.18 second*) in this lead II monitoring lead.
- The *ventricular* **rhythm** is *regular* at a rate *just over* **50/minute** (*the R-R interval is just under 6 large boxes in duration*).
- The **QRS** complex is *narrow*. For practical purposes — this means that the rhythm is **supraventricular** (*arising from either the SA node as in sinus rhythm — or from the AV node*).

- The **P waves** *preceding* **beats #3** and **#4** are definitely *not* conducting. They *can't* be — since the PR interval preceding these beats is clearly *too short* to conduct.
- The P wave preceding **beat #2** is also probably *not* conducting. Although the PR interval preceding beat #2 is *not* necessarily "too short to conduct" — it is clearly *less* than the PR interval preceding beat #1. Given that we *know* the P waves preceding beats #3 and #4 are not conducting — it is highly likely that the P wave preceding beat #2 is also *not* conducting.
- The **atrial rate** (*as defined by the P-P interval*) is **regular** at **50/minute** (*the P-P interval is precisely 6 large boxes in duration*).
- Regardless of whether the P wave preceding beat #2 is or is not conducting — **the *"theme"*** of the rhythm in Figure 20-8 is that there is **initial *sinus* bradycardia** (*beat #1*) at a rate of 50/minute — followed by a period of AV dissociation (*since P waves preceding subsequent beats are definitely* not *conducting*). This is **AV Dissociation *by* Default** (ie, *default from sinus node slowing that allows emergence of an appropriate junctional escape rhythm at 52/minute*).

▶ **KEY *Clinical* Point:** There is *no* evidence of any AV block at all in Figure 20-8. *None* of the P waves that fail to conduct have any reasonable chance to conduct (*since the PR interval is simply too short before an appropriate junctional escape rhythm supervenes*).

- What occurs in Figure 20-8 is commonly seen among healthy adolescents or young adults during sleep or undergoing anesthesia. The sinus rate temporarily slows — and an *appropriate* junctional escape rhythm intermittently supervenes. There is *no* AV block. There is *no* pathology. There is *no* need for intervention with optimal treatment being "benign neglect" (*the clinician is perhaps better off* not *knowing that transient AV dissociation may be occurring in such otherwise healthy and asymptomatic individuals*).

▶ **BOTTOM Line:** The **correct** diagnosis for the rhythm strip shown in Figure 20-8 is: *Sinus bradycardia with AV dissociation by default that results in an appropriate junctional escape rhythm at 52/minute.* Nothing more need be written in your interpretation.

- *Beyond-the-Core:* Although we assumed that beat #1 in Figure 20-8 is conducting — We actually do *not* know for certain that this is true. This is because we *never* see 2 beats in a row that conduct with the same PR interval. Therefore, *it could be* that the patient's *underlying* rhythm is sinus with *marked* 1st degree AV block – and that beat #1 also manifests AV dissociation. That said, *regardless* of whether or not beat #1 is conducting — the "theme" of this rhythm is still sinus bradycardia with AV dissociation by default. The need for clinical correlation to guide management remains the same (ie, *no immediate intervention is needed if the patient is asymptomatic and the setting benign*).

☞ We summarize pages 242-244 by **Figure 20-9** — in which *all* **3 Causes** of **AV Dissociation** are illustrated. Note the following:

- **Panel A** in Figure 20-9: The rhythm is sinus bradycardia with AV dissociation by *default* — resulting in an *appropriate* junctional *escape* rhythm at 52/minute (*See Answer to* Figure 20-8 — *pg 243*).

- **Panel B:** This is **AV dissociation** *by* **usurpation**. Beats #1 and #2 are sinus conducted with a normal PR interval. The PR interval then shortens. We *know* that P waves preceding beats #4 and #5 in Panel B are *not* conducting (*the PR interval is clearly too short to conduct*). No P waves at all are seen after beat #5. The reason is that an **accelerated** *junctional* **rhythm** (*at 78/minute*) has *"usurped"* the pacemaking function from the SA node (*that was beating at 75/min*). This situation is commonly seen in **digitalis toxicity**. Although *none* of the sinus P waves in Panel B are conducting — *none* of the P waves seen have any reasonable chance to conduct. Thus, *despite* noncomduction of P waves — there is *no* evidence of any AV block. It is likely that AV dissociation will spontaneously *resolve* if digoxin is held.

- **Panel C:** This is **AV dissociation** *due to* **3rd Degree** **AV Block** (*Panel C is reproduced from* Figure 20-7 — *on pg 240*). As opposed to Panels A and B, in which *nonconducting* P waves *do not have any reasonable chance* to conduct — P waves in Panel C occur at *all* points in the cardiac cycle. One would therefore anticipate that virtually *all* of the P waves indicated by *solid arrows* in Panel C should have a chance to conduct. Despite this — *none* of the P waves in Panel C conduct. Instead — **P waves *"march through"*** the **QRS** throughout the rhythm strip. In addition — the ventricular escape rhythm is *less* than 50/minute. The rhythm in **Panel C** therefore fulfills criteria for **complete AV block** as the cause of AV dissociation (*pp 240-242*).

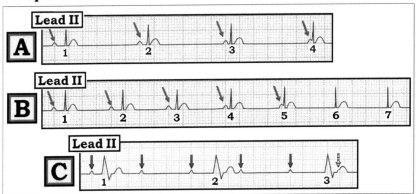

Figure 20-9: The 3 causes of AV dissociation. **Panel A:** AV dissociation by *default* of the sinus pacemaker (*that allows AV nodal escape to arise*); **Panel B:** AV dissociation by *usurpation* of the rhythm by another *accelerated* pacemaker (*which in this case arises from the AV node*); and **Panel C:** AV dissociation due to **AV block** — which could be *either* 2nd degree or as in Panel C, a **3rd degree AV block**.

High-Grade 2nd Degree AV Block

High-Grade AV Block:

● A term is needed to describe the situation in **Figure 20-10**.
• How would you interpret this rhythm?
• Is there AV block? IF so — Is the conduction disturbance likely to represent Mobitz I or Mobitz II 2nd degree? *Justify* your answer.

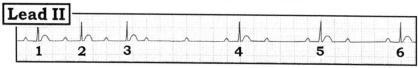

Figure 20-10: How might one *best* classify this type of AV block?

Answer to Figure 20-10: AV block is present in Figure 20-10. The QRS is narrow. The ventricular rhythm is irregular — but *regular* P waves do occur *throughout* the tracing (*arrows in* **Figure 20-11**).

• There is **2nd degree AV block**. We say this because *some* of the P waves in Figure 20-11 conduct — but others do not! For example — We see 2 P waves *in a row* following beat #3 that do *not* conduct. Single *nonconducted* P waves also follow beats #4 and 5.

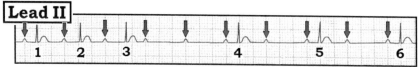

Figure 20-11: Arrows have been added to Figure 20-10 to indicate *regularly* occurring P waves *throughout* the tracing. Some P waves conduct whereas others don't (*the first 2 P waves after beat #3* — and *the P waves after beats #4 and #5 do not conduct*). This is **2nd degree AV block**. We know *at a glance* that this is *unlikely* to be 3rd degree AV block — because the ventricular rhythm is *not* regular (*See text*).

▶ **PEARL:** An easy way to recognize *at a glance* that Figure 20-10 is *unlikely* to represent 3rd degree AV block is to note that the ventricular rhythm is *not* regular. This strongly suggests that at least *some* P waves *are* conducting. We confirm that some P waves are conducting by noting that the PR interval preceding beats #4, 5 and 6 is constant.

High-Grade 2nd Degree AV Block

The rhythm strip in Figure 20-11 represents elements of *both* Mobitz I and Mobitz II forms of 2nd degree AV block:
• The **first 3 beats** represent a *definite* **Wenckebach cycle**. Note that the PR interval *progressively* increases from beat #1 — to beat #2 — to

beat #3. The P wave after beat #3 is nonconducted. The cycle then resumes with *shortening* of the PR interval prior to beat #4.

- What is *atypical* for AV Wenckebach (*Mobitz I 2nd degree AV block*) — is *nonconduction* of two P waves in a row. Although *not* impossible for successive nonconducted beats to occur with Mobitz I — it is far more common to see *successive* dropped beats with Mobitz II.

 Figure 20-11 concludes with 2:1 AV conduction for beats #4, 5 and 6. As discussed on pp 238-240 — **2nd degree AV block** <u>*with*</u> **2:1 AV conduction** could be due to <u>*either*</u> Mobitz I <u>or</u> Mobitz II AV block:

- Features in favor of **Mobitz I** as the explanation for the *entire* rhythm strip in Figure 20-11 include: **i)** that Mobitz I is much more common than Mobitz II; **ii)** that the QRS is narrow; **iii)** that the baseline PR interval for conducted beats is relatively long; <u>and</u> **iv)** that we see clear evidence of Mobitz I in the beginning of the tracing (*one usually does <u>not</u> switch back-and-forth between Mobitz I and Mobitz II block*).
- Features in favor of **Mobitz II** as *at least* a component of the conduction disturbance in Figure 20-11 include: **i)** the presence of 2:1 AV block with a *fixed* PR interval at the end of the tracing; <u>and</u> **ii)** successive *nonconducted* P waves following beat #3.

● **KEY *Clinical* Point:** In acknowledgement of these conflicting features between Mobitz I and Mobitz II forms of AV block (*as well as to reflect our increased clinical concern given successive nonconduction of P waves*) — we describe the conduction disturbance seen in Figure 20-11 as, *"High-Grade"* **2nd Degree AV Block.**

- There are *many* variations on the above "theme" — in which the degree of AV block is *not quite complete* <u>and</u> *not* necessarily conforming to either pure Mobitz I or Mobitz II — yet clearly of ***increased* clinical concern** due to nonconduction of *multiple* beats with resultant overly *slow* ventricular rate.

▶ *Clinical* **NOTE:** Much *more* important than the "degree" of AV block in assessing a patient with a rhythm as seen in Figure 20-11 — is assessment of the clinical situation (*pp 163-164*).

Ventricular Standstill vs *Complete AV Block*

Ventricular Standstill

● Confusion sometimes arises in the terminology used to describe certain ventricular or arrest rhythms related to complete AV block. The 4 rhythms illustrated in **Figure 20-12** will hopefully clarify the choice of terminology used:

- **Panel A** in Figure 20-12 — represents **complete AV block** at the *ventricular* level (*pp 240-242*). There is a regular *atrial* rhythm (*arrows*) and a regular *ventricular* rhythm — but *none* of the P waves are conducting (*P waves "march through" the QRS complex …*).

- **Panel B** in <u>Figure 20-12</u> — represents *ventricular* **standstill**. Atrial activity continues (*in the form of regularly-occurring P waves*) — but *no* QRS complexes are seen. Clinical implications of this rhythm are usually the same as for asystole. Patients with **Mobitz II** 2nd degree AV block sometimes suddenly go from minimal nonconduction of beats to ventricular standstill (*which is why pacing is almost always needed for patients with Mobitz II AV block*).
- **Panel C** — represents a **slow** *idioventricular* **rhythm** — seen here with an escape rate just over 30/minute. This is <u>not</u> a form of AV block — because there are *no* P waves. Instead, following sinus arrest (*and failure of an AV nodal escape pacemaker to arise*) — there *fortunately* is appearance of a **ventricular** *escape* **rhythm** (*without which there would have been asystole ...*).
- **Panel D** — represents **asystole**. There is *no* sign of any electrical activity (*No P waves; No QRS complexes = a flat line rhythm ...*).

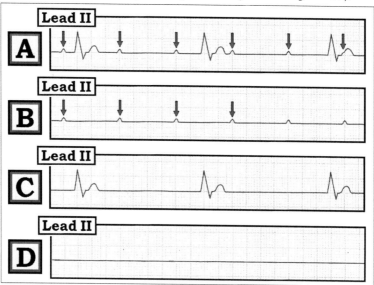

Figure 20-12: Clarification of *complete* AV block (**Panel A**) — ventricular *standstill* (**Panel B**) — slow *idioventricular* escape (**Panel C**) <u>and</u> the *flat line* rhythm of *asystole* in **Panel D** (*See text*).

Hyperkalemia **vs AV Block (*or VT*)**

☞ Hyperkalemia:

⬤ The incidence of *Hyperkalemia* has clearly increased in recent years. Reasons for this increase are multiple — but include the obesity epidemic with corresponding increase in the incidence of diabetes <u>and</u> improved treatment of diabetes resulting in increased longevity, such that many more patients with diabetes now live long enough to develop complications associated with *end-stage* kidney disease. **Hyperkalemia** is perhaps the most immediately *life-threatening* complication seen in this group of patients.

- Many more patients than ever before are now on **dialysis**. Hyperkalemia should *always* be thought of in such patients whenever they present with either an unusual (*or bizarre*) 12-lead ECG *and/or* a cardiac arrhythmia.

- Chronic kidney disease patients who are not yet on dialysis may also develop hyperkalemia — especially if any of a number of **predisposing situations** are present. These include: **i)** taking potassium-retaining medications (*ACE-inhibitors; angiotensin-receptor-blocking drugs; certain diuretics; potassium supplements*); **ii)** dehydration; **iii)** acidosis; **iv)** abrupt reduction in urine output; *and* **v)** cardiac arrest.

- **Hyperkalemia** is *notorious* for its ability to **mimic** *other* **ECG conditions**. Among ECG changes produced by more severe degrees of hyperkalemia (*common once serum potassium exceeds 6-6.5 mEq/L*) include: **i)** marked *peaking* of **T waves** in multiple leads; **ii)** **QRS widening**; **iii)** *reduced* **P wave** amplitude — sometimes with complete *loss* of **P waves** (*despite persistence of sinus conduction*); **iv)** bizarre frontal plane *axis* shifts; *and* **v)** **ST-T wave changes** that may mimic ischemia/acute infarction (*ST elevation or depression; T wave peaking and/or deep T wave inversion*).

⬤ Relevance of the above information on Hyperkalemia to this Section 20 on AV Block is highlighted by the rhythm in **Figure 20-13**.

- Should the patient whose rhythm is shown in Figure 20-13 be treated with Atropine *and/or* pacing?

- **HINT:** How might your answer to this question *change* IF told that this patient was alert <u>and</u> had a history of chronic kidney disease?

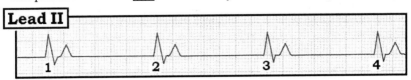

Lead II

1   2   3   4

Figure 20-13: Ventricular rhythm at ~40/minute. How should this patient be treated? (*See text*).

👉 **Answer to Figure 20-13:** A regular ventricular (*wide QRS*) rhythm is seen in Figure 20-13 at a rate of ~40/minute. There are no P waves. While our *initial* impression is that of a **ventricular escape rhythm** (*as might commonly occur in a setting of cardiac arrest*) — pending the need for *additional* information, there are *other* **possibilities** that should be entertained. For example — IF told that this patient was hemodynamically stable, alert <u>and</u> on longterm dialysis (*or that he/she had a history of chronic kidney disease*) — then a **stat potassium** value becomes essential for optimal management:

- QRS *widening* — the *slow* ventricular rate — *lack* of P waves — <u>and</u> suggestion of T wave *peaking* in **Figure 20-13** are all consistent with a *possible* diagnosis of hyperkalemia.

- IF the diagnosis is **hyperkalemia** — then ***immediate* treatment** will be very different than treatment of slow ventricular escape in a patient with cardiac arrest whose serum potassium is normal. As opposed to atropine, use of a pressor *and/or* pacing — **IV Calcium**, **Bicarb** *and/or* **D50 *plus* Insulin** may become the treatment(s) of choice.

⬤ A second example of what *initially* appears as a ventricular rhythm but is not — is shown in **Figure 20-14**:
- IF this rhythm was obtained from an unresponsive patient in cardiac arrest — We would interpret it as **AIVR** (*Accelerated IdioVentricular Rhythm*) at a rate of 100/minute (*page 195*).
- **IF instead** it was obtained from a *hemodynamically* stable patient with **chronic *kidney* disease** — We would be concerned that this *wide-complex* rhythm *without* P waves **might *reflect* hyperkalemia.**
- It should be obvious that knowing serum electrolytes of a patient in cardiac arrest is highly desirable <u>and</u> may be critical to optimal management. That said — emergency providers will unfortunately <u>not</u> always have access to this information. In such cases — *empiric* **management** may be needed until a serum potassium value can be obtained.
- IF the patient whose rhythm is shown in Figure 20-14 was *hemodynamically* stable — *no* immediate treatment may be needed. Even if the patient was hypotensive — it is *unlikely* that cardioversion of a ventricular rhythm this slow (*well under 140/minute*) would improve the situation. IF immediate treatment was needed *prior to* lab confirmation of *suspected* hyperkalemia — *empiric* **Bicarb** (1 amp) *and/or* **Calcium Chloride** (*250-500mg given by slow IV over 5-10 minutes*) may be reasonable to see if the QRS narrows and P waves return.

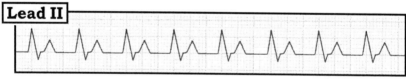

Figure 20-14: Wide QRS rhythm without P waves at 100/minute. Depending on the clinical situation — this could be AIVR in a patient with cardiac arrest or acute reperfusion – <u>or</u> – it this rhythm may be due to hyperkalemia (*See text*).

Section 20A – *AV Blocks / AV Dissociation* (*pp 251-287*)

 ⇒ <u>**PRACTICE**</u> **Examples:**

● What follows is a series of *Practice* **Rhythm Strips** with goal of reinforcing the essential arrhythmia concepts covered in this section on *AV Blocks/AV Dissociation*. Although clearly *not* an exhaustive compendium of clinical examples on this topic — our hope is that review of these examples will increase your appreciation <u>and</u> comfort level in recognizing and applying the principles summarized on pages 233-250.

 • For each of the *Practice* Tracings that follow (*pp 251-287*) — Assess the rhythm using the ***Ps,Qs,3R* Approach**.
  • **HINT #1:** Each tracing illustrates one or more of the important concepts regarding the *AV Blocks/AV Dissociation*.
  • **HINT #2:** Use of *calipers* will be **invaluable** for understanding (*and facilitating diagnosis*) of the AV blocks. Your ability to recognize the various AV blocks (*and distinguish them from "mimics" of AV block*) will be instantly enhanced as soon as you use calipers.
  • Our *explained* interpretations follow.

● ***Practice*** **Tracing #1:** Interpret the rhythm strips in <u>Figure 20A-1</u> using the *Ps,Qs,3R* Approach. The patient is *hemodynamically* stable.
• **Rhythm Strips A** and **B** in <u>Figure 20A-1</u> were obtained *sequentially* from a patient with syncope. — What type of AV block is present?
• Has the *degree* of AV block become *worse* in Tracing B?

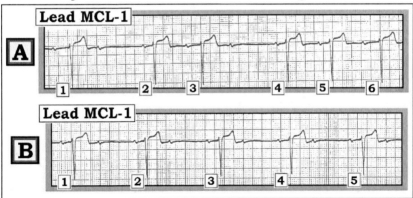

Figure 20A-1: *Practice* Tracing #1 (*sequential rhythm strips*).

 Answer to Rhythm A (*of Tracing #1*): There is group beating. The QRS complex is narrow. *Similar-looking* P waves occur at a slightly irregular rate of between **~60-70/minute** (*ventriculophasic sinus arrhythmia*). The PR interval gradually increases within groups until a beat is nonconducted (*the P waves that occur after beats #1 and #3 in*

Tracing A are not conducted). This is **2nd degree AV block, Mobitz Type I** (*AV Wenckebach*). Of interest — Note the following:

- The 2 pauses that contain dropped beats are of equal duration (*1.78 second for the interval between beats #1-2 and between #3-4*).
- Each pause ends with a P wave that conducts with the shortest PR interval (*0.23 second for the PR interval preceding beats #2 and #4 in Tracing A*). Progressive PR lengthening then begins anew.

☞ **Answer to Rhythm B** (*of Tracing #1*): The QRS complex is again narrow. The ventricular rhythm is fairly regular at a rate just under 40/minute. A slightly irregular sinus rhythm is again present — but this time at a faster rate (*range between **80-85/minute***). Every-*other*-P wave conducts — as determined by the presence of a fixed (*albeit prolonged*) PR interval preceding each QRS complex on the tracing. This is **2nd degree AV block _with_ 2:1 AV conduction**.

- Although fewer beats are conducted and the overall ventricular rate in Tracing B is slower — there has _not_ necessarily been any "worsening" in the degree of AV block between Tracing A and Tracing B.
- Instead — it may simply be that at the slightly faster atrial rate (*of 80-85/minute*) — fewer impulses are able to penetrate the AV node.

☞ **_Review_ of the 2nd Degree AV Blocks**

As emphasized on pages 236-240 – there are **3 types** of **2nd degree AV block**: i) **Mobitz I** (*AV Wenckebach*); ii) **Mobitz II**; _and_ iii) **2nd degree AV block _with_ 2:1 AV conduction**. This distinction is important because the clinical course and recommended management for the various types of 2nd degree AV block is quite different.

- **Mobitz I** is recognized by: **i)** Progressive lengthening of the PR interval until a beat is dropped; **ii)** Group beating; **iii)** A regular (*or almost regular*) atrial rate; _and_ **iv)** The pause that contains the dropped beat is *less* than twice the shortest R-R interval. These characteristics are all evident in **Tracing A**. Note that the pause containing the dropped beat (*the pauses between beats #1-2 and 3-4*) is *less* than twice the shortest R-R interval (*which is the R-R between beats #2-3 and #4-5*).
- **Mobitz II** is recognized by QRS widening and a *constant* PR interval for *consecutively* conducted beats _until_ one or more beats are dropped.
- By far — the most common form of 2nd degree AV block is **Mobitz I**. Because Mobitz I 2nd degree AV block usually occurs at the level of the AV node — the QRS complex is typically narrow — the conduction defect may respond to Atropine (*especially if due to acute inferior infarction and treated within the first few hours of onset*) — _and_ a permanent pacemaker is usually *not* needed.
- In contrast — the less common **Mobitz II** form is more likely to occur at a *lower* level in the conduction system (*below the AV node*) — often in association with large anterior infarction. As a result — the QRS complex is likely to be wide — Atropine will usually *not* work — and permanent pacing is much *more* likely to be needed.

- The reason for addition of a **3rd category** (= **2:1 AV conduction**) — is to acknowledge that because you *never* see 2 consecutively conducted beats in a row, you *cannot* tell IF the PR interval would progressively lengthen if given a chance to do so. As a result — one *cannot* be certain if 2nd degree AV block with 2:1 AV conduction represents Mobitz I or Mobitz II simply from looking at a single isolated rhythm strip such as Tracing B.

▶ *Clinical* **PEARLS:** The 2 sequential tracings in Figure 20A-1 serve to highlight the following points regarding the **2nd Degree AV blocks**:

- The atrial rate should be regular (*or almost regular*) when there is AV block. It is common to see slight variation (*known as* **ventriculophasic sinus arrhythmia**) in the setting of 2nd or 3rd degree AV blocks (*as is evident in Tracings A and B*). However — *marked* P wave irregularity — *change* in P wave morphology — or *prolonged* sinus pauses all suggest some phenomenon *other than* AV block is operative (*sick sinus; sinus arrest; blocked PACs; escape rhythms without AV block*).
- The *KEY* for diagnosing **Mobitz II** as the type of 2nd degree AV block is that the PR interval remains constant for *consecutively* conducted P waves. Because you *never* see 2 consecutively conducted complexes in Tracing B — you cannot tell if the PR interval would increase if given a chance to do so. Therefore — one could *not* diagnose Mobitz II from Tracing B alone — but instead should classify this rhythm as 2nd degree AV block with 2:1 AV conduction.
- That said — we can make an educated guess that **Tracing B** is *almost certain* to represent **Mobitz I** 2nd degree AV block because: **i)** Mobitz I is so much more common than Mobitz II; **ii)** The QRS is narrow; **iii)** The PR interval of conducting beats is prolonged (*far more common in Mobitz I*); *and* **iv)** Tracing A is definitely Mobitz I — *and* it is rare to go *back-and-forth* between Mobitz I and Mobitz II.
- Knowing that Tracing B is almost certain to be Mobitz I would support a trial of **Atropine** as an *initial* intervention IF this patient was symptomatic. Whether or not **pacing** would eventually be needed would be determined by *other factors* including the cause of the conduction block — how slow the ventricular response remained and symptoms.
- Although **Atropine** may be highly effective during the early hours of *vagally* induced Mobitz I 2nd degree AV block — this treatment is **not benign** (*pp 164-166*). In addition to improving AV conduction, Atropine may speed up the sinus rate. This in fact could be what happened between Tracing A and Tracing B — in which case this sequence of tracings would illustrate a potential *paradoxical* response from appropriate use of Atropine. That is, by increasing the atrial rate — use of Atropine may sometimes *slow* of the overall ventricular response.
- **Final Point:** Remember to **assess** the *atrial* **rate** whenever evaluating patients with AV block. Forgetting to do so may result in overlooking the reason for a change in AV conduction ratios (*as occurs here between Tracing A and Tracing B*).

Practice **Tracing #2:** *AV Block or Not?*

 ⇒ **PRACTICE Tracing:**

● Interpret the 2 rhythm strips below using the **Ps,Qs,3R Approach.** Each of these tracings was obtained from an *asymptomatic* young adult who was *hemodynamically* stable.

• Is there AV block or not? If so — Describe the type of block present.
• **HINT:** A *similar* mechanism is operative in each tracing.

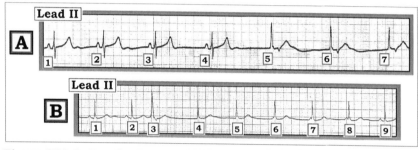

Figure 20A-2: *Practice* Tracing #2 (*Assess each rhythm strip*).

☞ **Answer to Rhythm A** (*of Tracing #2*): The first 4 beats in A are sinus conducted. The QRS complex is narrow throughout — although there is slight change in QRS morphology beginning with beat #5.

• Note that there is **gradual slowing** in the rate of the **sinus brady-cardia** seen for the **initial 4 beats**. That is, the R-R interval between sinus beats (*solid arrows in* **Figure 20A-3**) increases from 6.2 large boxes (*between beats #1-2*) — up to an R-R of 7.0 large boxes (*between beats #3-4*).

• No P wave precedes **beat #5**. This QRS complex is narrow (*albeit slightly different in morphology compared to the QRS for sinus conducted beats*). Beat #5 is **a junctional** *escape* **beat**.

• Note that the R-R interval preceding **beat #5** is a bit *over* 7 large boxes in duration. Thus, it is appropriate (*and downright fortunate*) that this AV nodal escape beat occurred — since the underlying sinus bradycardia rhythm has continued to slow down. Note also that the R-R interval for *each* of the junctional escape beats in Tracing A manifests the *same* R-R interval (*7.4 large boxes*) — which corresponds to an **appropriate AV nodal escape rate** at ~**40/minute**.

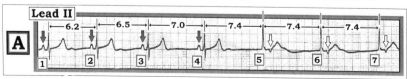

Figure 20A-3: Addition to **Tracing A** of arrows and intervals.

- Finally — note in <u>Figure 20A-3</u> that each junctional escape beat (*beats #5,6,7*) is followed by a *negative* P wave in this lead II (*open arrows*). This reflects **retrograde atrial conduction** from junctional beats that continually resets the sinus node and serves in this way to perpetuate the junctional escape rhythm.

☞ BOTTOM Line Regarding Tracing A in <u>Figure 20A-3</u>:

There is *no* evidence of any AV block at all in Tracing A. On the contrary, in view of the fact that this tracing was obtained from a presumably healthy and otherwise *asymptomatic* young adult — there is <u>not</u> necessarily any abnormality at all. We simply see progressive sinus bradycardia with an *appropriate* AV node escape rhythm arising once the sinus rate drops below 40/minute.

- *Marked* sinus bradycardia as seen here **could be normal** for this patient <u>IF</u> this young asymptomatic individual was an endurance athlete. In this case — no intervention would be needed. On the contrary — sinus bradycardia to this degree with need for an AV nodal escape rhythm to arise <u>would</u> be cause for concern <u>IF</u> the patient was an *older* adult with a history of weakness or syncope. *Clinical correlation is everything.*

▶ **NOTE:** There is **no evidence of** any **AV dissociation** in Tracing A. This is because *all* P waves seen on this tracing *are* related to neighboring QRS complexes (*either appearing before the QRS and conducting — or appearing after the QRS reflecting retrograde AV conduction from junctional escape beats*).

Review of Tracing B from Page 254 (<u>Figure 20A-4</u>):

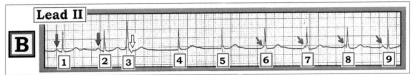

Figure 20A-4: Addition of arrows to **Tracing B**.

☞ **Answer to Rhythm B** (*of Tracing #2*): The *underlying* rhythm in Tracing B is **sinus** — as determined by the presence of an upright P wave with fixed PR interval preceding **beats #1** and **#2**.

- **Beat #3** is **premature**. It is slightly wider and quite different in morphology compared to other beats on this tracing. Beat #3 is <u>not</u> preceded by a premature P wave. We **suspect** that **beat #3** is a **PVC** (*although acknowledge that it could be a fascicular escape beat given that it is not overly wide*).
- <u>Regardless</u> of the origin of **beat #3** — this premature beat is *followed* by a **retrograde P wave** (*open arrow*). Just like the situation in

Tracing A — retrograde atrial conduction *resets* the sinus node. As a result — there is *no* P wave preceding beat #4. Given how similar QRS morphology of beat #4 is to the first two sinus beats — this defines **beat #4** as a **junctional *escape* beat**.

- The remaining beats in Tracing B (*beats #5,6,7,8,9*) represent a fairly regular albeit slightly *accelerated* **junctional escape rhythm** at **~65/minute**.

- Sinus node activity gradually returns toward the end of the tracing (*slanted arrows preceding beats #6,7,8 with a PR interval too short to conduct ...*).

➡ *Clinical* Note: We are *uncertain* if the P wave preceding beat #9 in Tracing B is or is not conducting. We suspect that it is not, because the PR interval preceding it appears to be *ever-so-slightly* shorter than the PR interval preceding sinus beats #1 and #2. Clinically — *it does not matter* if the P wave preceding beat #9 is conducting or not — since the "theme" of this rhythm remains unchanged. In either case — ***Our* Interpretation** for **Tracing B** is the following:

- Underlying ***sinus* rhythm** (*beats #1 and #2*). One **PVC** is seen (*beat #3 in Tracing B*).

- Resultant **AV dissociation *by default*** beginning with beat #4 — with a fairly regular (*albeit slightly accelerated*) junctional escape rhythm (*AV Dissociation was discussed on pp 242-245*).

- ***Bottom* Line:** Given that **Tracing B** was obtained from a presumably healthy and asymptomatic young adult — *no* intervention is needed.

Practice Tracing #3: *AV Block or Not?*

 ⇒ **PRACTICE Tracing:**

● Interpret the rhythm below using the **Ps,Qs,3R Approach.** The patient is *hemodynamically* stable.
• Is there AV block or not? If so — Describe the type of block present.
• **HINT #1:** Look *first* at this tracing *from a little distance* away.
• **HINT #2:** The patient was admitted with **recent *inferior* infarction.**

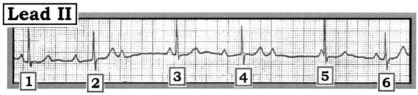

Figure 20A-5: *Practice* Tracing #3.

☞ **Answer to Figure 20A-5:** Full interpretation of the rhythm strip shown in Figure 20A-5 is challenging and a bit *beyond-the-scope* of the less experienced emergency care provider. That said — **basic interpretation** is **not** nearly as **difficult** as it may seem IF one simply keeps in mind the key concepts discussed in this Section 20.

• The overall rhythm is **not regular.** Looking *first* at the tracing *from a little distance* away — there appears to be **group beating.** That is — there are alternating *short-longer* cycles (*beats #1-2; 3-4; and 5-6*).
• Awareness that an arrhythmia manifests **"group beating"** — should at least *suggest* the possibility of **some type** of **Wenckebach** conduction disturbance. This is especially true in a patient with recent *inferior* infarction — since 2nd degree AV block, **Mobitz Type I** (*AV Wenckebach*) often occurs in this setting.
• We emphasize that *not* every rhythm with group beating will be the result of Wenckebach. For example, atrial or ventricular bigeminy or trigeminy (*every 2nd or every 3rd beat a PAC or a PVC*) — will also manifest group beating. That said — **recognition** that there is **group beating** may be *invaluable* for tuning in our diagnostic assessment!

☞ Continuing with the **Ps,Qs,3R Approach** in Figure 20A-5:

• The **QRS complex** is **narrow** for *all* beats on the tracing (*albeit some QRS complexes look slightly different from neighboring QRS complexes*). The fact that the QRS complex is narrow *confirms* that the mechanism of this rhythm is supraventricular.
• The **atrial rhythm** is at least **fairly regular** (*arrows in Panel B of* **Figure 20A-6**). There is slight variability in the P-P interval (*due to underlying sinus arrhythmia*) — but *all* P waves are *upright* and manifest *similar* morphology in this lead II.
• The most challenging aspect of this rhythm is determining IF there is **any relationship** between **P waves** and *neighboring* **QRS** complexes?

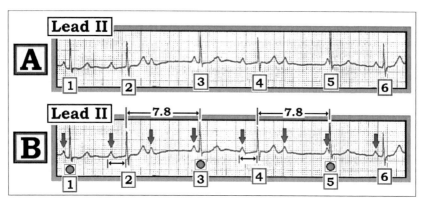

Figure 20A-6: To facilitate detection of whether any P waves may be conducting — We *add* intervals, arrows, and circles to Figure 20A-5.

▶ **PEARL:** Whenever you are confronted with a challenging rhythm strip — *START* with those aspects of the tracing about which you can be certain. Therefore, in Figure 20A-6 — we *know* that the P wave preceding beat #5 is *not* conducting. It can't be — since the PR interval preceding beat #5 is simply *too* short to conduct! Since the QRS complex of **beat #5** is *narrow* and *not* preceded by a P wave that conducts — it must be a **junctional *escape*** beat.

- There are *other* P waves in Figure 20A-6 that are *not* conducting. These include the P waves just after the T waves of beats #2 and #4.
- On the other hand — some P waves *do* conduct. Note in **Panel B** of Figure 20A-6 that the PR interval preceding beats #2 and #4 is *identical* — and that both of these beats end a short cycle. This is because **beats #2** and **#4** are ***sinus-conducted*** beats. These beats are conducted with **1st degree AV block** (*since the PR interval preceding beats #2 and #4 clearly exceeds one large box in duration*).
- Since the atrial rhythm is at least *fairly* regular — and some beats are conducted while others are not — the rhythm disturbance in Panel B of Figure 20A-6 must represent a form of **2nd degree AV block**.
- Given that the QRS complex in Panel B is narrow — and that there is group beating in this patient with recent *inferior* infarction — the odds overwhelmingly favor **Mobitz I** (*which is so much more common than the Mobitz II form of 2nd degree AV block*). In further support of Mobitz I — is the long PR interval preceding the 2 beats that we know are conducting (*pp 236-240*).

➡ ***Beyond-the-Core:*** IF your interpretation of Figure 20A-6 was simply 2nd degree AV block of *some* sort with *group* beating — therefore *possible* Mobitz I — We would be ecstatic. Exploring this premise further — We make the following ***advanced-level*** observations:

- Despite the fact that there are many *nonconducted* beats in Figure 20A-6 — the conduction disturbance for this rhythm is clearly *not* 3rd degree AV block. We can recognize *at a glance* that this is unlikely to be 3rd degree AV block — because the ventricular rhythm is *not* regular. Instead — beats #2 and #4 each occur *earlier-than-anticipated*, and are preceded by the *same* PR interval. These beats <u>are</u> conducted.

• Note the **subtle-but-real** difference in **QRS morphology** among various beats on this tracing. *This is not artifact.* Compared to beats #2,4,6 — **beats #1,3,5** all manifest slightly taller R waves and less deep S waves (*circles*). We have already established that **beat #5** is a **junctional** *escape* beat — since the PR interval preceding beat #5 is clearly *too short* to conduct. Recognition that *each* of the beats highlighted by the **circles** in Panel B (*beats #1,3,5*) manifest *similar* QRS morphology strongly suggests that **beats #1** and **#3** are also **junctional escape beats**. This is supported by the finding that beats #3 and #5 are each preceded by the *same* R-R interval (*of 7.8 large boxes in duration*) — which corresponds to an **escape** rate of **~40/minute**.

☞ We can now make sense of the complex events that are seen to occur in **Figure 20A-6**:

• **Beat #2** begins a Wenckebach cycle. This beat is conducted with a long PR interval.
• The P wave just after the T wave of beat #2 is nonconducted.
• The P wave just preceding beat #3 was about to begin the next Wenckebach cycle — but *before* it could do so, 7.8 *large* boxes in time (*1.56 second*) had elapsed. As a result — a **junctional** *escape* beat (*beat #3*) arises.
• **Beat #4** <u>is</u> conducted and begins the next Wenckebach cycle.
• The P wave immediately after the T wave of beat #4 is nonconducted.
• The P wave just before beat #5 was about to begin the next Wenckebach cycle — but *before* it could do so, 7.8 *large* boxes in time has elapsed, which results in another **junctional** *escape* beat (*beat #5*).
• The rhythm strip ends with beat #6. Despite the relatively short PR interval preceding beat #6 — **We *suspect*** that **beat #6** <u>is</u> **conducted** because it manifests the *same* QRS morphology as the other 2 beats on the tracing that we <u>know</u> are conducted (*beats #2 and #4*).

▶ **BOTTOM Line:** This is *not* an easy rhythm strip to interpret! Do *not* be concerned if you did not follow all aspects of our explanation. The point to emphasize is that **2nd degree AV block** is present — that in this patient with recent *inferior* infarction, a *narrow* QRS complex <u>and</u> *group* beating — most likely represents a form of **AV Wenckebach**.

• **P.S.:** We present a **laddergram** of this rhythm on **page 271** (*at the end of our 7-page Basic Laddergram Review on pp 266-272*).

Practice Tracing #4: *AV Block or Not?*

 ➡ **PRACTICE** Tracing:

● Interpret the rhythm below using the **Ps,Qs,3R Approach**. The patient is *hemodynamically* stable.
• Is there AV block or not? If so — Describe the type of AV block.

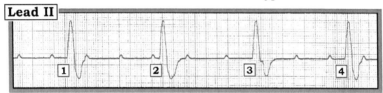

Figure 20A-7: *Practice* Tracing #4.

☞ **Answer to Figure 20A-7:** The QRS complex is wide. The ventricular rhythm is regular at a rate of ~35/min for the 4 beats shown on this tracing. Regular P waves are seen at an atrial rate of ~90/minute. However — *none* of the P waves are related to the QRS. Instead — the **P waves "march through"** the **QRS** complex.
• Note that the PR interval preceding each QRS *continually* changes.
• The rhythm is **complete AV block** at the **ventricular** level.

➡ **_KEY Clinical_ Point:** Definitive diagnosis of *complete* AV block requires the occurrence of P waves at *all* points in the cardiac cycle. **No P waves conduct _despite_ adequate opportunity to do so** (*pp 240-242*). We illustrate this in Figure 20A-8, in which arrows have been added to highlight the **regular atrial rate** at ~90/minute.

• Note that the **ventricular rhythm** is **regular** — as it most often is with complete AV block. The **ventricular rate** is **under 50/minute** — which usually ensures that *at least some P waves* will have an opportunity to conduct IF the degree of conduction block is *not* complete.
• We would *not* expect the P waves highlighted by *striped arrows* to conduct. This is because these P waves *either* occur during the *absolute* refractory period – or – with a *very short* PR interval (*as seen just before beat #2*) that may not allow adequate time for the impulse to be conducted to the ventricles.
• In contrast — we *would* expect *at least* one or more of the P waves highlighted by *solid* arrows to have adequate opportunity to conduct. *None of them do* — since the ventricular escape rhythm continues at its regular slow rate throughout the rhythm strip. Thus, there is **complete AV dissociation** — in this case due to **complete AV block**.

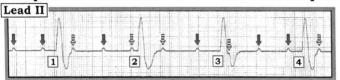

Fig. 20A-8:

Practice Tracing #5: *AV Block or Not?*

(?) ⇒ PRACTICE Tracing:

● Interpret the rhythm below using the **Ps,Qs,3R Approach**. The patient is *hemodynamically* stable.

• Is there AV block or not? If so — Describe the type of AV block.

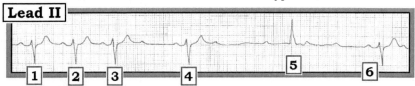

Figure 20A-9: *Practice* Tracing #5.

☞ **Answer to Figure 20A-9:** The first 3 beats show sinus rhythm. Thereafter the rate slows and many beats are nonconducted (*best seen in labeled* **Figure 20A-10**).

• There is *underlying* sinus arrhythmia (*often referred to as* **ventriculophasic sinus arrhythmia** *when associated with significant AV block*).
• The QRS complex of sinus-conducted beats is wide.
• The P wave after the T wave of beat #3 is nonconducted. Four nonconducted P waves follow beat #4 — interrupted only by a ventricular escape beat manifesting a *different* wide QRS morphology (*beat #5*).
• *All* **conducted beats** on this tracing (*beats #1,2,3; #4; #6*) — manifest a *fixed* (*albeit slightly prolonged*) **PR interval**. Given that this rhythm strip begins with consecutively conducted beats (*beats #1,2,3*) — criteria are satisfied for **Mobitz II** 2nd degree AV block (*page 238*). Failure to conduct *multiple* P waves in a row might further qualify as **"high-grade" AV block** (*pp 246-247*).
• Note that the QRS complex is wide, as it most commonly is with Mobitz II 2nd degree AV block. The reason for routine pacing (*or at least "standby" pacing*) with Mobitz II is also evident from the *multiple* consecutive *nonconducted* P waves seen.

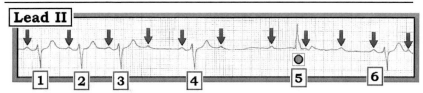

Figure 20A-10: Addition of *arrows* highlighting atrial activity to Figure 20A-9. *Consecutively* conducted beats begin the tracing (*beats #1,2,3*). Multiple P waves are nonconducted. The PR interval is *fixed* for those P waves that do conduct. This is **Mobitz II** 2nd degree AV block. Beat #5 (*circle*) is a ventricular escape beat (*See text*).

Practice Tracing #6: *The Cause of a Pause*

 ⇒ <u>PRACTICE</u> Tracing:

● Interpret the rhythm below using the ***Ps,Qs,3R* Approach**. The patient is *hemodynamically* stable.
• Is there AV block or not? If so — Describe the type of AV block.
• What is the cause of the *long* pause?

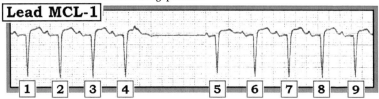

Figure 20A-11: *Practice* Tracing #6.

☞ **Answer to Figure 20A-11:** The rhythm in <u>Figure 20A-11</u> is **sinus** with **1st degree AV block**. Each beat in the beginning and end of this MCL-1 lead tracing is preceded by a *similar-morphology* P wave with fixed (*albeit slightly prolonged*) PR interval — that we estimate at 0.23 second (*slightly more than one large box in duration*).
• 2nd degree AV block is <u>not</u> present. The ***cause*** of the **1.66 sec. pause** (*between beats #4-5*) — is <u>not</u> the result of any form of AV block.
• **Beat #5** manifests an additional phenomenon that you are probably becoming increasingly aware of. (**<u>HINT</u>:** *What happens to the PR interval preceding beat #5?*).

⇨ **<u>KEY</u> Points:** Answers to the above questions become evident below in <u>Figure 20A-12</u>, to which we have added arrows *and* revealing labels.

• The ***commonest*** cause of a **pause** is a ***blocked* PAC** (*pg 233*). By repeating this mantra to yourself <u>whenever</u> you see anything more than the briefest of pauses — you will <u>not</u> overlook *blocked* PACs. Careful inspection of the ST-T waves of *each* beat in <u>Figure 20A-12</u> reveals that the *only* ST-T wave with a notched deformity is the ST-T wave at the beginning of the pause (*open arrow*). Thus the **cause** of this pause is a ***blocked* PAC**.
• Note that the PR interval preceding the beat that ends the pause (*beat #5*) — is slightly shorter (*0.17 second*) than the PR interval of all other beats on this tracing. This means that there was *not enough time* for the P wave preceding beat #5 to conduct to the ventricles — which tells us that **beat #5** must be a **junctional *escape* beat** (*pp 188-189*).

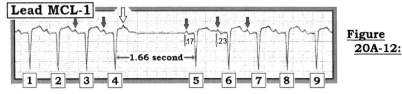

Figure 20A-12:

Practice Tracing #7: *Group Beating*

 ➡ **PRACTICE Tracing:**

● Interpret the rhythm below using the **Ps,Qs,3R Approach**. The patient is *hemodynamically* stable.

• Note **group beating**. Is it due to AV block? If so — What *type*?

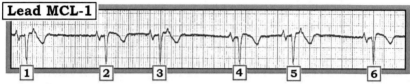

Figure 20A-13: *Practice* Tracing #7.

☞ **Answer to Figure 20A-13:** We have emphasized how the presence of **group beating** should *always* make one consider the possibility of a Wenckebach conduction disturbance (*pp 236-237*).

• **Alternate *short-long* cycles** of **group beating** are clearly present in Figure 20A-13 (*beats #2-3; beats #4-5*). While recognition of group beating in this tracing *should* make us consider the *possibility* of Wenckebach conduction — this is one instance in which group beating is *not* due to Wenckebach. *Why not?*

• **HINT:** What is the *most* common *cause* of a pause?

➡ **KEY Points:** There are a number of causes of **group beating**. In addition to Wenckebach conduction — group beating may be due to atrial/ventricular bigeminy or trigeminy — *and* other *less* common arrhythmia phenomena (*echo beats; escape capture bigeminy; Mobitz II; SA block*). While prompt recognition of *group* beating will facilitate more rapid diagnosis of Mobitz I 2nd degree AV block — awareness of **other causes** of **group beating** is essential for accurate diagnosis. The cause of group beating here becomes evident in labeled **Figure 20A-14**:

• There are groups of **2 sinus beats** in a row in Figure 20A-14 (*beats #2-3; beats #4-5*). Recognizing that each group of 2 beats is followed by a brief pause — *and repeating* the **mantra** that the **commonest cause** of a **pause** is a **blocked** PAC — allows us to identify *"tell-tale"* notching in the T wave of beats #1, 3 and 5 (*open arrows*). This notching is a PAC that occurs so early in the cycle (*within the absolute refractory period*) that it is nonconducted.

• There is *no* AV block in Figure 20A-14. Despite group beating — the reason there is *no* AV block is that the atrial rhythm is *not* regular. Instead — *every-third-P-wave* occurs *early* and is blocked. Thus, the rhythm is **atrial trigeminy** with **blocked** PACs.

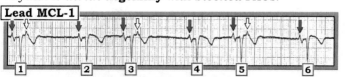

Figure 20A-14:

Practice **Tracing #8:** *More Group Beating*

 ➡ **PRACTICE Tracing:**

⬤ Interpret the *sequential* tracings below using the **Ps,Qs,3R Approach**. The patient is *hemodynamically* stable.

- Note **group** beating in **Tracing A**. Is this due to AV block? If so — What *type* of AV block?
- HINT: Interpretation of Tracing A becomes easier if you first interpret **Tracing B** obtained from the *same* patient a lit bit later. This is because the *same* phenomenon responsible for the abnormal findings is operative in *both* tracings.

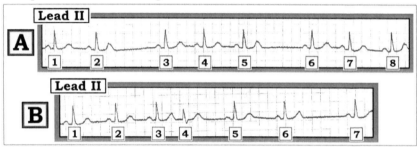

Figure 20A-15: Sequential tracings in a patient who initially manifests group beating (*Tracing A*) — and later manifests some irregularity with a brief pause following beat #6 (*Tracing B*). What is the cause of the abnormal findings seen in *both* tracings?

🐾 **Answer to Figure 20A-15:** As was the case for Figure 20A-13 (*on page 263*) — there once again is **group** beating in **Tracing A** that is **not** the result of **Mobitz I** 2nd degree AV block. This is because: **i)** The PR interval is *not* progressively increasing within the groups of beats (*from beat #1-to-2; from #3-to-4-to-5; from beat #6-to-7-to-8*); and **ii)** The atrial rhythm in Tracing A is clearly *not* regular.

- The *KEY* to interpretation of Tracing A resides in interpretation of **Tracing B**. The abnormal findings are easier to see in **Figure 20A-16** — in which we label atrial activity.

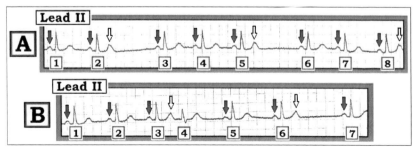

Figure 20A-16: Addition of arrows to highlight atrial activity.

☞ The *underlying* rhythm for both tracings in Figure 20A-16 is sinus arrhythmia. In **Tracing A** — a short pause follows each group of *sinus-conducted* beats. There is *subtle-but-real* peaking of the T wave of beats #2, 5 and #8 in Tracing A (*open arrows*). That this peaking is real and *not* due to artifact — is determined by the fact that the T wave *of all other beats* in Tracing A is smoother and of smaller amplitude. This peaking of T waves must therefore reflect *blocked* **PACs**.

- A *similar* phenomenon is operative in **Tracing B** — and much easier to see. Note that **beat #4** in Tracing B occurs early. The T wave just preceding beat #4 in Tracing B is again peaked — strongly suggesting that a **PAC** is *hidden* within this T wave. The reason the QRS complex of beat #4 looks slightly different — is that **beat #4** is a **PAC** conducted with **aberration**.
- A short pause follows beat #6 in Tracing B. The *commonest* **cause** of a **pause** is a *blocked* **PAC**. Once again — "telltale" notching of the T wave of beat #6 in Tracing B indicates this is due to another *blocked* **PAC**.

➡ *BOTTOM* **Line:** The 2 tracings in **Figure 20A-16** reflect the *same* phenomenon. There is *underlying* sinus arrhythmia that is punctuated by *multiple* PACs. Most of these PACs are blocked.
- The PAC that notches the T wave of beat #3 in **Tracing B** is conducted with aberration.
- The T wave of beat #6 in Tracing B is unmistakably peaked.
- Recognition that the "theme" for **Tracing B** is the occurrence of **PACs** alerts us to *carefully* focus on T wave morphology at the beginning of each pause in **Tracing A**. Doing so facilitates identifying the *subtle-but-real* deformity brought about by *hidden* **PACs** within the T waves of beats #2, 5 and 8 in Tracing A.

⇨ **How to *Read* a Laddergram**

● Mastering laddergrams is <u>not</u> essential for attaining competency in arrhythmia interpretation. This is fortunate — since it may literally take *months-to-years* to become comfortable and proficient at drawing laddergrams. That said — being able to *understand* a laddergram that is already drawn for you is <u>not</u> difficult. This goal is readily *achievable* in the few minutes it takes to read this brief sub-section. Our discussion will focus on review of the basic principles needed to read a laddergram. Please keep in mind the following:

- Do <u>not</u> be intimidated by laddergrams!
- You do <u>not</u> have to learn to draw laddergrams unless you are completely *impassioned* by arrhythmias <u>and</u> have true desire to put the mechanism of arrhythmia events on paper.
- ***Reading a laddergram is easy.*** Doing so reveals a *sequential* tale of precisely what is happening at which level of the heart's conduction system. After a while — *reading* laddergrams becomes fun.
- Even the experts occasionally disagree. As the acclaimed electrocardiographer Rosenbaum once said, *"Every self-respecting arrhythmia has at least 3 possible interpretations".*

☞ What is a Laddergram?

A laddergram is merely a graphic tool used to illustrate the conduction pathway for a series of cardiac beats or a cardiac rhythm.

- **3 Tiers** are usually drawn on a ***standard* laddergram** to represent the path of conduction *through* the atria — AV node — and the ventricles (**Figure 20A-17**).

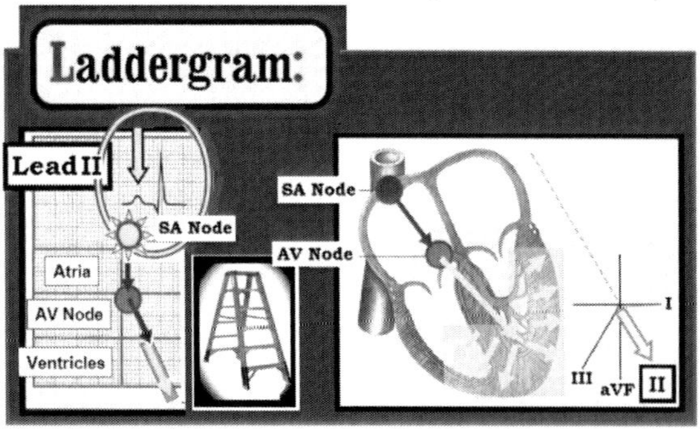

Figure 20A-17: Laddergram illustration of normal sinus conduction (*See text*).

- **Time** is conveyed along the ***horizontal* axis**.
- The **SA nodal tier** (*where the impulse begins with normal sinus rhythm*) **is *implied*** and usually *not* drawn on a standard laddergram. Exceptions exist with rare conduction defects such as SA block (*in which delay and failed conduction results from disease <u>within</u> the SA node itself*) — but the **3 *Standard* Tiers** (*for the **Atria – AV Node –***

and ***Ventricles***) are all that is needed to explain events for the overwhelming majority of arrhythmias encountered.
- What could be simpler than the graphic depiction in **Figure 20A-17** of a normal *sinus-conducted* beat?

☞ *Key* Points about Laddergram Basics

Much information is integrated within (*and implied by*) events shown on a laddergram. We highlight the following *KEY* points from our *schematic* depiction of a normal *sinus-conducted* beat in **Figure 20A-17**:
- The impulse for a normal sinus beat originates from the SA node. We illustrate this on the laddergram schematically with onset of the impulse at the beginning of the P wave at the top of the Atrial Tier.
- Travel through the atria is fast, owing to conduction over *specialized* intra-atrial pathways. We schematically depict rapid conduction through the atria by means of a **vertical line** through the **Atrial Tier**. Life is far simpler approximating the time required to traverse the atria as a vertical line — although in reality (*since some finite time is required*) — there should be a very slight decline conveyed to this vertical line in the Atrial Tier.
- **Conduction** *slows down* significantly *within* the **AV Nodal Tier**. This is schematically depicted by the definite decline attributed to the slanted line traveling through the AV Nodal Tier. With 2nd degree AV block of the Wenckebach type — a progressively *increasing* slant is conveyed to this line within the AV Nodal Tier, corresponding to the progressively *increasing* PR interval until a beat is dropped.
- **Conduction** *through* the **Ventricles** is generally conveyed by a slanted line with a **downward** arrow to indicate the direction of conduction. The degree of slant is subject to variation depending on width of the QRS complex — presence of bundle branch block or aberrant conduction — <u>and</u> personal preference of the laddergram artist. Regardless of these potential slight variations in format — *what counts* is that sinus beat conduction through the ventricles is conveyed by a *downward* slanted line with *downward* arrow. This is important for distinguishing sinus beats from beats or rhythms that originate <u>in</u> the ventricles (*PVCs, VT, ventricular escape*) — in which the slant and arrow point upward.
- **In Practice** — the circles we added to <u>Figure 20A-17</u> to depict the SA and AV nodes are *implied* and <u>*not*</u> drawn in.

☞ *Laddergram* Basics of AV Nodal Beats

Armed with the basics — We devote the remainder of this Sub-section to illustrating how *easy* it is to interpret laddergrams already drawn for you. Consider **Figure 20A-18** — which illustrates the **3 *possible* manifestations** of ***atrial* activity** in **lead II** for AV nodal beats or AV nodal rhythms:
- With **normal** <u>*sinus* **rhythm**</u> — the P wave in lead II should always be upright. The reason for this is that the path of depolarization from the

SA node (*in the upper right atrium*) to the AV node (*located at approximately +60 degrees in the frontal plane*) is oriented directly *toward* standard lead II.

> ▶ **PEARL:** The *only* exception to the above general rule in which there may be sinus rhythm with a *negative* P wave in lead II is when there is *either* dextrocardia *or* lead misplacement.

• With **AV Nodal beats** or an **AV nodal rhythm** — the impulse originates from the AV node. This is schematically depicted *within* the AV Nodal Tier by a circle with starburst for Panels A, B and C in Figure 20A-18. Conduction of the impulse is then transmitted back (*retrograde*) to the atria *at the same time* as it is transmitted down to the ventricles.

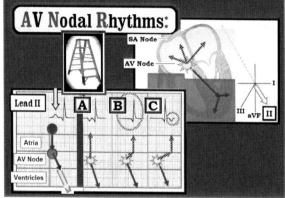

Figure 20A-18: Laddergram depiction of atrial activity with AV nodal beats *and/or* AV nodal rhythms. (*See text*).

> ▶ **Clinical Note:** Because the atria are activated in *retrograde* fashion with AV nodal beats or rhythm — the **P wave** will be *negative* in **lead II**. Whether this negative P wave occurs *before* the QRS complex — *within* the QRS — or *after* the QRS will depend on the *relative* speed of conduction backward (*from the AV node*) compared to the forward speed of conduction through the ventricles.

• In **Panel A** of Figure 20A-18 — A *negative* **P wave** occurs **before** the **QRS** in lead II because the speed of conduction back to the atria is *faster* than the speed of conduction down to the ventricles.

• In **Panel C** — A *negative* **P wave** occurs **after** the **QRS** in lead II (*either within the ST segment or T wave*) because the speed of conduction back to the atria is considerably *slower* than the speed of conduction down to the ventricles. This situation is by far the *least* common clinically; it is only rarely seen.

• In **Panel B** — *No* **P wave** at all is seen in lead II. Presumably, the speed of conduction back to the atria is *about equal to* the speed of conduction down to the ventricles. This situation is by far the *most* common clinically.

☞ *Schematic* Laddergram Examples

We schematically illustrate the most common laddergram elements in <u>Figure 20A-19</u> and <u>Figure 20A-20</u>. Reading laddergrams that have already been drawn for you is largely intuitive. A picture is worth a thousand words:

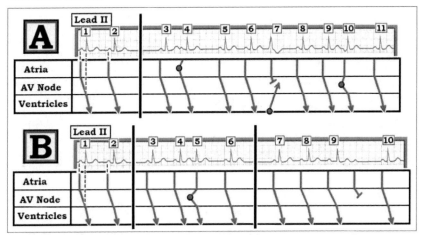

<u>Figure 20A-19:</u> Schematic depiction of basic laddergram elements.

☞ **Panel A** in **<u>Figure 20A-19</u>:**

- **Beats #1** and **#2** are *sinus* **conducted.** Note that the *vertical* line in the Atrial Tier begins at the *onset* of the P wave. The *downsloping* line in the Ventricular Tier begins at a point corresponding to the onset of the QRS complex.
- **Beat #3** is another sinus P wave. **Beat #4** is a **PAC** — with the premature P wave notching the terminal portion of the T wave of beat #3. Note depiction of this PAC as a small *circle* within the Atrial Tier positioned slightly before the onset of the premature P wave. The PAC depolarizes the rest of the atria *at the same time* as it travels downward to depolarize the ventricles.
- **Beats #5,6; 8,9;** and **11** are all normal sinus beats. **Beat #7** is a **PVC** that is sandwiched within 2 normal sinus beats. Note origin of beat #7 in the laddergram at the *bottom* of the Ventricular Tier, with an upward inclining line <u>and</u> arrow that ends within the AV Nodal Tier.
- The **PVC** depicted by **beat #7** manifests a **full *compensatory* pause.** That is — the pause containing this PVC is exactly equal to *twice* the R-R interval. This schematic laddergram illustrates why. The next sinus P wave after beat #6 occurs precisely on time (*vertical line in the Atrial Tier that occurs at about the same time as the PVC*). This P wave is *prevented* from conducting down to the ventricles because the PVC has rendered the ventricles refractory (*schematically depicted by the butt ending of the P wave line within the AV Nodal Tier*). The ventricles

recover by the time the following sinus P wave arrives at the AV node — leading to normal conduction for beat #8.

- **Beat #10** is a **PJC**. A *negative* P wave *precedes* the QRS in this lead II rhythm strip because conduction back (*retrograde*) to the atria takes less time than conduction down to the ventricles (*corresponding to Panel A in* Figure 20A-18 — *on page 268*).

☞ **Panel B** in **Figure 20A-19** (*page 269*):

- The initial beats in **Panel B** are *sinus* conducted. **Beat #5** in Panel B is a **PJC**. No P wave is seen preceding this PJC. The laddergram explains why: schematic time for conduction back (*retrograde*) to the atria takes *about the same amount of time* as conduction down to the ventricles (*corresponding to Panel B in* Figure 20A-18 — *on page 268*).
- Second degree AV block, **Mobitz Type I** (*AV Wenckebach*) is illustrated for **beats #7-thru-10** in Panel B. Note persistence of regular sinus P waves throughout (*constant P-P interval*). The PR interval *progressively* lengthens from beat #7 — to #8 — to #9 — until *nonconduction* of the regularly occurring P wave after beat #9. The cycle then resumes with **beat #10** showing *normal* conduction with a PR interval equal to the PR interval preceding beat #7.

☞ **Figure 20A-20:** We finish this brief series of basic *schematic* laddergram elements with illustration of the onset and offset of a *reentry* tachycardia.

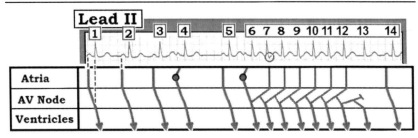

Figure 20A-20: *Additional* laddergram elements. The 2nd PAC in this tracing (*beat #6*) initiates a run of a *reentry* SVT (*See text*).

⬤ **Figure 20A-20:** The laddergram begins with 3 sinus beats.

- **Beat #4** is a **PAC**. A brief pause follows as the sinus node is reset. Normal sinus rhythm resumes with beat #5. ***Another*** **PAC** occurs with **beat #6**. This time, however — there is *retrograde* conduction back to the atria within the AV Nodal Tier. When conditions for reentry are *just right* such that a *critically* timed premature impulse (*beat #6*) occurs at precisely the moment that retrograde conduction out of the AV node is possible — a **reentry circuit** may be set up that *sustains* the **tachycardia**, as it does here for **beats #7-thru-12**.

- Sometimes with SVT *reentry* rhythms — you will be able to see evidence of this retrograde conduction back to the atria in the form of a notch in the terminal portion of the QRS complex (*open circle at the end of the QRS of beat #7*). Normal sinus beats in Figure 20A-20 do *not* manifest this terminal notch. Instead — this terminal notch representing *retrograde* atrial activity is *only* seen for beats #7-*thru*-12 during the reentry tachycardia.
- The laddergram in Figure 20A-20 also illustrates why the reentry tachycardia ends. Note slight prolongation of the R-R interval between beats #12-to-13 compared to the R-R interval during the tachycardia. Slowing of retrograde conduction out of the AV Nodal Tier results in a *change* in timing for one of the limbs of the reentry circuit — such that conduction back to the atria is no longer possible. Normal sinus rhythm resumes with beat #14.

☞ Clinical Applications: *Demystifying* Arrhythmias

We conclude this Subsection on *How to Read a Laddergram* with a laddergram drawing of the complex arrhythmia previously presented in Figure 20A-5 (*pp 257-259*). Our purpose in showing **Figure 20A-21** is not to repeat our detailed analysis — but rather to demonstrate that when *given* a laddergram — even IF the rhythm is challenging to interpret (*as this one is!*) — that it becomes surprisingly *easy to under-stand* the mechanism of the arrhythmia from simple review of an accompanying laddergram. *Verify this* for yourself:
- Are there regular (*or almost regular*) P waves in **Figure 20A-21**?
- Which P waves are conducting? — Which are *not* conducting?
- Does the PR interval *prolong* for successive beats within the AV Nodal Tier? — Are there any AV nodal *escape* beats?

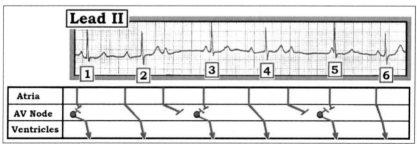

Figure 20A-21: Laddergram of Figure 20A-5 (*from pp 257-259*).

☞ **Answer to Figure 20A-21:** The following observations should be *immediately* apparent from seeing the laddergram in Figure 20A-21:

- The *underlying* rhythm is sinus arrhythmia. It is easy to appreciate *slight* variation in the P-P interval from viewing slight *irregularity* in the distance between the vertical lines within the Atrial Tier.

- The P waves preceding beats #1, 3 and 5 are *not* conducted. The reason for this nonconduction — is that junctional *escape* beats (*small circles within the AV Nodal Tier*) arise just before each of these P waves — and this renders the ventricles *refractory* to conduction.
- The PR interval *prolongs* in two separate areas *within* the AV Nodal Tier. Specifically, note *within* the AV Nodal Tier — that the degree of slant *increases* for the P waves following beats #2 and #4 *compared to* the degree of slant for the P waves arising before beats #2 and #4. This indicates Wenckebach conduction. As a result of this Wenckebach conduction — the P waves following beats #2 and #4 are nonconducted.

➡️ ***Bottom* Line:** Reading basic laddergrams is *not* difficult. Becoming more comfortable in your ability to read laddergrams that have already been drawn for you greatly facilitates understanding complex arrhythmias such as the one shown in Figure 20A-21.

Practice Tracing #9: *Acute MI and AV Block?*

⑦ ⇨ PRACTICE Tracing:

● The patient whose 12-lead ECG is shown below in <u>Figure 20A-22</u> presented to the ED with *new-onset* chest pain. The patient was *hemo-dynamically* stable at the time this ECG was recorded.
- Is there evidence of **acute STEMI** (<u>ST</u> <u>E</u>levation <u>M</u>yocardial <u>I</u>nfarction)?
- Based on the lead II rhythm strip at the bottom of the tracing — **What is the cardiac rhythm?** — *Is there AV block?*

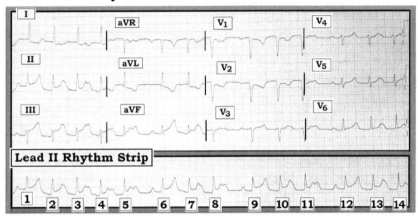

Figure 20A-22: *Practice* Tracing #9.

☞ **Answer to Figure 20A-22:** Initial assessment of the **lead II rhythm strip** at the bottom of <u>Figure 20A-22</u> reveals a somewhat *irregular* supraventricular (*narrow QRS*) rhythm at a rate slightly under 100/minute. Some *sinus-conducting* P waves appear to be present (*beats #6, 9 and 12*). That said, we defer momentarily further analysis of the rhythm given this patient's presentation with *new-onset* chest pain. Instead — we focus first on important **12-lead ECG** findings:
- There is **marked ST elevation** in the **inferior leads** (*II,III,aVF*).
- There is equally marked *reciprocal* ST depression in leads aVL; V1,V2 — and to a lesser extent in lead I.
- QS complexes are seen in leads V1,V2 (*with no more than tiny r waves in V3,V4*). Transition is *delayed* until V4-to-V5 in the precordial leads.
- The overall picture is highly suggestive of **acute infero-postero STEMI**. Acute **RCA** (<u>R</u>ight <u>C</u>oronary <u>A</u>rtery) **occlusion** is suspected given more ST elevation in lead III compared to lead II — <u>and</u> more ST depression in lead aVL compared to lead I.

☞ **A Closer Look at the RHYTHM (**<u>*Figure 20A-22*</u> **):**

● Analysis of the rhythm in <u>Figure 20A-22</u> is indeed a *challenging* task. That said — there *are* several clues to the etiology of the rhythm — which together with a pair of **calipers** should allow definitive diagnosis. We make the following observations and comments regarding determination of the rhythm in this case (**Panel A** of **Figure 20A-23**):

- The first clue to the rhythm lies in the ***clinical* setting**. That is — this patient presents within the *early* hours of acute *inferior* infarction.
- There is ***group* beating**. It is often helpful to step back a short distance to overview regularity of the entire tracing. Note that the fairly rapid supraventricular rhythm in **Panel A** is punctuated by 3 brief pauses (*between beats #5-6; 8-9; and 11-12*). The duration for each of these brief pauses is virtually identical (*5 large boxes separate beats #5-6; 8-9; and 11-12*). This is *unlikely* to be due to chance.
- Awareness that a patient is in the *early* hours of acute *inferior* infarction – <u>and</u> – presents in a rhythm with *group* beating — should *alert us* to the possibility of **AV Wenckebach**. While there clearly are other reasons for group beating — keeping the possibility of AV Wenckebach at the forefront will serve us well as we complete systematic assessment of this arrhythmia.

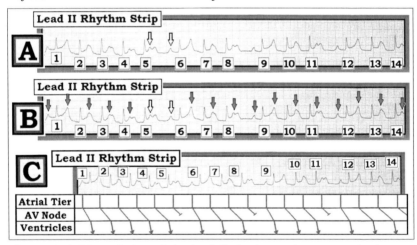

Figure 20A-23: Isolation of the lead II rhythm strip seen at the bottom of Figure 20A-22 (*from page 273*). Accompanying laddergram (*See text*).

☞ *Systematic* **Assessment of the Rhythm in** **Figure 20A-23:**

● Given that the patient in this case is *hemodynamically* stable — we assess the arrhythmia in **Panel A** of Figure 20A-23 in the *same* manner we approach any cardiac arrhythmia = By the *Ps,Qs & 3R approach*:
- The **QRS** complex is narrow — so the rhythm is supraventricular.
- The ventricular rhythm is fairly rapid (*just under 100/minute*) — and slightly irregular. As noted — there is ***group* beating**.
- **P waves** are *not* readily visible in all parts of the tracing. That said — we <u>can</u> identify a definite *upright* P wave with consistent (*albeit slightly prolonged*) PR interval immediately preceding the 1st beat at the end of each pause. That is — a constant PR interval is seen preceding

beats #6, 9, and 12. Therefore, the **underlying rhythm** is **sinus** with **1st degree AV block**.

- We next look to see <u>IF</u> the atrial rhythm is regular. **Calipers** greatly facilitate this assessment. The best way to map out P waves is to identify a place in the rhythm strip where you *clearly* see 2 P waves in a row (*open arrows in* **Panel A** *of* <u>Figure 20A-23</u>). Setting calipers to this P-P interval allows us to walk out *regular* P waves for the *entire* tracing (*solid arrows in* **Panel B**).

- Having walked out *regular* P waves (*Panel B*) — We can now recognize *nonconduction* of the P waves at the beginning of each pause (*P waves notching the T waves of beats #5, 8, and 11*). This observation establishes the diagnosis of **2nd degree AV block** — since there <u>are</u> *regular* sinus P waves — <u>and</u> *some* P waves conduct but *others* do not! The degree of AV block is <u>not</u> complete because some of the P waves <u>do</u> conduct (*fixed PR interval preceding beats #6,9,12*).

▶ *Putting* **Together** our observations thus far, we have: **i)** Acute *inferior* infarction; **ii)** 2nd degree AV block with a *narrow* QRS complex; **iii)** Group beating; <u>and</u> **iv)** Definite conduction of some P waves with 1st degree AV block.

- This *combination* of observations *overwhelmingly* favors **Mobitz I (***AV Wenckebach***)** as the diagnosis for the conduction disturbance.

- This observation is supported by the clinical reality that Mobitz I is *by far* the most common form of 2nd degree AV block — especially in patients with acute *inferior* infarction <u>and</u> baseline 1st degree AV block as seen here.

- *Beyond-the-Core:* An additional ***"footprint of Wenckebach"*** present in **Panel A** is that the pause containing the dropped beat is *less* than twice the shortest R-R interval (*pp 236-237*).

▶ *Use of the* <u>**Laddergram:**</u> *Confirmation* of **Mobitz I** is forthcoming from the laddergram depiction of events in **Panel C** of <u>Figure 20A-23</u> (*on page 274*). Note how much *easier* the laddergram makes it to track the progressively *increasing* PR intervals within the AV Nodal Tier until a beat is dropped.

- Although <u>not</u> essential for making the diagnosis of AV Wenckebach — Use of a laddergram *confirms* our diagnosis <u>and</u> tremendously *facilitates* understanding our explanation.

Practice Tracing #10: *Acute MI* and *AV Block?*

 ➡ PRACTICE Tracing:

● The tracing in <u>Figure 20A-24</u> represents a final example of a 12-lead ECG obtained from a patient with *new-onset* chest pain. Development of Q waves and *marked* ST-T wave abnormalities are consistent with **acute STEMI** (*ST* <u>E</u>levation <u>M</u>yocardial <u>I</u>nfarction). The patient was *hemodynamically* stable at the time this ECG was recorded.
- What is the rhythm?
- **HINT:** Why do we include this tracing in this Section on AV block?

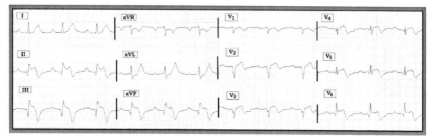

Figure 20A-24: *Practice* Tracing #10.

🖙 **Answer to Figure 20A-24:** As noted — *definite* Q waves and *marked* ST-T wave abnormalities in this patient with *new-onset* chest pain clearly indicate **acute STEMI**. That said — Determination of the rhythm is made difficult by: **i)** lack of a long lead II rhythm strip; <u>and</u> **ii)** the *marked* ST-T wave abnormalities that may easily mask underlying atrial activity.
- One might be *tempted* to diagnose the rhythm in <u>Figure 20A-24</u> as sinus at 65-70/minute with 1st degree AV block. *This is a mistake ...*
- It is well to be aware of the sometimes **subtle forms** that **AV block** may take in the setting of acute MI (*pp 273-275*). Be especially *alert* for this possibility whenever you see a relatively *long* PR interval (*as in lead II of* <u>Figure 20A-24</u>). Seeing a *longer-than-expected* PR interval may mean that *another* P wave is *in hiding* within the ST-T wave.
- Use of **calipers** is essential to prevent overlooking subtle forms of AV block. Did you consider the possibility that an **extra P wave** might be **hiding** in the tail portion of each QRS complex on this tracing?

🖙 **Looking for *Extra* P Waves**

The possibility of an *extra* P wave within each R-R interval is most evident from inspection of **lead II** (*open arrows in* **Figure 20A-25**).
- Setting **calipers** to a *proposed* P-P interval suggested by the *open* arrows in lead II of <u>Figure 20A-25</u> — allows one to march out a **surprisingly *regular* atrial rhythm** at ~**140/minute** throughout the entire tracing (*solid arrows in selected leads*). Thus, there <u>is</u> underlying **atrial tachycardia**.

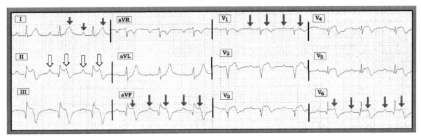

Figure 20A-25: Addition of *arrows* to Figure 20A-24 indicating regular atrial activity is present throughout the tracing (*See text*).

☞   Notching in each T wave in lead II of **Figure 20A-25** is obvious in hindsight (*open arrows*). Sometimes, subtle extra P waves in hiding are *not* as obvious. In such cases — we set our **calipers** to precisely *half* the R-R interval — *and* then determine if *subtle* deflections are seen when we walk out this *pre-set* interval throughout the tracing. Solid arrows in selected leads of Figure 20A-25 suggest that consistent atrial activity is present *and* persists.

- Note that the **PR interval** preceding each QRS complex is **fixed** (*albeit prolonged to 0.26 second*). Thus, *every-other-P-wave* is conducting — and the rhythm is **2nd degree AV block *with* 2:1 AV conduction**.

➡ **KEY Clinical Point:** As discussed on pp 238-240 — 2nd degree AV block with 2:1 AV conduction could be *either* Mobitz I or Mobitz II. That said — the conduction disturbance in Figure 20A-25 is **more likely** to be **Mobitz I** because: **i)** Mobitz I is far more common than Mobitz II; **ii)** The QRS complex is narrow; and **iii)** The PR interval for beats that conduct is prolonged.

- *Beyond-the-Core:* Localization of infarct is *less* helpful for determining the type of AV block for this tracing because ST elevation is noted diffusely (*in the inferior, anterior and lateral precordial leads*). This distribution could result from acute occlusion of *either* the RCA (*Right Coronary Artery*) or the LAD (*Left Anterior Descending*) coronary artery depending on coronary anatomy (*possible "wraparound" LAD lesion vs a dominant RCA that also supplies parts of the anterior wall*).

▶ *Bottom* Line: The 12-lead ECG in Figure 20A-25 is **diagnostic** of a large **acute STEMI *with* 2:1 AV block**. As a result — acute reperfusion is urgently needed at the *earliest* opportunity!

Beyond-the-Core: *SA Block*

  ⇒ *Beyond-the-Core ...*

● Interpret the rhythm below using the **Ps,Qs,3R Approach**. The patient is *hemodynamically* stable.
• There is **group** beating. Is this the result of AV block?
• *Beyond-the-Core:* If not AV block — Is there another type of Wenckebach block that might account for the *group* beating seen?

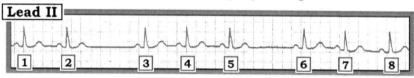

Figure 20A-26: There is group beating. Is this due to AV block?

☞ **Answer to Figure 20A-26:** The rhythm in Figure 20A-26 is unusual in several regards. There is **group** beating — but this is *not* due to Mobitz Type I 2nd degree AV block because: **i)** the atrial rhythm is *not* regular (*with no P wave at all within the pauses between beats #2-3 and 5-6*); and **ii)** the PR interval is *not* progressively increasing within groups of beats.
• The P-P interval *does* vary slightly from conducted beat to conducted beat. That said — it would be distinctly unusual for simple sinus arrhythmia to produce such *patterned* beating with disproportionately long pauses (*between beats #2-3 and #5-6*) punctuating an otherwise fairly regular rhythm.
• This is *not* atrial trigeminy or atrial quadrigeminy — since P wave morphology is the *same* for *all* P waves – and – there is absolutely *no* deformity of the T wave at the onset of each pause (*as occurs when a PAC is in hiding and nonconducted*).
• By the process of elimination — we are left with **SA Wenckebach** as the most likely explanation for this arrhythmia.

☞ **SA (*SinoAtrial*) Wenckebach/SA Block**

Wenckebach phenomena are *not* limited to the Mobitz I 2nd degree AV block kind. The physiologic phenomenon of *progressive* lengthening of conduction time *until* an impulse is nonconducted may be seen in response to a variety of *other* intrinsic rhythms including: **i)** rapid atrial rhythms (*AFib, AFlutter, or atrial tachycardia with Wenckebach conduction out of the AV node to the ventricles*); **ii)** retrograde in response to accelerated junctional rhythms or even ventricular tachycardia (*with progressive lengthening of retrograde R-P' interval out of the accelerated junctional or ventricular focus*); and **iii)** with **SA nodal *exit* block**.
• Recognition of the various types of Wenckebach phenomena *other than* Mobitz I extends beyond the scope of this book. These rhythms are not common — and their mechanisms are often complex. That

said — it is nevertheless helpful to be aware that **unexplained *group* beating** may indicate the presence of *some type* of Wenckebach conduction. The ***laddergram*** in **Figure 20A-27** illustrates the mechanism implicated in this case.

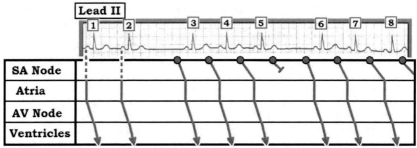

Figure 20A-27: Laddergram of the rhythm shown in Figure 20A-26. The *mechanism* of **SA block** is best illustrated by *adding* the SA Nodal Tier to the traditional laddergram. Doing so makes clear the *progressive* prolongation in conduction time *within* the SA Nodal Tier until a sinus impulse is blocked (ie, *the SA nodal impulse after beat #5 never gets out of the SA node*). Beats #3,4,5 therefore illustrate **4:3 SA block** (*4 sinus impulses — but only 3 are conducted to the atria*). The cycle then resumes with the next group of beats (*beginning with beat #6*) that again show *progressive* conduction time *within* the SA Nodal Tier.

➡ **SA Block** — is an ***Exit* Block** that occurs at the level of the SA node. It reflects *impaired* conduction after generation of the impulse *within* the SA node until arrival of the impulse to atrial tissue.

- In theory — **SA nodal block** may be 1st degree — 2nd degree — or 3rd degree (*similar to the 3 degrees of AV block*). That said — **1st degree SA block** is ***clinically* undetectable** on the surface ECG (*since we only see a P wave after the sinus node has successfully fired*). We are unable to detect any *delay* in conduction that might be occurring *within* the SA node.
- Complete (*3rd degree*) SA block — implies that *no* sinus impulse is successful in leaving the SA node. As a result — *no* P waves are seen. Rather than "3rd degree SA block" — we generally describe the event as a ***sinus* pause** or ***sinus* arrest**, depending on duration of time until sinus node recovery (*if the sinus node recovers at all*).
- In between — is **2nd degree SA block**, that may be *either* of the Mobitz I or Mobitz II type. That said — our purpose in presenting the example of SA block in Figure 20A-26 is *not* to discuss fine differences between Mobitz I vs Mobitz II SA block (*the above example is not completely typical*). Instead — Our Goals are: **i)** to make you aware that **unexplained *group* beating** (*as seen in* Figure 20A-26) may result from *some* type of ***Wenckebach* conduction** *other than* Mobitz I; and **ii)** to again illustrate (*in follow-up to our Laddergram subsection on pp 266-272*) how a **laddergram** may facilitate understanding the mechanism of complex rhythm disturbances.

ADDENDUM: *Sick Sinus Syndrome and Sinus Pauses*

AV Block: ⟹ Addendum:
— *Sick Sinus / Sinus Pauses*

● Sick Sinus Syndrome (**SSS**) — is an extremely common entity among the elderly. The arrhythmias encountered in SSS are easily recalled by considering its name. *Think of the arrhythmias that might be expected IF the SA node was "sick".* One might see the following (**Figure 20A-28**):

- **Slowing** and **irregularity** of the heart rate (*resulting in sinus bradycardia and/or sinus arrhythmias*).
- Progressive **deterioration** of **SA node function** (*leading to sinus pauses, varying degrees of sinus exit block — and even sinus arrest*).
- Emergence of **escape pacemakers** *and/or* alternative rhythms (*junctional rhythm/AFib*) — usually with a **slow ventricular response** (*since the AV node is often also "sick" and dysfunctional*).

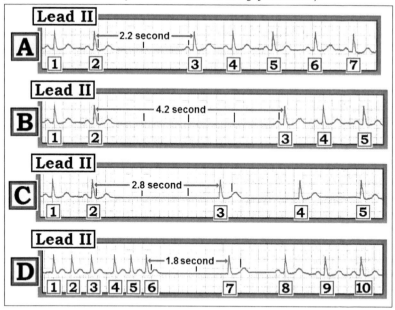

Figure 20A-28: Arrhythmias commonly encountered in Sick Sinus Syndrome. **Panel A** — relatively *brief* sinus pauses (*lasting just over 11 large boxes in Panel A = 2.2 second*); **Panel B** — *longer* sinus pauses (*here lasting 21 large boxes = 4.2 second*); **Panel C** — sinus pause followed by a slow and irregular AV nodal escape rhythm (*beats #3-5 in Panel C*); and **Panel D** — initial *rapid* AFib (*beats #1-to-#6*) followed by a 1.8 second pause that is terminated by a junctional escape beat (*beat #7*) — and finally resumption of sinus rhythm (*beats #8-to-10*). Delay in sinus node recovery (*often for longer than the pause seen between beats #6-7*) is characteristic of SSS (*See text*).

▶ ***"Tachy-Brady"* Syndrome:** A significant percentage of patients with Sick Sinus Syndrome also manifest the *other* extreme to SA node dysfunction (*namely* **tachycardia**). The common forms of tachycardia that are seen with SSS include ***rapid* AFib** (Panel D in **Figure 20A-28**); AFlutter; PSVT; *and* various types of atrial tachycardia (*hence the other name for this entity, which is the "Tachy-Brady" syndrome*).

☞ Sick Sinus Syndrome: *KEY Clinical Points*

The natural history of SSS is typically one of slow, *gradual* progresssion — often with *minimal* symptoms for *many* years ...

* The *initial* rhythm disturbance is most commonly **sinus bradycardia** — often with associated **sinus arrhythmia**. Sinus bradycardia and arrhythmia may persist with stable heart rates in the 45-to-60/min range in some elderly subjects for *over* a decade *before* the **symptoms** of **weakness**, **syncope** or **presyncope** become evident. At what point an older subject with persistent bradycardia *transcends* the definition of *age-related* heart rate slowing/sinus bradycardia to development of "sick sinus syndrome" is often unclear.
* In addition to weakness and syncope/presyncope — ***other* signs/ symptoms *associated*** with **SSS** include: **i)** hypotension (*from the slow heart rate*); **ii)** palpitations (*from alternating fast-then-slow arrhythmias*); *and* **iii)** heart failure, angina, *and/or* mental status changes (*from reduced cardiac output due to bradycardia and inability to increase heart rate normally in response to activity*).
* Essential to the **Work-Up** of *any* elderly subject who presents with symptoms or arrhythmias potentially due to SSS are the following: **i)** Careful ***drug* history** for use of any potential **rate-slowing medications** (*See NOTE below*); **ii)** Consideration of **recent infarction** (*obtain a 12-lead ECG; consider troponins if/as clinically indicated*); *and* **iii)** Rule out **hypothyroidism** (*an uncommon cause, but one that is easily diagnosed and treated*).

▶ **NOTE:** Use of one or more ***Rate-Slowing* Medications** is *by far* the most common cause of bradyarrhythmias in the elderly. Inquire about: **i) AV nodal blocking agents** (*verapamil-diltiazem; β-blockers; amiodarone; digoxin*); **ii) Eye drops** (*β-blocker eye drops are absorbed systemically and may cause bradycardia*); **iii) Clonidine** (*may cause rate slowing*); *and* **iv) Herbals** (*some herbals cause rate slowing, so Look Up physiologic effects of any herbal preparations the patient is taking*).

* IF your patient is older (*over 60-to-70 years of age*) and presents with *symptomatic* bradyarrhythmias — Once you *rule out* medication effect, ischemia/infarction, and hypothyroidism — You have virtually made the diagnosis of Sick Sinus Syndrome.
* ***Permanent* Pacing** is indicated *only* for **symptomatic bradycardia**. Pacing is *not* indicated for symptoms from tachycardia (ie, *palpitations from rapid AFib*) — unless the *only* way to control tachyrhythms is with *rate-slowing* drugs that *then* produce symptomatic bradycardia.

▶ **NOTE:** Once the patient has a pacemaker — *rate-slowing* drugs to control tachycardia may be *added* again.

- <u>Clinically</u> — The challenge in treating a patient with **"tachy-brady"** **syndrome** is that drugs used to control *rapid* heart rates from tachy-arrhythmias such as AFib or AFlutter (*verapamil-diltiazem-digoxin-amiodarone*) — are likely to overly *slow* the ventricular response in these older patients with intrinsic SA and AV nodal disease. While AV nodal *blocking* drugs may initially control tachycardia symptoms — with time, many (*most*) patients with SSS will eventually need pacing because of *medication-induced* excessive bradycardia.

☞ Sinus Pauses: *How Long is "Long"* ?

Sinus pauses are an important part of the symptom complex of SSS. To facilitate assessment of pauses on short-term or long-term ECG monitoring — We emphasize the following points:

- We define **"<u>brief</u>" pauses** as the *absence* of a QRS complex for **less** than a **2 second period** (ie, *for less than 10 large boxes on ECG grid paper*). Brief pauses are common in the general population — <u>and</u> many otherwise healthy individuals manifest one or more **short-lived** **pauses** (*of less than 2 seconds*) over 24 hours of monitoring. There are many potential causes of such *short* pauses — including sinus bradycardia and arrhythmia; medication effect; vasovagal effect; PACs (*especially blocked PACs*); PVCs (*post-ectopic pause until the next sinus P wave is able to conduct*); <u>and</u> SA node or AV node disease. Even if the cause of a brief (*less than 2 second*) pause is pathologic — this rarely (*if ever*) requires treatment.

- We define **"<u>significant</u>" pauses** as lasting for **more** than **3 seconds** (ie, *for more than 15 large boxes on ECG grid paper*). This duration is usually considered the *minimum* to qualify a patient with SSS as having **"symptomatic bradycardia"** severe enough to merit perma-nent pacing (*See* **Panel B** *in* <u>Figure 20A-28</u> — *on page 280*).

- **Pauses <u>between</u> 2.0-to-3.0 seconds** constitute a **"gray zone"** area within which our concern rises for *possible* "symptomatic brady-cardia". Such patients may *not yet* qualify for permanent pacing (ie, **Panel A** — *pg 280*) — but they clearly deserve closer monitoring.

➡ **<u>KEY Clinical</u> Point:** The **need for pacing** may be enhanced when pauses of *less* than 3.0 seconds in duration are associated with *other* features of concern. For example — even though pause duration in **Panel C** (*pg 280*) is *less* than 3 seconds (*it is 2.8 seconds*) — this pause is associated with *lack of sinus node recovery* necessitating a junctional escape rhythm to prevent asystole (*with the junctional rate being slow and irregular*). <u>IF</u> symptomatic — this patient would almost certainly qualify for permanent pacing.

☞ Sinus Node *Recovery* Time: *Delayed with SSS*

Another common feature of SSS is *delay* in sinus node recovery time. Many patients with SSS alternate between fast and slow rhythms (*AFib being the most common tachyarrhythmia seen*). In patients with normal sinus node function — the period from the last beat of a tachycardia until the next *sinus-conducted* beat is relatively brief. In contrast — the **post-tachycardia** pause in patients with SSS may be *prolonged* because the *diseased* sinus node requires more time to recover following repetitive stimulation from a run of tachycardia.

- **Panel D** in Fig. 20A-28 (*pg 280*) — shows a **post-tachycardia pause** of 1.8 seconds following an episode of *rapid* AFib. The *post-tachycardic* pause may be much *longer* than this in patients with more *advanced* sinus node dysfunction.
- Keep in mind that *repetitive* sinus node stimulation during tachycardia may be *retrograde* from tachyarrhythmias originating *outside* the sinus node. Constant resetting of the SA node in this manner produces an **overdrive** suppression that may result in *prolonged* pauses after the tachycardia is over.

☞ Sinus *Pause* vs Sinus *Arrest*

The semantics for distinguishing between a *prolonged* sinus pause and sinus "arrest" may be confusing. While *shorter* pauses that are *less* than 3.0 seconds in duration (**Panel A** in Fig. 20A-28) should *not* be labeled as sinus "arrest" — consensus is lacking as to whether a *longer* pause (*as seen in* Panel B) should qualify.

- *Regardless* of whether one calls the pause in **Panel B** a *prolonged* sinus "pause" or sinus "arrest" — **specifying** pause duration (*in this case, to 4.2 seconds*) clarifies what the clinician needs to know.
- *True* sinus "arrest" implies *permanent* cessation of sinus impulses. This may be what has happened in **Panel C** — in which there fortunately has been emergence of an AV nodal *escape* rhythm (*pg 280*).

☞ Sinus *Pause* vs SA *Exit* Block

The various forms of **SA (**<u>Sino</u><u>A</u>trial**) Block** were discussed on pages 278-279. The common denominator for *each* of the forms of SA block is *impaired* conduction after generation of the impulse within the SA node until arrival of the impulse to atrial tissue. Semantically — there <u>is</u> a difference between SA block (*in which a sinus impulse does occur, but has difficulty getting out of the SA node*) <u>vs</u> sinus "arrest" (*in which the sinus node "dies" and sinus impulses no longer arise*). That said — this difference is much *less* important clinically than appreciation of the patient's response to sinus node dysfunction.

- *Beyond-the-Core:* **SA Node *Exit* Block** — may either be of the Mobitz I or Mobitz II type. In its *pure* form — one can distinguish between the two because the R-R interval for normal sinus beats is a *precise* fraction of pause duration. For example — with **2:1 SA *Exit* Block** of the **Mobitz II** type — the pause should be exactly *twice* the R-R interval. In contrast, with the Mobitz I form of SA block — the pause will be *less* than twice shortest R-R interval (*pp 278-279*).

➡️ ***Clinical* Point:** Practically speaking — It will often be *impossible* to tell with any certainty <u>IF</u> the cause of a pause from sinus node dysfunction is due to a sinus pause — true sinus "arrest" — <u>or</u> some form of SA exit block. This is especially true if there is underlying sinus arrhythmia, as is so often the case.

• Clinically the distinction between a sinus "pause" — sinus "arrest" — *and/or* SA node *exit* block will usually <u>not</u> matter. Instead, it generally suffices to specify what is seen. Thus, for the rhythm in **Panel A** of <u>Figure 20A-28</u> (*pg 280)*— a **2.2 second *sinus* pause** is seen following beat #2, with resumption of normal sinus rhythm at 70/minute beginning with beat #3.

Beyond-the-Core: *Vagotonic AV Block*

  ➡ *Beyond-the-Core ...*

● We conclude this Section 20 on AV Block with a series of 3 tracings obtained from a previously healthy young adult following recent noncardiac surgery. How would you interpret the 3 rhythm strips shown in **Figure 20A-29**?

• What type of AV block is present? *Is a permanent pacemaker needed?*
• **HINT #1:** What features are *atypical* for Mobitz I and Mobitz II block?
• **HINT #2:** Consider the clinical scenario (*a previously healthy young adult with recent noncardiac surgery*). What is the *title* of this Section?

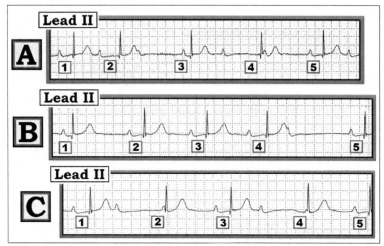

Figure 20A-29: Series of 3 lead II rhythm strips obtained post-surgery.

☞ **Answers to Figure 20A-29:** Clinical assessment of what we are seeing in this interesting series of 3 *successive* lead II rhythm strips is best accomplished by first *noting* all findings — and *then putting them together* into a single cohesive explanation:

● **Panel A** (*in* Figure 20A-29) — The QRS complex is narrow. The R-R interval is the *same* between beats #2-3 and #3-4 — but it *varies* for other beats on this tracing. This suggests that **beats #3** and **#4** (*which each end a longer R-R interval cycle*) may be **junctional *escape* beats**.

• In support of the premise that beats #3 and #4 are junctional *escape* beats — is the finding of at least ***transient* AV dissociation** (*there seems to be no relationship between P waves and the QRS in the middle portion of* Panel A).

• The **P-P interval *varies greatly*** throughout Panel A. This *continual* variation in P-P duration is more easily seen in **Figure 20A-30**, in which we add **arrows** to highlight sinus P waves. The degree of P-P variability is *much more* than expected for simple sinus arrhythmia.

- **Beats #1** and **#5** in **Panel A** may be **conducting**, albeit with a *long* PR interval (*the PR interval appears to be the same for <u>both</u> beat #1 and beat #5*). If this were true (*that beats #1 and #5 in <u>Panel A</u> are conducting*) — then what we see in Panel A would constitute a **Wenckebach cycle** with *progressive* lengthening of the PR interval preceding beat #2 compared to #1 — with <u>non-conduction</u> of the following P wave (*that notches the T wave of beat #2*). That said — interpretation of **Panel A** in <u>Figure 20A-30</u> is complex and **clearly atypical** from the usual appearance of **Mobitz I** 2nd degree AV block.

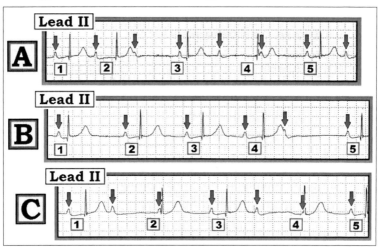

Figure 20A-30: Arrows have been added to highlight sinus P waves.

⬤ **Panel B** (*in* <u>Fig. 20A-29</u>) — Interpretation of the rhythm in Panel B is equally challenging as was the rhythm in Panel A.

- The **P-P interval** in <u>Panel B</u> is **even more** **irregular** than it was in Panel A. Yet P wave morphology appears constant — suggesting this is due to marked variability in sinus rate discharge.
- It is difficult to determine <u>IF</u> **beats #2, #3** and **#4** in <u>Panel B</u> make up a **Wenckebach cycle** (*with progressive PR interval lengthening until a beat is dropped*) <u>vs</u> some *random* occurrence accounting for marked P-P interval variation and the *unpredictable* change in PR intervals (*note the surprisingly short PR interval preceding beat #1*). More questions are raised by Panel B than are answered.

⬤ **Panel C** (*in* <u>Fig. 20A-29</u>) — We <u>know</u> **beat #2** is **<u>not</u> conducting** (*the PR interval preceding beat #2 in Panel C is clearly too short to conduct*).

- By the same token — We <u>know</u> **beat #4** is also **<u>not</u> conducting**.
- We wonder <u>IF</u> **beats #3** and **#5** in Panel C are *sinus* conducted with 1st degree block (*both beats preceded by similar but long PR intervals*).
- Although at first glance, one might think **beat #1** in Panel C is conducted in the same manner — measurement (*with calipers*) of the

PR interval preceding beat #1 reveals *slight-but-real* lengthening compared to the PR interval preceding beats #3 and 5. The cause for this is *uncertain* from assessment of Panel C alone.

☞ *Bottom-Line* Impression of the **3 Rhythms** in **Figure 20A-30:**

● The usual rules for rhythm interpretation and assessment of AV blocks and AV dissociation are *not* closely followed for the 3 rhythm strips shown in **Figure 20A-30**. Instead, we see: **i)** *dramatic* variation in P-P interval; <u>and</u> **ii)** elements resembling Mobitz Type I AV block — *higher-grade* 2nd degree AV block — <u>and</u> AV dissociation.

- There <u>is</u> one phenomenon that *readily* explains <u>all</u> findings seen in this series of 3 tracings — which is ***Vagotonic* <u>AV</u> <u>Block</u>**.
- The literature is scant regarding *vagotonic* AV block. This *unusual* conduction disturbance occurs *far less often* than other forms of AV block — which may in part account for the difficulty in recognizing it.
- The ***clinical* scenario** in this case is **consistent** with what may be expected for *vagotonic* AV block (ie, *this patient was an otherwise healthy young adult with recent surgery that may predispose to an increase in vasovagal tone*).

☞ *Recognition* of *Vagotonic* AV Block

Clinical characteristics of ***vagotonic* AV block** include the following:
- Presence of a condition *consistent* with **increased vagal tone** (*the patient in this case presented in the early post-operative period*). **Other situations** in which **enhanced vagal tone** may be seen include *persistent* vomiting; performance of a medical procedure; <u>and</u> athletic training. *Vagotonic* AV block may also be seen healthy adults during normal sleep (*and especially in individuals with sleep apnea*).
- ***Sinus* arrhythmia** which may be **marked** — <u>and</u> which especially *slows* just *prior to* <u>and</u> *during* periods of AV block.
- ***Mixed* forms** of **AV block** including Mobitz I 2nd degree AV block — 2nd degree AV block <u>*with*</u> 2:1 AV conduction — Mobitz II — periods of *high-grade* <u>and</u> *even* complete AV block.
- ***Frequent* switching *back-and-forth*** between *several* of the *above* forms of AV block — which is often punctuated by periods of P-P irregularity, sinus rate slowing, <u>and</u> *unexpected* change in PR interval.

☞ *Clinical* Course of *Vagotonic* AV Block

Fortunately the course of *vagotonic* AV block in otherwise healthy adults without underlying heart disease is ***most often* benign**. It usually does <u>not</u> progress to AV conduction system disease — <u>and</u> pacing is generally *not* needed. That said — more severe, symptomatic cases not responding to simple measures should be referred.

- Be aware of ***vagotonic* AV block**. This conduction disturbance may be *transiently* seen during Holter monitoring of otherwise healthy individuals during sleep <u>or</u> in a situation of *increased* vagal tone (ie, *persistent vomiting*). The overall course is usually benign.

Basics of Rhythm Diagnosis

🔴 The *KEY* to effective arrhythmia interpretation is to utilize a **Systematic Approach**. The system we favor is based on assessing for the following **5 Parameters:**

▶ *P* waves ?

  ▶ *QRS* width ?

    ▶ *Regular* rhythm ?

      ▶ Are P waves *Related* to the QRS ?

        ▶ Heart *Rate* ?

> It does *not* matter in what sequence you look at the 5 parameters — as long as you check *all* 5 of them!

⇒ *Remember the following Memory Aid:*

👉 *"**Watch** your **P**'s and **Q**'s — and the 3 **R**'s".*

🔴 First — *Ensure* the **patient** is **stable** (*pp 51-52*).

• IF there is normal **sinus rhythm** — then **P** waves should be present and clearly **upright** in **lead II**.

• The **QRS** is defined as **narrow** — IF it is **≤0.10 second** (ie, *not* more than *HALF* a *large* box in duration).

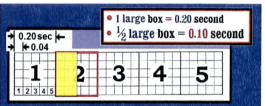

• 1 large box = 0.20 second
• ½ large box = 0.10 second
0.20 sec
0.04

• *Regularity* — Look to see IF the rhythm is *regular* ?
• Determine if P waves are *"Related"* to QRS complexes (ie, *conducting*) — Look *in front* of each QRS to see IF there is a P wave present with a *fixed* PR interval.
• *Rate* — is most easily calculated by the **Rule** of **300** (*Provided that the rhythm is regular* — the heart rate can be *estimated* IF you **divide 300** by the **number** of *large* **boxes** in the **R-R interval**).

🔴 **NOTE:** Use the ***Every-other-Beat*** **Method** when the rate is fast and the rhythm is regular. The R-R interval of *half* the rate below = 3 large boxes (= *100/min*). Therefore, the *actual* rate = 100 X 2 = ~ 200/minute.

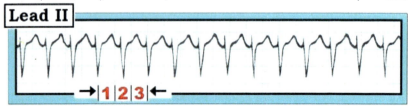

Lead II